T0382451

We all have beliefs, even strong convictions, about what is just and fair in our social arrangements. How should these beliefs and the theories of justice that incorporate them guide our thinking about practical matters of justice? This wide-ranging collection of essays by one of the foremost medical ethicists in the United States explores the claim that justification in ethics, whether concerning matters of theory or practice, involves achieving coherence or "reflective equilibrium" (as Rawls has called it) between our moral and nonmoral beliefs. Among the practical issues the volume addresses are the design of health-care institutions, the distribution of goods between the old and the young, and fairness in hiring and firing practices.

Justice and justification

Cambridge Studies in Philosophy and Public Policy

GENERAL EDITOR: Douglas MacLean

Justice and justification

REFLECTIVE EQUILIBRIUM IN THEORY AND PRACTICE

NORMAN DANIELS
TUFTS UNIVERSITY

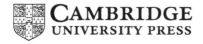

Published by the Press Syndicate of the University of Cambridge
The Pitt Building, Trumpington Street, Cambridge CB2 1RP
40 West 20th Street, New York, NY 10011-4211, USA
10 Stamford Road, Oakleigh, Melbourne 3166, Australia

First published 1996

Library of Congress Cataloging-in-Publication Data
Daniels, Norman, 1942–
Justice and justification: reflective equilibrium in theory and
practice/Norman Daniels.
p.   cm. – (Cambridge studies in philosophy and public policy)
Includes bibliographical references.
ISBN 0-521-46152-9. – ISBN 0-521-46711-x (pbk.)
1. Justice (Philosophy)   2. Justification (Ethics)   3. Medical ethics.
4. Applied ethics.   I. Title.   II. Series.
B105. J87D36   1996
174'.2 – dc20   96-3888
                                                     CIP

A catalog record for this book is available from the British Library.

ISBN 0-521-46152-9 Hardback
ISBN 0-521-46711-x Paperback

Transferred to digital printing 2004

For Hugo Bedau and John Rawls
friends and mentors
whose lives, work, and support
helped me learn about
ethical theory and practice

Contents

Contents

Preface

When I was an undergraduate at Wesleyan University in the early 1960s, I majored in English and dabbled in science and philosophy. (We had in those days more luxury than students have now to "find ourselves" in a liberal arts curriculum.) In my senior year, I wrote a thesis on the distinction between prose and poetry and the role that distinction played in the "objectivist" literary criticism of Ransom, Tate, and Brooks, still fashionable in that period. My real concern, as I gradually became aware, was philosophical: What is a "literary theory"? What is it about? What does it really explain? What makes one such theory better than another? What is the relationship between a literary theory and good literary criticism, or good creative writing, for that matter? How was theory connected to practice? I could not answer these questions. The net result of my undistinguished senior thesis was that I abandoned my career plans to study literature and went into philosophy instead. Philosophy, and in particular, philosophy of science, I hoped, would help me understand what makes one theory a better theory than an alternative. Armed with that understanding, I thought, I might then go back to answer the questions that plagued me as an undergraduate.

The essays in this volume grow out of those early interests in the nature of theory and its relationship to practice, but the focus is on ethical, not literary, theory and practice. I suppose it would be nice to report that the shift in focus was the result of some insight that I had while pursuing these questions over the years, but I cannot claim that kind of intellectual integrity. The shift in focus is, like many key elements of our lives, largely serendipitous, a manifestation of chaos, the result of being in a certain place at a cerain time, in my case, Harvard in the late 1960s.

As a graduate student at Harvard in that period, I did continue my interest in those questions about the nature of theory. I even wrote my dissertation under Hilary Putnam on the relationship between Thomas Reid's mathematical discovery of a non-Euclidean geometry and the philosophical practice that explains how he made it. But the late 1960s were a time of political ferment, at Harvard as at many universities. Issues of race, class, and social justice were made vivid by the struggle against the war in Vietnam, by the aftermath of rebellions in black ghettos, and by the emerging environmental and feminist movements. The times demanded engagement and commitment. There was no refuge: the graduate student offices in the philosophy department became the headquarters of the Harvard student strike in April 1969. The demand for engagement created considerable tension with my quite abstract interests in the nature of theories and how we come to accept them. For me, as for many others with emerging academic careers, the search for "relevance" in our work and lives was not the cliché it later became but as necessary as water for the thirsty.

More serendipity. "Relevance" for me was given a focus by Hugo Bedau, then philosophy chair at Tufts, who hired me to teach a course in "radical social philosophy" in the fall of 1969. Fortunately, he tolerated on-the-job learning, since I had no preparation to teach in this area other than my political activism. More than that, I read his *Death Penalty in America* (1964) and saw in a new way how work in ethical theory and in practical ethics could be related. His work seemed a model of "relevance." It was a rigorous exercise in connecting ethical theory and empirical knowledge about the death penalty and its effects. To my mind, it boldly flew in the face of all the ethics I had studied and provided me with a new model for what philosophical work might be.

It is hard to explain to students today, familiar with yards of bookshelf space devoted to anthologies in "applied ethics," how paradigm-shattering Bedau's work and other work that began to emerge in that period were. This was a period when ethics was solely the study of the language and logic of moral discourse. The dominant theory held that ethical discourse was primarily expressive or emotive and not cognitive. (Though the dominance of the grip of logical positivism on philosophy of language and science had already ended as a result of work by Quine and Putnam, the implications of positivism for ethics lingered through much of the 1960s; its power did not wain until Rawls' work provided a full-blown model of an alternative approach.) Practical examples in the literature were as unimaginative as the promise to return a book to the library, or the damage done by walking across the grass in the quad. In Bedau's work, the full complexity of the act of the state taking lives was revealed in all its horrifying detail, and whether or not justification was possible depended on understanding the whole context and all the consequences.

Preface

The publication of John Rawls' *A Theory of Justice* in 1971 did more to topple the old paradigm of work in ethics than any other single intellectual event. Here was a truly substantive work in ethics and political philosophy. It talked about principles we should adopt and use to govern the institutions under which we live. It clarified moral commitments to equality in opportunity and other social goods, and it did so by building on avowed commitments to basic liberties. Rawls was willing to talk about our moral convictions and commitments. He gave them weight in moral argument, and not merely as evidence of a linguistic practice. In fact, Rawls barely mentioned the language or logic of ethics. This work was about the big issues in social justice, not just returning books to the library or not walking on the grass. It was relevant and yet highly respectable. Not coincidentally, I believe, that same year the journal *Philosophy and Public Affairs* began publication. The respectability and importance of work in practical ethics were institutionalized in what rapidly became a leading journal in the field.

In Rawls' work, I began to see the shape of answers to the questions I had been unable to answer about literary theory and had set aside. The very structure of his book posed the central issues: how can we choose among alternative theories of justice? which is the most acceptable theory? how can we justify our choice? Not only did Rawls articulate his own theory of justice as fairness as an alternative to the dominant theory, utilitarianism, but he articulated, albeit quite briefly, a general account of justification in ethics. My debt to Rawls is not only to his work, but to the generous, gentle collegial encouragement he has offered me over the twenty-five years in which I have been trying to understand and extend his work.

My debts in this volume go well beyond those to Bedau and Rawls. Joshua Cohen has spent many hours with me over the years deepening my understanding of Rawls' work and political philosophy more generally. My colleagues, especially George Smith and Stephen White, have provided important insights and generous criticism. Many others are cited in the acknowledgements for particular articles.

My debts are also institutional. Support for my early work on reflective equilibrium was provided by the National Endowment for the Humanities and a Tufts sabbatical leave in 1977–78. Subsequent work on justice and health care has been supported by the National Institutes of Health, the National Endowment for the Humanities, the Retirement Research Foundation, and the Robert Wood Johnson Foundation. I was prompted to think more about method in bioethics by the stimulation of other Fellows in the Harvard Program for Ethics and the Professions, where I spent a sabbatical leave in 1992–93.

Preface

I also wish to thank publishers of articles incorporated in this volume for permission to reprint them, as follows:

Chapter 2. "Wide Reflective Equilibrium and Theory Acceptance in Ethics." *Journal of Philosophy* 76 (1979):5:256–82.
Chapter 3. "Reflective Equilibrium and Archimedean Points." *Canadian Journal of Philosophy* 10 (1980):1:83–103.
Chapter 4. "On Some Methods of Ethics and Linguistics." *Philosophical Studies* 37 (1980):21–36. Reprinted by permission of Kluwer Academic Publishers.
Chapter 5. "Two Approaches to Theory Acceptance in Ethics," in D. Copp and D. Zimmerman (eds.), *Morality, Reason and Truth* (Totowa, NJ: Rowman & Littlefield, 1985), pp. 120–40 [based on "Can Cognitive Psychotherapy Reconcile Reason and Desire?" *Ethics* 93 (July 1983):772–85, published with the permission of *Ethics* and the University of Chicago Press].
Chapter 6. "An Argument about the Relativity of Justice." *Egalitarian Ethics*, special issue of *Revue Internationale de Philosophie* 3 (1989):170:361–78.
Chapter 7. "Moral Theory and the Plasticity of Persons." *Monist* 62 (1979):3:267–87.
Chapter 9. "Health-Care Needs and Distributive Justice." *Philosophy and Public Affairs* 10 (1981):2:146–79.
Chapter 10. "Equality of What: Welfare, Resources, or Capabilities?" *Philosophy and Phenomenological Research* 50 (Fall 1990), Supplement: 273–96.
Chapter 11. "Determining 'Medical Necessity' in Mental Health Practice: A Study of Clinical Reasoning and a Proposal for Insurance Policy." Coauthored with James Sabin, MD. *Hastings Center Report* 24 (November–December):6:5–13. Reproduced by permission. © The Hastings Center.
Chapter 12. "The prudential Lifespan Account of Justice Across Generations," in Lee M. Cohen (ed.), *Justice across Generations: What Does It Mean?* (Washington, D.C.: Public Policy Institute, AARP, 1993), pp. 197–213, 243–46, with changes © 1993, American Association of Retired Persons. Reprinted with permission. This chapter also includes pages 87–91 of *Am I My Parents' Keeper? An Essay on Justice between the Young and the Old* (New York: Oxford, 1988) by Norman Daniels. Copyright © 1988 by Norman Daniels. Reprinted by permission of Oxford University Press, Inc.
Chapter 13. "Problems with Prudence." Appendix to *Am I My Parents' Keeper? An Essay on Justice between the Young and the Old* (New York: Oxford, 1988), pp. 157–76, with changes.

Chapter 14. "Merit and Meritocracy." *Philosophy and Public Affairs* 7 (1978):3:206–23.
Chapter 15. "Rationing Fairly: Programmatic Considerations." *Bioethics* 7:2–3(April 1993):224–33.
Chapter 16. "Wide Reflective Equilibrium in Practice" is being published simultaneously in L. W. Sumner and Joseph Boyle (eds.), *Philosophical Perspectives in Bioethics* (Toronto: University of Toronto Press, in press).

Chapter 1

Introduction:
Reflective equilibrium in
theory and practice

The title proclaims that the essays in this volume are all either about justice or about the justification of beliefs about justice. That is enough unity to warrant collecting them together in this way, at least if there is merit enough to the individual essays. My task in this introduction, however, is to persuade the reader that there is more than this titular unity to this collection of essays and that the whole is something more than the sum of its parts. This may take some persuasion. These essays, mostly previously published, were written over an eighteen-year period, and, with the exception of the two newest ones, they were never intended to be part of this volume. Nevertheless, the themes that link them, and not just their overlapping subject matter, led me to assemble them in this way. Although they do not form a systematic study of those themes, lacking the sustained, exhaustive argument of a monograph, together they suggest an understanding that separately they cannot convey.

The central idea behind this collection is that the broadly coherentist view or "method" of justification that Rawls (1974) calls "wide reflective equilibrium" not only offers a promising account of the justification of ethical theories but also gives us guidance about philosophical method in practical ethics. All of us are familiar with the process of working back and forth between our moral judgments about particular situations and our effort to provide general reasons and principles that link those judgments to ones that are relevantly similar. Sometimes we use this process, which is what Rawls (1974) calls "narrow reflective equilibrium," to justify our judgments, sometimes our principles. We can still ask about the principles that capture our considered judgments: why should we accept them? To answer this question, we must widen the circle of justificatory beliefs. We must show why it is reasonable to hold these principles and beliefs, not just that we happen to do so. Seeking wide reflective equilibrium is thus the process of bringing to bear the broadest evidence and critical scrutiny we can, drawing on all the different moral and nonmoral beliefs and theories that arguably are relevant to our selection of principles or adherence to our moral judgments. Wide reflective equilibrium is thus a theoretical account of justification in ethics and a process that is relevant to helping us solve moral problems at various levels of theory and practice.

The main division of the essays reflects this central idea. The essays in Part I, focusing primarily on Rawls' work, elaborate and consider objections to reflective equilibrium as an account of theory justification in ethics. The new essay concluding Part I discusses the role of reflective equilibrium in Rawls' most recent work, where justice as fairness is seen as a "political" conception of justice. The essays in Part II are largely about justice in more specific, practical contexts, with an emphasis on the distribution of health care. They illustrate and sometimes comment on the implications of taking the method of reflective equilibrium seriously in solving practical ethical problems. The new concluding essay in Part II, about methodological debates in bioethics, develops some of the implications of reflective equilibrium for work in practical ethics. I single out a few of these implications for comment in the remainder of this introduction, but before turning to these unifying themes of the book, I want to say more about reflective equilibrium itself.

1. WIDE REFLECTIVE EQUILIBRIUM IN THEORY

The key idea underlying the method of reflective equilibrium is that we "test" various parts of our system of moral beliefs against other beliefs we hold, seeking coherence among the widest set of moral and non-moral beliefs by revising and refining them at all levels. For example, we might test the appropriateness of a purported principle of justice by seeing whether we can accept its implications in a broad range of cases and whether it accounts for those cases better than alternatives. Rawls appeals to such a test in *A Theory of Justice* when he imposes a condition of adequacy on the principles chosen in his contract situation, requiring that they match our considered moral judgments in reflective equilibrium. (Coherence involves more than mere logical consistency. As in the sciences, for example, we often rely on inference to the best explanation and arguments about plausibility and simplicity to support some of our beliefs in light of others.)

Our moral beliefs about particular cases count in this process. They have justificatory weight. Yet, they are not decisive. Even firmly held beliefs about particular cases may be revised. For example, if a principle incompatible with such a firmly held belief about a particular case accounts better than alternatives for an appropriate range of cases we

2

seem equally confident about, and if the principle also has theoretical support from other parts of our belief system, we may revise our particular belief and save the principle. Unless we are willing to appear dogmatic and to abandon all claim to reasonableness, we cannot dogmatically insist on the particular belief without supplying reasons for our view, and we must show that those reasons are superior to the reasons we have for the alternative.

This coherentist account of justification is intended to be quite general and not limited to moral justification. Rawls (1971, 20n) says the "mutual adjustment of principles and considered judgments is not peculiar to moral philosophy." He cites Goodman (1955) for "parallel remarks concerning the justification of the principles of deductive and inductive inference." The general account, of course, is not uncontroversial (see Stich 1990, Ch. 4).

To explain why Rawls' application of the idea of reflective equilibrium to justification in ethics was both so striking and so controversial, it will help to consider the standard form of criticism of utilitarianism and the response to it by utilitarians. (Similar points might be made about testing other principles or theories, including the adequacy of Kant's categorical imperative.) Classical act utilitarianism appeals to a single general moral principle, that an act or policy is right if and only if it produces at least as much utility as any alternative. ("Utility," the generic term for intrinsic goodness, is explained in different ways by different utilitarians, e.g., as the net of pleasure minus pain or happiness or the satisfaction of desires.) This principle, however, produces notorious counterexamples to our ordinary moral beliefs. It seems to permit, indeed to require, actions that ordinary morality prohibits outright, such as the punishment of the innocent whenever doing so would avoid greater harm or the direct killing of some to save more. Anti-utilitarians count these cases as decisive counterexamples to the principle of utility and conclude the principle and the theory supporting it are untenable.

Utilitarians respond to this appeal to ordinary moral judgments in several ways. Sometimes they try to show that a careful accounting of the actual consequences in specific cases actually yields a result not far from what our ordinary moral judgments require. The alleged counterexamples are dismissed as resulting from a poor calculation of utility. Other times they might modify the theory into an "indirect" form, such as rule or code utilitarianism, in which the principle of utility is not applied directly to an act but directly to rules (or even dispositions) and thus indirectly to the classes of acts governed by those rules (or produced by those dispositions). The hope is that the indirect version of the theory better matches our ordinary views. For example, on the indirect view, we cannot kill the innocent in those cases where we might maximize utility by doing so because the rule prohibiting killing the innocent produces more utility than a rule permitting it, if it is generally complied with. In this case, and whenever utilitarians are inclined to give some credence to common moral views, it will be because those views are credited with reflecting the wisdom of people over time who have roughly determined how to promote utility.

A more forceful utilitarian response, and the one most relevant to us, is to reject the appeal to ordinary moral judgments as a "test" with any justificatory force at all (see the detailed discussion of this issue in Chapters 2 and 5). On this view, such moral judgments have no evidentiary credentials. Indeed, these judgments are dismissed as the results of cultural training, mere historical accidents, containing a legacy of various prejudices and social biases.

The charge that there is no reason to give justificatory weight to these moral judgments is an important one, especially since two standard ways of supplying credentials for these judgments are not available. One traditional way to support the reliability of these judgments is to claim that they are the result of a special moral faculty that allows us to "intuit" particular moral facts or universal principles. Proponents of wide reflective equilibrium do not resort to any such mysterious faculty, however. As I noted earlier, moral judgments are revisable in wide reflective equilibrium, and such revisability is not compatible with positing any traditional version of such a faculty. Rawls suggests that there is an analogy between the way reflective equilibrium allows us to uncover moral principles underlying our moral judgments and the way in which syntacticians use native speakers' judgments about grammaticality to uncover the grammatical rules underlying their linguistic capacity. This comparison might seem to suggest he is thinking of a moral faculty and not simply about the analogy between moral principles and rules of grammar. I argue in Chapter 4, however, that the analogy is overdrawn, especially if we think about wide and not narrow reflective equilibrium. Moral judgments, but not native speakers' judgments about grammaticality, are in general revisable.

The second way to support the reliability of such judgments would be to draw an analogy between considered moral judgments and "observations" in science or everyday life. We use observations based on our senses and on instruments to test hypotheses, laws, or theories. If we accept this analogy (I raise questions about it in Chapter 2), then we seem to owe an explanation of why these judgments standardly have reliability, just as we might invoke causal theories to tell us why our senses are generally reliable. Whether or not the analogy to sense observations is appropriate, we cannot supply the needed story about the reliability of considered moral judgments, at least not with the

4

current development of ethical theory. So these objections have some force (see Sencerz 1986). They force us to explain why systematizing our considered moral judgments and making them cohere with our other moral and nonmoral beliefs should make us think we are any closer to believing or knowing what is morally right or true.

The concern that our considered judgments are tainted by historical accident and prejudice is legitimate and adds urgency to the appeal that we supply some reasons to give these judgments justificatory weight. It is important, however, when facing any problem, including a philosophical one, to consider the alternatives. If we cannot appeal to moral judgments in the process of trying to arrive at justifiable ones, what else should we appeal to?

One alternative proposed by Brandt (1979) is that we undertake selecting moral principles without any prior appeal to moral judgments at all, since they have no demonstrable reliability. He proposes instead that we adopt the moral code that, if we generally abided by it, would be rational to choose, provided that our desires are themselves "rational." To make our desires rational, we must subject them to a process ("cognitive psychotherapy") of extinction and reinforcement using maximal criticism by facts and logic alone. The choice of moral principles, then, rests on the fact that we have the set of rational desires we do, and no explicit moral judgments have played a role in making the desires rational or motivating the choice of principles.

A crucial problem with Brandt's alternative (see Chapter 5) is that making our choice depend in this way on a cleaned-up (maximally criticized) system of desires still means that we are relying on desires that have already been structured by social institutions. These institutions, in turn, have themselves been shaped by moral practices and principles. Unfortunately, these practices and principles are themselves the results of the sort of accidents of history that Brandt and others object to when deploring considered moral judgments because they are "tainted" by historical and cultural accident. The utilitarian thus smuggles the effects of our conforming to those moral principles and practices into the process, and there is no real escape from prior moral "intuitions" after all. Our rationalized desires are not a bedrock of morally neutral facts. It is therefore better to lay all our moral cards on the table, where they can be assessed, as wide reflective equilibrium proposes, than to pretend we can end up justifying moral beliefs without appealing in any way to other moral beliefs.

If there were a better alternative to appealing to our moral judgments and then criticizing them as much as we can, then we should consider it. We seem to lack, however, a plausible alternative to appealing to some moral judgments. Moreover, if we are to appeal to them, then we should do so in a way that brings the most evidence and critical scrutiny to bear, that is, we should do so by seeking wide reflective equilibrium. To be sure, it would be good if we could supply a philosophically satisfactory set of credentials for the reliability of considered moral judgments. But, failing that, the remedy is not to abandon them but to submit them to the most extensive critical scrutiny possible. This means seeking coherence with all our other moral and nonmoral beliefs – all the other evidence we can bring to bear through empirical and philosophical argument.

This marshaling of the broadest evidence and critical scrutiny is the attraction of *wide* as opposed to *narrow* reflective equilibrium. We not only must work back and forth between principles and judgments about particular cases, the process that characterizes narrow equilibrium, but we must bring to bear all theoretical considerations that have relevance to the acceptability of the principles as well as the particular judgments. These theoretical considerations may be empirical or they may be moral. One task of ethical theory, then, is to show how work in the social sciences, for example, has a bearing on moral considerations. Ethical theory helps us to expand the kinds of considerations that count as evidence for or against our moral views at all levels of generality. Wide reflective equilibrium, then, forces us to elaborate moral theory in many directions and to attend to the broadest range of considerations and arguments that could count as evidence for our moral beliefs; it forces us to examine the structure of this far-flung system of beliefs and theories.

It is important that we see how diverse the types of beliefs included in wide reflective equilibrium are, as well as the kinds of arguments that may be based on them. They include our beliefs about particular cases; about rules, principles, and virtues and how to apply or act on them; about the right-making properties of actions, policies, and institutions; about the conflict between consequentialist and deontological views; about partiality and impartiality and the moral point of view; about motivation, moral development, strains of moral commitment, and the limits of ethics; about the nature of persons; about the role or function of ethics in our lives; about the implications of game theory, decision theory, and accounts of rationality for morality; about human psychology, sociology, and political and economic behavior; about the ways we should reply to moral skepticism and moral disagreement; and about moral justification itself. As is evident from this broad and encompassing list, the elements of moral theory are diverse. Moral theory is not simply a set of principles.

A central issue in ethics and in any account of justification in ethics is the fact of moral disagreement and the prospects for resolving moral disputes. One suggestion I make early in the volume (see Chapter 2) is that attention to wide reflective equilibrium as a method of justification may make theory acceptance in ethics a more tractable problem. By forcing us to attend to various kinds of theoretical considerations that bear on moral issues, wide reflective equilibrium may make it more possible to resolve moral disputes that otherwise might seem to rest on entrenched, conflicting moral judgments about particular cases.

Rawls' own argument for justice as fairness is supposed to make this claim about improved tractability plausible. Consider the problem of how to choose among competing conceptions of justice, say the utilitarian principle versus Rawls' two principles of justice. (His principles provide for equal basic liberties, equal opportunity, and inequalities only if they work to the maximal advantage of those who are worst off.) If we simply considered the alternative, utilitarian principles and their match to our moral judgments, Rawls might claim support from our ordinary beliefs, while the utilitarian might challenge the relevance of those unsupported "intuitions." That seems like a standoff, especially if we get some divergence among our considered moral judgments about particular cases, as we do among liberals who disagree about the relative importance of liberty and equality.

Rawls tries to break the standoff through the construction of an apparatus that gives us a "fair procedure" for selecting among principles, and then showing that his principles are chosen by that procedure over the principle of utility. This extra layer of theory seems to add justificatory support for the principles only if there is some independent reason to accept his account of a fair procedure. If the contract situation is itself designed (and redesigned) just so that it yields the principles that match our considered moral judgments about particular cases, then there is no extra support to the additional layer of theory. Critics of Rawls suggested that he "rigged" the contract situation and that it therefore added no justificatory force to the selection of principles. On their view, the whole construction just collapses into an exercise in narrow reflective equilibrium. At best the exercise only tells us what we happen to believe – a kind of moral anthropology – and fails to justify our beliefs.

This criticism misses its target (see Chapters 2 and 3). The argument for Rawls' fair procedure rests on the acceptability of some other morally laden views, for example, about the nature of persons as "free and equal," about the role of justice in a society, and about procedural fairness. These other (moral) ideas are not simply reducible to our considered judgments about justice in particular cases. A central point behind Rawls' construction is that, by appealing to the power of these other ideas and the way in which these other ideas provide support for points of agreement, for instance, agreement about the value of equal basic liberties, people may leverage further agreements on basic questions of justice (see Joshua Cohen 1989). Thus, people who might have disagreed in their judgments about the balance of equality and liberty might be moved to agreement on Rawls' principles through the force of their agreement on matters of procedural fairness and the view that a process of selecting principles must model the freedom and equality of people. Consequently, the extra layer of theory does add justificatory force to the selection of the principles. In addition, by compelling us to think in this way about aspects of moral theory and about other empirical and moral considerations that bear on what is right, wide reflective equilibrium offers some chance to improve on the intractability of moral disagreement that may otherwise seem to reduce to dogmatic disagreements about particular cases.

The suggestion that pursuing the elaboration of theory involved in wide reflective equilibrium can lead to more tractability for moral disputes is easily overstated. Walzer (1983) argues that views about what is just depend on the "shared meanings" that particular cultures develop for different categories ("spheres") of goods, and that we should expect considerable relativity about justice as a result. In Chapter 6 I examine how much relativity about justice is warranted by the kinds of intercultural considerations Walzer raises. I argue that Walzer too closely ties people's ultimate disagreements in wide reflective equilibrium to differences in these "shared meanings" because he underestimates our abilities to detach ourselves from some of our values while assessing them in light of our other beliefs. Still, the prospects of divergence in wide reflective equilibrium remain significant.

In his recent work, Rawls (1993) pays much greater attention to the forces that make pluralism about moral views a persistent fact of life in modern societies. He argues that, under conditions of freedom, we are likely to arrive at very different "comprehensive" views about philosophical, religious, and moral issues. This variation in our views results from the complexity of these issues ("the burdens of judgment") and does not imply moral skepticism.

Given this diversity, how can a society form a stable commitment to a conception of justice that specifies fair terms of cooperation among its members? The answer (see Chapter 8) is that the same conception of justice can form a "module" that is in turn justified in different ways in wide reflective equilibrium by people holding different comprehensive moral views. In this "overlapping consensus," convergence is only partial. It is limited to the (political) conception of justice; there is no shared wide reflective equilibrium, as was suggested in his earlier work. Since people continue to diverge in their other views, the publicly shared political conception of justice must be rich enough in its content to provide reasons for resolving disputes about constitutional essentials and basic questions of justice. For public discussion of these matters, the political conception thus defines the content of what Rawls calls "public reason." The idea that in discussion of certain questions of justice we should limit reasons to those we converge on, setting aside other areas of dispute, has a bearing on the use of ethics in public policy, a point I return to in the next section of this introduction.

Wide reflective equilibrium implies that the acceptability of particular conceptions of justice or of other ethical views must be reconciled with many of our other beliefs, including metaphysical and other philosophical views. This reconciliation is not part of "public reason" (see Chapter 8), but it must be possible for groups of reasonable people who hold these metaphysical views to make them cohere with the political conception of justice that forms the overlapping consensus. Parfit (1973, 1984) has proposed that our metaphysical views about such issues as personal identity have an important bearing on the acceptability of different views of distributive justice and other ethical concerns. Specifically, he suggests that justice as fairness, which emphasizes the "separateness of persons," seems to presuppose a Cartesian view of the identity of persons through time, whereas utilitarianism, which cares less how goods are distributed across the boundaries between persons, might be more compatible with contemporary arguments that construe persons as varying in psychological connectedness over time. If personal identity is a less deep metaphysical fact, Parfit contends, then the separateness of persons may be a less important moral one.

Parfit's general point, that metaphysical beliefs will have some bearing on the acceptability of different moral beliefs, is certainly true. If when we awoke each morning, we had few of the memories or intentions we had when we went to sleep, this deep fact about our nature would clearly affect the notion of cooperation over time and the very possibility of morality as we know it. Nevertheless, Parfit's specific claims about personal identity and their bearing on the choice of theories of justice are disputed in Chapters 7 and 13 and briefly in Chapter 8.

Two points are worth highlighting here. The first is that the kinds of "intuitions" or beliefs Parfit appeals to in making his metaphysical arguments about the identity of persons may ignore important factors or facts relevant to our concept of persons. For example, the intuitions about brain switching and other cases may ignore important social facts about how we must interact with people in order to accomplish cooperative goals over time (see also White 1991 for a similar, clearer development of this claim). This point raises interesting general questions (see Chapter 7) about the nature of the philosophical intuitions we commonly appeal to both in metaphysics and in doing ethics, especially when we use highly idealized or stylized hypothetical examples.

The second point is that Rawls' (1974) insistence that considerations of justice are "independent" of metaphysics has been refined as a result of the "politicization" of justice in his more recent work. The "political" conception of persons as "free and equal" over their whole lives models widely held ideas about how we treat citizens in a democratic society and how we should continue to do so. These political ideas must be thought of as compatible with a broad array of divergent views about the metaphysics of persons, even if some one of these views turns out to be true. Though this point is touched on in Chapter 8, I cannot discuss in detail how politicization affects Parfit's main claim (see Cohen 1994).

I want to conclude this introduction to the notion of wide reflective equilibrium and the essays in Part I with a reminder of my earlier disclaimer. The essays consider some main objections to this coherence account of justification, but they do not consider in detail all the issues raised in the substantial literature on this topic (see also Sencerz 1986; Holmgren 1989; Brink 1987; De Paul 1986). For example, an important matter not discussed in any of the essays is the idealization that is involved in talking about coherence among all our moral and nonmoral beliefs. Most people have no such systematic unity or comprehensiveness in their systems of beliefs (cf. Rawls 1993, 1995 for comments on the "looseness" of our comprehensive views). Work in ethics thus sometimes forces the elaboration of beliefs that had never been considered. In some cases this may provide the basis for further critical pressure to revise views. In any case, the great idealization about the scope of reason raises serious questions about what justification means in the ordinary, non-ideal case (cf. Cherniak 1986; Stich 1990).

2. WIDE REFLECTIVE EQUILIBRIUM IN PRACTICE

Wide reflective equilibrium, we have seen, requires that we develop support for our moral beliefs by working back and forth among judgments about particular cases, moral principles, and other theoretical considerations, both moral and nonmoral. We are to revise them wherever appropriate, aiming for the system of strongest mutual support among them. If we take this account seriously, then we must abandon some of the strong divisions that exist in the field between work in ethical theory and work in practical ethics. The ramifications of this quite simple point are the rationale for assembling the essays in practical ethics together with the more theoretical discussion of reflective equilibrium in this volume.

In what follows, I suggest how the essays in Part II illustrate several important implications of taking wide reflective equilibrium seriously as an account of justification in ethics. I want to emphasize five such lessons (there are others), without turning them into homilies: (1) The view that "applied ethics" results from merely plugging in the details or facts to theory or principles is an obstacle to solving problems at any level. (2) We should reject the "spinning wheels" view of ethical theory, as it has little bearing on practical matters. (3) The revision of moral judgments and elements of theory produces moral surprise and discovery. (4) Solutions to some ethical problems, especially matters of policy, do not require agreement on everything, and sometimes solutions preclude trying to agree on everything. (5) "Principled" solutions to some practical problems may not be possible in real time, and work in theoretical and practical ethics must attend more to issues of process and not just principle. These introductory comments supplement points made in Chapter 16, which adds to the rationale I offer here. There I discuss how some of these implications can be used to defuse methodological disputes in bioethics or practical ethics more generally.

When I began work on practical problems in ethics, I held what I believe is a fairly common view, namely, that we solve practical problems in ethics by supplying a description of a particular situation that allows us to subsume it under a relevant moral principle. The principles are ready-at-hand, perhaps delivered to us through work in ethical theory. The details of seeing how to fit them to the relevant facts is a complex but not philosophically challenging task. For example, I thought the problem of "applying" Rawls' theory of justice to health care was just such a problem (Daniels 1979), even though I was aware he had simplified his theory by presupposing everyone was fully functional over a whole life. My interest was in "testing" the theory by seeing whether the resulting application yielded more plausible judgments about the distribution of health care than, say, libertarian or utilitarian theories.

I quickly learned that my working picture of "applied ethics" was useless. To make progress on justice and health care, I had to answer basic questions about why the things that health care does for us are so important morally. From studying examples, including insurance practices, I came to believe that the health-care services we think we owe people as a matter of obligation are ones that work to keep them functioning as close to normally as possible. Normal functioning, I gradually concluded, was itself important because it served to keep open to us a reasonable range of opportunities. But if this account of the importance of health care is plausible, then extending Rawls' theory to cover the case where people are not fully functioning requires modest modifications of aspects of the theory (cf. Rawls 1993, 184, n. 14). Specifically, the account of equal opportunity has to be broadened so that it addresses more than capabilities affecting only access to jobs and careers. If the arguments of Chapter 9 are correct, then this effort at solving a problem in practical ethics about the distribution of health care *adds support* to the revised or extended version of Rawls' general theory of distributive justice.

Chapter 10 illustrates a similar point, that work in practical ethics can have important implications for ethical theory. In the 1980s, a debate emerged about the appropriate "target" of our concerns about equality or justice more generally. (The two concerns are distinct; see Chapter 10 and the postscript to Chapter 11.) What is it we want to make more equal or equitable among people: How happy they are? Their opportunities for welfare? The resources they have available to them? Or the capabilities to do or to be what they want? A key complaint about Rawls' theory, which emphasizes the distribution of primary social goods, is that it leaves unacceptable inequalities among people incapable of converting those resources into capabilities or "positive freedom" (Sen 1990, 1992) or equal opportunities for welfare (Arneson 1988; Joshua Cohen 1989). Chapter 9, however, which shows how to extend Rawls' theory to health care, provides a way to defuse some of the criticisms advanced from both of these perspectives. There is much less distance between Sen's views and Rawls' than at first appears.

The second lesson is that ethical theory does not (always) spin its wheels in ways irrelevant to solving practical problems. The dispute about the "target" of concerns regarding equality or justice discussed in Chapter 10 illuminates a widespread controversy in the practice of mental health care, which is described in Chapter 11. What kinds of mental health care services do we owe it to each other to provide in cooperative schemes, including health insurance schemes? Do we owe any assistance that simply reduces unhappiness? Do we owe services that contribute to opportunities for welfare? Are we interested in any services that improve or help equalize capabilities? Or is our goal really just the more modest one of preserving normal functioning? Chapter 11 is coauthored with a psychiatrist, James Sabin, and represents our analysis of the results of case studies we developed over a two-year period from interviews with clinicians. Their disagreements about what kinds of services ought to be covered in an HMO turn out to reflect the underlying dispute about the target of our concerns about equality or justice. In this case, the underlying theoretical controversy seemed to clarify the basis of the practical disagreement. The policy recommendation at which we arrive draws on our understanding of that dispute. In a postscript to Chapter 11 I add some further points challenging the degree to which Sen's account actually offers a more egalitarian view than the approach I defend in Chapter 9; these comments in effect are another illustration of the first lesson, that attending to the concerns of practical ethics helps to clarify theory.

The relevance of theory to the solution of practical problems in ethics is also illustrated by issues surrounding my approach to the problem of justice between age groups. It will help to provide a little background. When I first concluded that an account of the just distribution of health-care services required appeal to a principle of equal opportunity (see Chapter 9), I was immediately faced with an objection. If the opportunities of the elderly are in their past, then my account seemed to imply we give too much (beneficial) health care to the elderly (Daniels 1985). To address this objection, I had to consider what justice required in the distribution of various goods between age groups. My solution to the problem (described in Chapter 12, but more fully in Daniels 1988) is that differential treatment by age is different from differential treatment by race or sex, if it is done systematically over a whole life. Because we age, but do not change race or (typically) sex, objectionable inequalities between persons over their whole lives are not created by age-specific policies. Some such policies in fact make our lives go better: they are prudent. My proposal is that we view a distributive scheme as fair between age groups if it is prudent from the perspective of a whole life.

This account relies on commonly held views that lead us to think about prudence over a whole life-span. These views, however, have come under challenge, notably through Parfit's (1984) work on personal identity and the related work of McKerlie (1989a, b, 1992) on equality and time. Our standard view that it is acceptable for us to impose sacrifices on one stage of our lives in order that other stages do much better rests on a particular view of the identity of persons through time. We think this is acceptable because it is still "us" at all times making the sacrifices and getting the benefits. If persons should not be viewed as identical in this way through time, because, for example, the degree of their psychological connectedness varies over time, then prudence may face the same problems of distributive fairness that distributions across persons typically face.

McKerlie raises some related concerns about the fairness of viewing whole lives, rather than temporal stages of lives, as the appropriate units for thinking about issues of equality. He claims we should be troubled about inequalities between the temporal stages of persons and not, or at least not solely, about inequalities between whole lives. An approach such as mine must not simply rely on our ordinary or familiar intuitions about persons but must be justifiable in light of everything we learn from theory about personal identity and related issues. At least that is what taking reflective equilibrium seriously means.

In Chapter 7, as I noted earlier, I object to Parfit's arguments about personal identity and the nature of persons through time, and in Chapter 13 I argue that the widely held view of prudential reasoning I appeal to can be defended against his objections. In Chapter 12 I also defend the appeal to whole lives as the units of concern for issues of distributive justice. These challenges from theory must be taken seriously by work in practical ethics, whether or not specific challenges ultimately are sustained.

The work on justice between age groups serves to illustrate the relevance of work in ethical theory in yet another way, namely that it forced me to revise some moral judgments I had held about the permissibility of pure rationing by age. Much of our anti-age discrimination legislation in this country is directly modeled on anti-race and anti-gender discrimination legislation, and most people when asked are adamantly opposed to taking age alone into account in distributive matters. The argument sketched in Chapter 12 (see Daniels 1988, Ch. 5 for more detail), however, says that age works differently from race or gender, and it even justifies rationing by age under certain resource constraints. For me, this led to a gradual revision of my moral judgments about the permissibility of rationing by age, at least under special circumstances of scarcity. The revision was a slow surprise. My argument about the permissibility of rationing by age is quite distinct from Callahan's (1987) and Kamm's (1993).

Chapter 14 is included to illustrate the same point but from a distributive context outside health care. In the debate on affirmative action and reverse discrimination, it is often assumed – I began with this assumption myself – that people who have higher capabilities for performing a job or office have a claim to merit that job more than competitors with lesser capabilities. Of course, we must rely on some measurements of capabilities, and those may be inaccurate or biased, and so objectionable, but that is not the focus of this chapter. Rather, once we try to understand the grounds for thinking that greater capability might give rise to a claim to merit a particular position, we see that broader social concerns about productivity are really what does the work. These concerns may under many conditions actually work against the very merit claims people think they can make. The moral surprise for me was the degree to which my confidence in my earlier judgments about merit were undercut by these theoretical arguments.

The fourth lesson is not actually illustrated by any of the papers I have included (but see Brock and Daniels 1994 and Daniels 1994), but it is alluded to in Chapter 8 and discussed explicitly in Chapter 16. I noted earlier that Rawls politicizes his account of justice by treating justice as fairness as a "module" that might be incorporated within different wide reflective equilibria. To agree about justice as fairness, then, does not require agreeing on all moral matters. Nevertheless, justice as fairness is justified for people only if it is the view they accept in wide reflective equilibrium. People can then agree to restrict themselves to the reasons allowed by "public reason" without being morally schizophrenic because public reasons are justified for them from within their wider views. It is an interesting question whether a similar point may be made about other "middle-level" moral principles that people can all accept, even for somewhat different reasons. In Chapter 16 I develop this point with reference to what is sometimes called "public ethics" and with reference to the specific example of the kinds of principles that were developed and agreed to by the Ethics Working Group of the Clinton Health Care Task Force. The point, here, is that it is not necessary to look at such principles as merely a "compromise" among people who, had they greater numbers and more power, would really prefer some other principles. It is possible for people to find principles that they can accept and find justified for various reasons; such convergence is not merely a moral compromise but a principled moral solution to a policy problem.

The fifth lesson is that principled solutions to some important moral issues, including matters of public policy, may not be available to us at all, and in any case they are often not available to us in "real time," that is, within the time the problem has to be addressed. This point became clear to me when I saw the practical limitations of my equal opportunity account of justice and health care. I had originally hoped that we could get guidance on a broad range of resource allocation questions, including the rationing of beneficial medical services, by thinking about the relative impact on the range of opportunities different treatments provide. In Chapter 15, however, I explain why this account will not give determinate answers to a cluster of key, unsolved rationing problems. I do not think these problems are necessarily unsolvable; we may over time find persuasive philosophical solutions to them. Principled solutions to them are not available to us now, however, and there is also the chance that solutions would not be acceptable to everyone, at least in the short run, even if we found them.

Since the kinds of rationing problems I describe are not peripheral but very widespread, this conclusion has important implications for ethical theory (first lesson again). If general principles of distributive justice fail to guide us in the design of institutions, then it is not enough to say, "This is a matter for the political process to resolve." We need a more specific account of when a decision-making process is a fair one for addressing the kind of distributive problem involved in these rationing problems. A postscript to Chapter 15 adds some further thoughts on one line of solution to this problem.

As I noted above, in Chapter 16 I discuss further the implications of wide reflective equilibrium for moral problem solving in various practical contexts. My goal in that paper is to defuse the claims of various people who have argued that certain specific methodologies must be used if practical ethics is to progress effectively. Some, for example, insist we should adopt a "casuistical" approach; others emphasize the importance of relying on a general theory, or at least a framework of a few principles. I claim these "methods" generally focus on one type of problem and too narrowly understand the variety of work that is involved in solving ethical problems. Each might be seen as having a contribution to make, but none should be viewed as a general methodology for doing ethics or even practical ethics. Their relationships to each other, and their shortcomings when they are deployed exclusively, are all clarified by taking wide reflective equilibrium seriously as a method of justification. It is encouraging that a number of the disputants seem to support some version of reflective equilibrium as a general approach to justification.

I said early in this introduction that my task was to suggest some of the ways in which this volume was more than the sum of its parts. I have tried to do that by showing that taking wide reflective equilibrium seriously illuminates both practical and theoretical work in ethics. Even if I have delivered what I promised, my claim should not be understood to be stronger than it is. These essays, apart or together, do not provide the systematic defense of wide reflective equilibrium that some may expect or desire or that I would like to develop in future work. Each chapter is a piece of a larger discussion, and the discussion is far from complete. In addition, the lessons that I illustrate in this introduction and in the volume are ones that we could learn without any commitment to accepting wide reflective equilibrium as an account of justification. They are compatible with that account, and some of them seem to be implied by it, but they may also be accepted independently of it. Therefore the lessons are only weakly supportive of that account. My goal in this volume is to suggest a basis for future work, not to settle all the questions these essays raise.

REFERENCES

Arneson, Richard. 1988. "Equality and Equal Opportunity for Welfare," *Philosophical Studies* 54:79–95.

Brandt, Richard. 1979. *A Theory of the Good and the Right*. Oxford: Oxford University Press.

Brink, David. 1987. "Rawlsian Constructivism in Moral Theory," *Canadian Journal of Philosophy* 17:1(March):71–90.

Brock, Dan, and Daniels, Norman. 1994. "Ethical Foundations of the Clinton Administration's Proposed Health Care System," *JAMA* 271:15:1189–96.

Callahan, Daniel. 1987. *Setting Limits*. New York: Basic Books.

Cherniak, Christoper. 1986. *Minimal Rationality*. Cambridge, MA: MIT Press.

Cohen, G. A. 1989. "On the Currency of Egalitarian Justice," *Ethics* 99:906–44.

Cohen, Joshua. 1989. "Democratic Equality," *Ethics* 99:727–51.
Cohen, Joshua. 1994. "A More Democratic Liberalism," *Michigan Law Review* 92:6(May):1503–46.
Daniels, Norman. 1979. "Rights to Health Care and Distributive Justice," *Journal of Medicine and Philosophy* 4:2:174–91.
Daniels, Norman. 1985. *Just Health Care*. New York: Cambridge University Press.
Daniels, Norman. 1988. *Am I My Parents' Keeper? An Essay on Justice between the Young and the Old*. New York: Oxford University Press.
Daniels, Norman. 1994. "The Articulation of Principles and Values Involved in Health Care Reform," *Journal of Medicine and Philosophy* 19:425–33.
De Paul, Michael. 1986. "Reflective Equilibrium and Foundationalism," *American Philosophical Quarterly* 23:1:59–69.
Goodman, Nelson. 1955. *Fact, Fiction, and Forecast*. Cambridge, MA: Harvard University Press.
Holmgren, Margaret. 1989. "The Wide and Narrow of Reflective Equilibrium," *Canadian Journal of Philosophy* 19:1(March):43–60.
Kamm, Frances. 1993. *Morality and Mortality*. Vol 1. Oxford: Oxford University Press.
McKerlie, Dennis. 1989a. "Equality and Time," *Ethics* 99: 475–91.
McKerlie, Dennis. 1989b. "Justice between Age Groups: A Comment on Norman Daniels," *Journal of Applied Philosophy* 6:227–34.
McKerlie, Dennis. 1992. "Equality between Age Groups," *Philosophy and Public Affairs* 21:275–95.
Parfit, Derek. 1973. "Later Selves and Moral Principles." In A. Montefiori, ed., *Philosophy and Personal Relations*, pp. 137–69. London: Routledge and Kegan Paul.
Parfit, Derek. 1984. *Reasons and Persons*. Oxford: Oxford University Press.
Rawls, John. 1971. *A Theory of Justice*. Cambridge, MA: Harvard University Press.
Rawls, John. 1974. "The Independence of Moral Theory," *Proceedings and Addresses of the American Philosophical Association* 47:5–22.
Rawls, John. 1993. *Political Liberalism*. New York: Columbia University Press.
Rawls, John. 1995. "Reply to Habermas," *Journal of Philosophy* 92:3:132–80.
Sen, Amartya. 1990. "Justice: Means vs. Freedoms." *Philosophy and Public Affairs* 19:111–21.
Sen, Amartya. 1992. *Inequality Reexamined*. Cambridge: Harvard University Press.
Sencerz, Stefan. 1986. "Moral Intuitions and Justification in Ethics," *Philosophical Studies* 50:77–95.
Stich, Stephen. 1990. *The Fragmentation of Reason*. Cambridge, MA: MIT Press.
Walzer, Michael. 1983. *Spheres of Justice*. New York: Basic Books.
White, Stephen. 1991. *The Unity of the Self*. Cambridge, MA: MIT Press.

PART I

Chapter 2

Wide reflective equilibrium and theory acceptance in ethics

There is a widely held view that a moral theory consists of a set of moral judgments plus a set of principles that account for or generate them. This two-tiered view of moral theories has helped make the problem of theory acceptance or justification[1] in ethics intractable, unless, that is, one is willing to grant privileged epistemological status to the moral judgments (calling them "intuitions") or to the moral principles (calling them "self-evident" or otherwise a priori). Neither alternative is attractive. Nor, given this view of moral theory, do we get very far with a simple coherence view of justification. To be sure, appeal to elementary cohence (here, consistency) constraints between principles and judgments sometimes allows us to clarify our moral views or to make progress in moral argument. But there must be more to moral justification of both judgments and principles than such simple coherence considerations, especially in the face of the many plausible bases for rejecting moral judgments; e.g., the judgments may only reflect class or cultural background, self-interest, or historical accident.

I shall argue that a version of what John Rawls has called the *method of wide reflective equilibrium*[2] reveals a greater complexity in the structure of moral theories than the traditional view. Consequently, it may render theory acceptance in ethics a more tractable problem. If it does, it may permit us to recast and resolve some traditional worries about objectivity in ethics. To make this suggestion at all plausible, I shall have to defend reflective equilibrium against various charges that it is really a disguised form of moral intuitionism and therefore "subjectivist." First, however, I must explain what wide equilibrium is and show why seeking it may increase our ability to choose among competing moral conceptions.

Justice and justification

The method of wide reflective equilibrium is an attempt to produce coherence in an ordered triple of sets of beliefs held by a particular person, namely, (a) a set of considered moral judgments, (b) a set of moral principles, and (c) a set of relevant background theories. We begin by collecting the person's initial moral judgments and filter them to include only those of which he is relatively confident and which have been made under conditions conducive to avoiding errors of judgment. For example, the person is calm and has adequate information about cases being judged.[3] We then propose alternative sets of moral principles that have varying degrees of "fit" with the moral judgments. We do *not* simply settle for the best fit of principles with judgments, however, which would give us only a *narrow* equilibrium.[4] Instead, we advance philosophical arguments intended to bring out the relative strengths and weaknesses of the alternative sets of principles (or competing moral conceptions). These arguments can be construed as inferences from some set of relevant background theories (I use the term loosely). Assume that some particular set of arguments wins and that the moral agent is persuaded that some set of principles is more acceptable than the others (and, perhaps, than the conception that might have emerged in narrow equilibrium). We can imagine the agent working back and forth, making adjustments to his considered judgments, his moral principles, and his background theories. In this way he arrives at an equilibrium point that consists of the ordered triple (a), (b), (c).[5]

We need to find more structure here. The background theories in (c) should show that the moral principles in (b) are more acceptable than alternative principles on grounds to some degree independent of (b)'s match with relevant considered moral judgments in (a). If they are not in this way independently supported, then there seems to be no gain over the support the principles would have had in a corresponding narrow equilibrium, where there never was any appeal to (c). Another way to raise this point is to ask how we can be sure that the moral principles that systematize the considered moral judgments are not just "accidental generalizations" of the "moral facts," analogous to accidental generalizations which we want to distinguish from real scientific laws. In science, we have evidence that we are not dealing with accidental generalizations if we can derive the purported laws from a body of interconnected theories, provided these theories reach, in a diverse and interesting way, beyond the "facts" that the principle generalizes.

This analogy suggests one way to achieve independent support for the principles in (b) and to rule out their being mere accidental generalizations of the considered judgments. We should require that the background theories in (c) be more than reformulations of the same set of considered moral judgments involved when the principles are matched to moral judgments. The background theories should have a scope reaching beyond the range of the considered moral judgments used to "test" the moral principles. Some interesting, nontrivial portions of the set of considered moral judgments that constrains the background theories and of the set that constrains the moral principles should be disjoint.

Suppose that some set of considered *moral* judgments (a') plays a role in constraining the background theories in (c). It is important to note that the acceptability of (c) may thus in part depend on some *moral* judgments, which means we are not in general assuming that (c) constitutes a reduction of the moral [in (b) and (a)] to the nonmoral. Then, our *independence constraint* amounts to the requirement that (a') and (a) be to some significant degree disjoint.[6] The background theories might, for example, not incorporate the same type of moral notions as are employed by the principles and those considered judgments relevant to "testing" the principles.

It will help to have an example of a wide equilibrium clearly in mind. Consider Rawls' theory of justice.[7] We are led by philosophical argument, Rawls believes, to accept the contract and its various constraints as a reasonable device for selecting between competing conceptions of justice (or right). These arguments, however, can be viewed as inferences from a number of relevant background theories, in particular, from a theory of the person, a theory of procedural justice, general social theory, and a theory of the role of morality in society (including the ideal of a well-ordered society). These *level* iii theories, as I shall call them, are what persuade us to adopt the contract apparatus, with all its constraints (call it the *level* ii apparatus). Principles chosen at level ii are subject to two constraints: (i) they must match our considered moral judgments in (partial) reflective equilibrium; and (ii) they must yield a feasible, stable, well-ordered society. I will call *level* i the *partial* reflective equilibrium that holds between the moral principles and the relevant set of considered moral judgments. *Level* iv contains the body of social theory relevant to testing level i principles (and level iii theories) for "feasibility."

The independence constraint previously defined for wide equilibrium in general applies in this way: the considered moral judgments [call them (a')] which may act to constrain level iii theory acceptability must to a significant extent be disjoint from the considered moral judgments [call them (a)] which act to constrain level i partial equilibrium. I argue elsewhere that Rawls' construction appears to satisfy this independence constraint, since his central level iii theories of the person and of the role of morality in society are probably not just recharacterizations or systematizations of level I moral judgments.[8] If I am right, then (supposing soundness of Rawls' arguments!), the detour of deriving the principles from the contract adds justificatory force to them, justification not found simply in the level I matching of principles and judgments. Notice that this advantage is exactly what would be lost if the contract and its defining conditions were "rigged" just to yield the best level I equilibrium.[9] The other side of this coin is that the level II apparatus will not be acceptable if competing theories of the person or of the role of morality in society are preferable to the theories Rawls advances. Rawls' Archimedean point is fixed only against the acceptability of particular level III theories.

This argument suggests that we abstract from the details of the Rawlsian example to find quite general features of the structure of moral theories in wide equilibrium. Alternatives to justice as fairness are likely to contain some level II device for principle selection other than the contract (say a souped-up impartial spectator). Such variation would reflect variation in the level III theories, especially the presence of alternative theories of the person or of the role of morality. Finally, developed alternatives to justice as fairness would still be likely to contain some version of the level I and level IV constraints, though the details of how these constraints function will reflect the content of component theories at the different levels.

By revealing this structural complexity, the search for wide equilibrium can benefit moral inquiry in several ways. First, philosophers have often suggested that many apparently "moral" disagreements rest on other, nonmoral disagreements. Usually these are lumped together as the "facts" of the situation. Wide equilibrium may reveal a more systematic, if complex, structure to these sources of disagreement, and, just as important, to sources of agreement as well.

Second, aside from worries about universalizability and generalizability, philosophers have not helped us to understand what factors *actually do* constrain the considerations people cite as reasons, or treat as "relevant" and "important," in moral reasoning and argument. A likely suggestion is that these features of moral reasoning depend on the *content* of underlying level III theories and level II principle selectors, or on properties of the level I and IV constraints. An adequate moral psychology, in other words, would have to incorporate features of what I am calling "wide equilibrium." Understanding these features of moral argument more clearly might lead to a better grasp of what constitutes evidence for and against moral judgments and principles. This result should not be surprising: as in science, judgments about the plausibility and acceptability of various claims are the complex result of the whole system of interconnected theories already found acceptable. My guess – I cannot undertake to confirm it here – is that the type of coherence constraint that operates in the moral and nonmoral cases functions to produce many similarities: we should find methodological conservatism in both; we will find that "simplicity" judgments in both really depend on determining how little we have to change in the interconnected background theories already accepted (not to more formal measures of simplicity); and we will find in both that apparently "intuitive" judgments about how "interesting," "important," and "relevant" puzzles or facts are, are really guided by underlying theory.[10]

A third possible benefit of wide equilibrium is that level III disagreements about theories may be more tractable than disagreements about moral judgments and principles. Consequently, if the moral disagreements can be traced to disagreements about theory, greater moral agreement may result.

Some examples may perhaps make this claim more plausible. A traditional form of criticism against utilitarianism consists in deriving unacceptable moral judgments about punishment, desert, or distributive justice from a general utilitarian principle. Some utilitarians then may bite the bullet and reject reliance on these "pretheoretical" intuitions. Rawls has suggested an explanation for the class of examples involving distributive justice. He suggests that the utilitarian has imported into social contexts, where we distribute goods between persons, a principle acceptable only for distributing goods between life-stages of one person. Derek Parfit urges a different explanation: the utilitarian, perhaps supported by evidence from the philosophy of mind, uses a weaker criterion of personal identity than that presupposed by, say, Rawls' account of life plans. Accordingly, he treats interpersonal boundaries as metaphysically less deep and morally less important. The problem between the utilitarian and the contractarian thus becomes the (possibly) more manageable problem of determining the acceptability of competing theories of the person, and only one of many constraints on that task is the connection of the theory of the person to the resulting moral principles.[11]

A second example derives from a suggestion of Bernard Williams.[12] He argues that there may be a large discrepancy between the dictates of utilitarian theory in a particular case and what a person will be inclined to do given that he has been raised to have virtues (e.g., beneficence) that in general optimize his chances of doing utilitarian things. We may generalize Williams' point: suppose any moral conception can be paired with an *optimal* set of virtues, those which make their bearer most likely to do what is right according to the given conception. Moral conceptions may differ significantly in the degree to which acts produced by their optimal virtues tend to differ from acts they deem right. Level III and IV theories of moral psychology and development would be needed to determine the facts here. Since we want to reduce such discrepancies (at least according to some level III and IV theories), we may have an important scale against which to compare moral conceptions.

More, and better developed, examples would be needed to show that the theory construction involved in seeking wide equilibrium increases our ability to choose rationally among competing moral conceptions. But there is a general difficulty that must be faced squarely: level III theories may, I have claimed, depend in part for their acceptability on some considered moral judgments, as in Rawls' level III theories. (If the independence constraint is satisfied, however, these are not primarily the level I considered judgments.) If the source of our disagreement about competing moral conceptions is disagreement on such level III considered judgments, then it is not clear just how much increase in tractability will result. The presence of these judgments clearly poses some disanalogy to scientific-theory acceptance. I take up this worry indirectly, by first considering the charge that reflective equilibrium is warmed-over moral intuitionism.

2. THE REVISABILITY OF CONSIDERED MORAL JUDGMENTS

A number of philosophers, quite diverse in other respects, have argued that the method of reflective equilibrium is really a form of moral intuitionism, indeed of subjective intuitionism.[13] If we take moral intuitionism in its standard forms, then the charge seems unfounded. Intuitionist theories have generally been foundationalist. Some set of moral beliefs is picked out as basic or self-warranting. Theories differ about the nature or basis of the self-warrant. Some claim self-evidence or incorrigibility; others innateness; others some form of causal reliability. A claim of causal reliability might take, for example, the form of a perceptual account which even leaves room for perceptual error. Some intuitionists want to treat principles as basic. Others begin with particular intuitions and then attempt to find general principles that systematize the intuitions, perhaps revealing and reducing errors among them. Still, and this is the central point, the justification for accepting such moral principles is that they systematize the intuitions, which carry the epistemological privilege.[14]

No such foundationalism is part of wide reflective equilibrium as I have described it. Despite the care taken to filter initial judgments to avoid obvious sources of error, no special epistemological priority[15] is granted the considered moral judgments. We are missing the little story that gets told about why we should pay homage ultimately to those judgments and indirectly to the principles that systematize them. Without such a story, however, we have no foundationalism and so no standard form of moral intuitionism.

Nevertheless, it might be thought that reflective equilibrium involves an attempt to give us the *effect* of intuitionism without any fairy tales about epistemic priority. The effect is that a set of principles gets "tested" against a determinate and relatively fixed set of moral judgments. We have, as it were, foundationalism without foundations. Once the foundational claim is removed, however, we have nothing more than a person's moral opinion. It is a "considered" opinion, to be sure, but still only an opinion. Since such opinions are often the result of self-interest, self-deception, historical and cultural accident, hidden class bias, and so on, just systematizing some of them hardly seems a promising way to provide justification for them or for the principles that order them.

This objection really rests on two distinct complaints: (1) that reflective equilibrium merely systematizes some relatively determinate set of moral judgments; and (2) that the considered moral judgments are not a proper foundation for an ethical theory. I will return in section III to consider (2) in a version that abstracts from the issue of the revisability of considered judgments. Here I shall consider objection (1).

Wide reflective equilibrium does not merely systematize some determinate set of judgments. Rather, it permits extensive revision of these moral judgments. There is no set of judgments that is held more or less fixed as there would be on a foundationalist approach, even one without foundations. It will be useful to see just how far from the more traditional view of a moral intuition the considered moral judgment in wide reflective equilibrium has come.

The difference does not come at the stage at which we filter *initial* moral judgments to arrive at *considered* moral judgments. Sophisticated forms of intuitionism leave room for specifying optimal conditions for avoiding errors of judgment. Nor does the difference come at the stage at which we match principles to judgments, "smooth out" irregularities, and increase the power of the principles. Again, sophisticated intuitionism is willing to trade away some slight degree of unrevisability for the reassurance that errors of judgment are further reduced. It is because *narrow* reflective equilibrium allows no further opportunities for revision than these two that it is readily assimilated to the model of a sophisticated intuitionism.

But *wide* reflective equilibrium, as I have described it, allows far more drastic *theory-based* revisions of moral judgments. Consider the additional ways in which a considered moral judgment is subject to revision in wide equilibrium. Suppose the considered judgment is about what is right or wrong, just or unjust, in particular situations, or is a maxim that governs such situations. In that case, it is a judgment relevant to establishing partial reflective equilibrium with general moral principles. Consequently, we must revise it if background theories compel us to revise our general principles or if they lead us to conclude that our moral conception is not feasible. Suppose, in contrast, the considered moral judgment plays a role in determining the acceptability of a component level III theory. Then it is also revisable for several reasons. Feasibility testing of the background theory may lead us to reject it and therefore to revise the considered judgment. The judgment may be part of one background theory that is rendered implausible because of its failure to cohere with other, more plausible background theories, and so the considered judgment may have to be changed. The considered judgment may be part of a system of background theories that would lead us to accept principles, and consequently some other level I considered judgments, which we cannot accept. If we can trace the source of our difficulty back to a level III considered judgment that we can give up more easily than we can accept the new level I judgment, then we would probably revise the level III judgment.

In seeking wide reflective equilibrium, we are constantly making plausibility judgments about which of our considered moral judgments we should revise in light of theoretical considerations at all levels. No one type of considered moral judgment is held immune to revision. No doubt, we are not inclined to give up certain considered moral judgments unless an overwhelmingly better alternative moral conception is available and substantial dissatisfaction with our own conception at other points leads us to do so (the methodological conservatism I referred to earlier). It is in this way that we provide a sense to the notion of a "provisional fixed point" among our considered judgments. Since all considered judgments are revisable, the judgment "It is wrong to inflict pain gratuitously on another person" is, too. But we can also explain why it is so hard to imagine not accepting it, so hard that some treat it as a necessary moral truth. To imagine revising such a provisional fixed point we must imagine a vastly altered wide reflective equilibrium that nevertheless is much more acceptable than our own. For example, we might have to imagine persons quite unlike the persons we know.

Wide reflective equilibrium keeps us from taking considered moral judgments at face value, however much they may be treated as starting points in our theory construction.[16] Rather, they are always subjected to exhaustive review and are "tested," as are the moral principles, against a relevant body of theory. At every point, we are forced to assess their acceptability relative to theories that incorporate them and relative to alternative theories incorporating different considered moral judgments.[17]

3. COHERENCE AND JUSTIFICATION

A. No justification without credibility

Consider now the claim (2) that wide equilibrium uses inappropriate starting points for the development of moral theory. Here the accusation of neo-intuitionism seems to take the opposite tack, suggesting that considered judgments are not foundational enough. The traditional intuitionist seemed to have more going for him. With some pomp and circumstance, the earlier intuitionist at least outfitted his intuitions with the regal garb of epistemic priority, even if this later turned out to be the emperor's clothes. The modern intuitionist, the proponent of reflective equilibrium, allows his naked opinions to streak their way into our theories without benefit of any cover story. Richard Brandt has raised this objection in a forceful way which avoids the mistake about revisability noted earlier.

Brandt characterizes the method of reflective equilibrium as follows. We begin with a set of initial moral judgments or intuitions. We assign an *initial credence level* (say from 0 to 1 on a scale from things we believe very little to things we confidently believe). We filter out judgments with low initial credence levels to form our set of considered judgments. Then we propose principles and attempt to bring the system of principles plus judgments into equilibrium, allowing modifications wherever they are necessary to produce the system with the highest over-all credence level.[18] But why, asks Brandt, should we be impressed with the results of such a process? We should not be, he argues, unless we have some way to show that "some of the beliefs are initially *credible* – and not merely initially believed – for some reason other than their coherence" in the set of beliefs we believe the most ([Brandt 1979], *op. cit.*, chapter 1). For example, in the nonmoral case, Brandt suggests that an initially believed judgment is also an initially credible judgment when it states (or purports to state) a fact of observation. "In the case of normative beliefs, no reason has been offered why we should think that initial credence levels, for a person, correspond to *credibilities*."[19] The result is that we have no reason to think that increasing the credence level for the system as a whole moves us closer to moral truth rather than away from it. Coherent fictions are still fictions, and we may only be reshuffling our prejudices.[20]

If Brandt's "no credibility" complaint has force, a question I take up shortly, it has such force against wide, and not just narrow, reflective equilibrium. In my reconstruction, considered moral judgments *may* play an ineliminable role constraining the acceptance of background (level III) theories in wide reflective equilibrium. (In general, level III theories do not reduce the moral to the nonmoral, and level IV constraints do not select only one feasible system.) But level III considered moral judgments seem to be as open as level I considered judgments to the objection that they have only initial credence and not initial credibility. At least it would take a special argument to show why worries that initial level I considered judgments about justice lack initial credibility fail to carry weight against initial level III judgments about fair procedures or about which features of persons are morally central or relevant. The problem is that all such initial judgments are still "our" judgments.[21] The fact that wide equilibrium provides support for the principles independent from that provided by level I partial equilibrium does not imply that this support is based on considered judgments that escape the "no credibility" criticism. The criticism does not go away just because wide reflective equilibrium permits an intratheory gain in justificatory force not provided by narrow equilibrium.

B. Credibility and coherence

Much of the plausibility of the "no credibility" objection derives from the contrast between nonmoral observation reports and considered moral judgments or "intuitions." A minimal version[22] of the claim that initial credibility attaches to observation reports must do two things. It must allow for the revisability of such reports. It must also treat them as generally reliable unless we have specific reasons to think they are not. Observation reports seem to satisfy these conditions because we can tell some story, perhaps a causal story, that explains why the reports are generally reliable, though still revisable. In contrast, moral judgments are more suspect. We know that even sincerely believed moral judgments made under conditions conducive to avoiding mistakes may still be biased by self-interest, self-deception, or cultural and historical influences.[23] So, if we construe a considered moral judgment as an attempt to report a moral fact, we have no causal story to tell about reliability[24] and many reasons to suspect unreliability.

I would like to suggest three responses to this way of contrasting considered moral judgments and observation reports. First, the assumed analogy between considered moral judgments and observation reports is itself inappropriate. A considered moral judgment, even in a particular case, is in many ways far more like a "theoretical" than an "observation" statement. (I am not assuming a principled dichotomy here, at most a continuum of degree of theory dependence.) Evidence comes from the way in which we support considered moral judgments as compared to observation reports: we readily give reasons for the moral judgments, and our appeal to theoretical considerations to support them is not mainly concerned with the conditions under which the judgments are made. Further evidence for my claim would require that we carry out the programmatic suggestion made earlier: see whether we can explain the features of reason giving by reference to features of wide equilibrium.

On the other hand, some may cite other evidence to support the analogy between observations and moral judgments. They might point, for example, to language-learning contexts, in which children are taught to identify actions as wrong or unjust much as they are taught to identify nonmoral properties. Or they may point to the fact that we often judge certain acts as right or wrong with great *immediacy* – the "gut reaction," so called. But such evidence is not persuasive. One thing that distinguishes adult from childish moral reasoning is the ready appeal to theoretical considerations.[25] Similarly, we are often impatient with the person who refuses to provide moral reasons or theory to support his immediate moral judgments, much more so than we are with the person who backs up "It is red" with nothing more than "It sure looks red."

Consequently, I conclude, though I have not fully argued the point here, that the comparison of moral judgments to observation reports is misleading. Rightness and wrongness, or justice and injustice, are unlikely to be simple properties of moral situations. Consequently, they are unlikely to play a role analogous to that played by observational properties in the causal-reliability stories we tell ourselves concerning observation reports. But the "no credibility" argument gains its plausibility from the assumption that the analogy to observation reports *should* hold and then denigrates moral judgments when it is pointed out they differ from observation reports. If they *should* and *do* function differently – because they are different kinds of judgments – that is not something we should hold against the moral judgments.

Secondly, the "no credibility" criticism is at best premature. It is plausible to think that only the development of acceptable moral theory in wide reflective equilibrium will enable us to determine what kind of "fact," if any, is involved in a considered moral judgment. In the context of such a theory, and with an answer to our puzzlement about the kind of fact (if any) a moral fact is, we might be able to provide a story about the reliability of initial considered judgments. Indeed, it seems reasonable to impose this burden on the theory that emerges in wide reflective equilibrium. It should help us answer this sort of question. If we can provide a reasonable answer, then we may have a way of distinguishing initially credible from merely initially believed types of moral judgments.

The "no credibility" criticism gains initial plausibility because we *are* able to assign initial credibility to nonmoral observation reports, but not to moral judgments. The credibility assignment, however, draws implicitly on a broadly accepted body of theory which explains why those judgments are credible. Properly understood, the credibility story about nonmoral observation reports is itself only the product of a nonmoral wide reflective equilibrium of relatively recent vintage. In contrast, we lack that level of theory development in the moral case. What follows from this difference is that the "no credibility" argument succeeds in assigning a burden of proof. *Some* answer to the question about the reliability of moral judgments must be forthcoming. But the argument is hardly a demonstration that no plausible story is possible.

Thirdly, a more positive – though still speculative – point can be made in favor of starting from considered moral judgments in our theory construction. It is commonplace, and true, to note that there is variation and disagreement about considered moral judgments among persons and cultures. It is also commonplace, and true, to note that there is much uniformity and agreement on considered moral judgments among persons and cultures. Philosophers of all persuasions cite one or the other commonplace as convenience in argument dictates. But moral philosophy should help us to *explain both* facts.

What wide equilibrium shows us about the structure of moral theories may help us explain the extensive agreement we do find. Such agreement on judgments may reflect an underlying agreement on features of the component background theories. Indeed, people may be more in agreement about the nature of persons, the role of morality in society, and so on, than is often assumed. Of course, these other points of agreement might be discounted by pointing to the influence of culture or ideology in shaping level III theories. But it may also be that the agreement is found because some of the background theories are, roughly speaking, true – at least with regard to certain important features. Moreover, widely different people may have come to learn these truths despite their culturally different experiences. The point is that moral *agreement* – at levels III and I – may not be just the result of historical accident, at least not in the way that some moral *disagreements* are. Consequently, it would be shortsighted to deny credibility to considered judgments just because there is widespread disagreement on many of them: there is also agreement on many. Here moral anthropology *is* relevant to answering questions in moral theory.

I conclude that the "no credibility" objection reduces either to a burden-of-proof argument, which is plausible but hardly conclusive, or to a general foundationalist objection to coherence accounts of theory acceptance (or justification). It becomes a burden-of-proof argument as soon as one notices that the credibility we assign to observation reports is itself based on an inference from a nonmoral reflective equilibrium. We do not yet have such an account of credibility for the moral case, but we also have no good reason to think it impossible or improbable that we can develop such an account once we know more about moral theory. On the other hand, the "no credibility" argument becomes a foundationalist objection if it is insisted that observation reports are credible independently of such coherence stories.

My reply to the "no credibility" criticism points again to a strong similarity in the way coherence constraints on theory acceptance (or justification) operate in the two domains, despite the disanalogy between observation reports and considered moral judgments. The accounts of initial credibility we accept for observation reports (say, some causal story about reliable detection) are based on inferences from various component sciences constrained by coherence considerations. Observation reports are neither self-warranting nor unrevisable, and our willingness to grant them initial credibility depends on our acceptance of various other relevant theories and beliefs. Such an account is also owed for some set of moral judgments, but it too will derive from component theories in wide equilibrium. Similarly, in rejecting the view that wide equilibrium merely systematizes a determinate set of moral judgments, and arguing instead for the revisability of these inputs, I suggest that wide equilibrium closely resembles scientific practice. Neither in science nor in ethics do we merely "test" our theories against a predetermined, relatively fixed body of data. Rather, we continually reassess and reevaluate both the plausibility and the relevance of these data against theories we are inclined to accept. The possibility thus arises that these pressures for revision will free considered moral judgments from their vulnerability to many of the *specific* objections about bias and unreliability usually directed against them.

4. OBJECTIVITY AND CONVERGENCE

I would like to consider what implications, if any, the method of wide equilibrium may have for some traditional worries about objectivity in ethics. Of course, objectivity is a multiply ambiguous notion. Still, two senses stand out as central. First, in a given area of inquiry, claims are thought to be objective if there is some significant degree of intersubjective agreement on them. Second, claims are also said to be objective if they express truths relevant to the area of inquiry. Other important senses of "objectivity" reduce to one or both of the central uses [e.g., "free from bias" (said of methods or claims) and "reliability" or "replicability" (said of methods or procedures of inquiry)]. The two central senses are not unrelated. The typical realist, for example, hopes that methods or procedures of inquiry that tend to produce intersubjective agreement do so because they are methods that give us access to relevant truths. In contrast, there are also eliminative approaches which try to show that one or the other notion of objectivity is either confused, reducible to the other, or irrelevant in a given area of inquiry. Thus some have suggested that knowledge of moral truths is unattainable (perhaps because there are no moral truths) and we should settle for the objectivity of intersubjective agreement (based on rational inquiry) if we can achieve it. Does the method of wide reflective equilibrium commit us to one or another of these approaches to objectivity in ethics?

One traditional worry, that moral judgments are not objective because there is insufficient agreement about them, may be laid to rest by seeking wide equilibrium. I have suggested that seeking wide equilibrium may render problems of theory acceptance in ethics more tractable and may thus produce greater moral agreement. Specifically, it may lead us to understand better the sources of moral agreement and disagreement and the constraints on what we count as relevant and important to the revision of moral judgments. It may allow us to reduce moral disagreements (about principles or judgments) to more resoluble disagreements in the relevant background (level III and IV) theories. None of these possibilities guarantees increased agreement. How much convergence results remains an empirical question. But I think I have made it at least plausible that wide equilibrium could increase agreement and do so in a *nonarbitrary* way. At least, it could provide us with a clearer picture of how much agreement we already have (I return to this point later). And if it does, then there are implications for how objective, at least in the minimal sense of intersubjective agreement, ethics is.

To be sure, many who point to the lack of intersubjective agreement on many moral issues do so to raise a more robust worry about lack of objectivity in ethics. They point to moral disagreement as if it were strong *evidence* for the deeper claim about objectivity, that there are no moral truths for us to agree about. The inference from lack of agreement to the absence of truths to be acquired is generally unpersuasive, however. Sometimes there is the buried assumption that *if* there were such truths, we would probably have enough access to them to produce more agreement than we have. I see no way, however, to formulate this assumption so that it does not rule out the existence of truths in most areas of scientific inquiry, at least at some time in their history. Sometimes there is the qualification that it is not the disagreement about moral claims that is important, but the "fact" that we cannot agree about what would produce resolution of the disagreement. This is likely to be more true in science and less true in ethics than is usually claimed. Still, there is a kernel of truth behind the inference, though it is insufficient to warrant it: agreement, *when it is produced by methods we deem appropriate in a given area of inquiry*, does appear to have some evidential relation to what is agreed on.

What has troubled critics of reflective equilibrium, however, is an opposite worry. Anyone who believes that there *are* objective moral truths will want to leave room for the possibility that there may be consensus on moral falsehoods. The worry is clearly reasonable when we suspect that the factors that led to consensus have little, if anything, to do with rational inquiry (and we need not have in mind anything so drastic as the Inquisition). And if one thought the method of wide equilibrium fell far short of rational inquiry, the worry would again be reasonable. Moreover, it is not obviously unreasonable even if one takes wide equilibrium to be the best method available but wants to acknowledge the possibility that it may lead to justified acceptance of moral falsehoods. The fear here is that intersubjective agreement will be taken as *constitutive* of moral truth or as eliminative of any full-blown (realist) notion of objective moral truth.[26]

The worry might be put this way. Suppose that when diverse people are induced to seek the principles they would accept in wide reflective equilibrium, only one shared equilibrium point emerges. Can we still ask, Are these principles objective moral truths? Is the proponent of wide equilibrium committed to the view that such intersubjective agreement *constitutes* the principles and judgments as moral truths? Or is it at best *evidence* that we have discovered objective moral truths? Or is it any evidence at all that we have found some? I shall suggest that though convergence in wide equilibrium is neither a necessary nor a sufficient condition for claiming we have found objective moral truths, such convergence may constitute *evidence* we have found some.

To see that convergence in wide equilibrium is not a sufficient condition for claiming we have found objective moral truths, suppose we actually produced such convergence among diverse persons. Whether or not the principles and judgments they accept would count as such truths would depend on *how* we come to explain the convergence. Suppose, for example, we find that we can *explain* the convergence by pointing to a psychological feature of human beings that plays a *causal* role in producing their agreement. Suppose, to be specific, that, under widespread conditions of child rearing in diverse cultures, people tend to group others into "in groups" and "out groups" and that the effect of this mechanism is that moral judgments and principles in wide equilibrium turn out to be inegalitarian in certain ways.[27] Suppose we discover, further, that these child-rearing practices are themselves changeable and not the product of any deep features of human biology and psychology. We might begin to feel that the convergence we had found in wide equilibrium was only a fortuitous result of a provincial feature of human social psychology. Convergence would thus not by itself be sufficient grounds for constituting the principles as moral truths.

We can turn the example around to question the necessity of convergence for constituting the principles as objective moral truths. Suppose we find, after attempting to produce wide equilibria among diverse persons, that there is no actual convergence in wide equilibrium. Different families of equilibria emerge. Suppose also that we can *explain* the failure of convergence by pointing again to a provincial feature of human psychology or biology. But suppose further that we can abstract from this source of divergence. We can construct a modified and *idealized* "agreement" on principles. Such an idealization might, depending on other factors, be a good candidate for containing objective moral truths, even though it is *not* accepted in any actual wide equilibrium.

Which way we should go in either of these cases will have something to do with how fundamental we think the source of divergence or convergence is. But what we count as "fundamental" is itself determined by the view of the nature of moral judgments and principles which emerges in wide equilibrium. For example, if the convergence producing feature of human psychology turned out to be a central fact about the emotions or motivations, say, some fact about the nature of (Humean) sympathy, which proved invariant to all but the strangest (pathological) child-rearing practices, then we might think we had reached a fundamental fact (related at least to the *feasibility* of moral conceptions). Still, even here, I do not want to assume that metaethical considerations embedded in the background theories would force us to reject a more Kantian stance. To follow up our earlier discussion, we are here concerned with factors that may affect the "credibility" of initial considered judgments, leading us to discount some and favor others; how we weigh these factors will depend on complex features of our background theories.

In short, divergence among wide reflective equilibria does not imply that there are no such things as objective moral truths;[28] nor does convergence imply that we have found them; nor need "moral truth" be replaced by "adopted in wide equilibrium." How we will be motivated, or warranted, in treating the facts of divergence or convergence depends on the kinds of divergence or convergence we encounter and the kinds of explanation we can give for it. This result should not surprise us: wide reflective equilibrium embodies coherence constraints on theory acceptance or justification, not on truth.[29]

Actually, it is necessary to qualify my conclusion that wide reflective equilibrium need not be viewed as constitutive of moral truth.[30] My argument that convergence is neither necessary nor sufficient to establish the discovery of moral truths depends on bringing theoretical considerations to bear which seem sufficient to destabilize the actual equilibrium in some way. Suppose we now throw back into the ring these destabilizing considerations and seek a new wide equilibrium. If we can enrich wide equilibrium in this way, so that it adds up to something like "total rational considerations," then perhaps we can revive in a strengthened form the constitutive view. We would have here, perhaps, the analogue of Putnam's "empirical realist" rejection of objective (metaphysical) moral truths.[31] This version of the eliminative view is not open to the most reasonable worries of those who feel simple moral agreement should not be taken to constitute moral truth. In any case, on its form of verificationism, ethics may be no worse off than science!

A more modest way of putting the same objection is this. My reply to the eliminative view is compatible with the following claim: there is a sense in which the question, Do we really have moral truth, given convergence in wide reflective equilibrium? is an *idle* worry in the absence of any *specific* research capable of destabilizing the equilibrium. In the absence of some particular, plausible way to challenge the convergence, the question is tantamount to strong and unfruitful skepticism.

Despite these qualifications, my inclination is not to treat wide reflective equilibrium as constitutive of moral truth (assuming convergence) and to leave room instead for a weaker *evidential* relation holding between agreement in wide equilibrium and moral truth. What we would need to support this possibility is reason to think that the methods of inquiry in ethics that tend to produce convergence do so *because* they bring us close to moral truth. I can offer only a highly qualified and indirect argument to this conclusion.

Consider for a moment a general argument of this form.[32] (1) In a given area of inquiry, the methods used are successful in the sense that they produce convergence and a growth of knowledge; (2) the only plausible account of the success of these methods is that they lead us to better and better approximations to truths of the kind relevant to the inquiry; (3) therefore, we should adopt a realist account of the relevant objects of inquiry. Arguments of this form have been advanced to defend platonism with regard to mathematical objects and realism with regard to the referents of theoretical terms in the empirical sciences. To establish the second premise of such an argument, one must not only show that alternatives to the realist account (say intuitionist accounts in mathematics and verificationist or positivist accounts in science) will not explain the success of the methods used, but that the realist account has some independent plausibility of its own. Otherwise, it may simply seem to be a residual, *ad hoc* account. In mathematics, proponents of platonism, whatever the merits of their refutations of other accounts, have not provided accounts, aside from perceptual metaphors, which make it plausible that we can come to know anything about mathematical objects. In contrast, however, there are some interesting and promising arguments of this form in defense of scientific realism.[33] In these, a version of a causal theory of knowledge and reference is used to satisfy the requirement that we lend plausibility to the realist account of methodology independent of the refutation of alternative accounts.

Suppose a version of such an argument for scientific realism is sound – a supposition I shall not defend here at all. Then we would be justified in claiming that certain central methodological features of science, including its coherence and other theory-laden constraints on theory acceptance (e.g., parsimony, simplicity, etc.), are consensus producing *because* they are *evidential* and lead us to better approximations to the truth. I have been defending the view that coherence constraints in wide equilibrium function very much like those in science. If I am right, this suggests that we may be able to piggyback a claim about objectivity in ethics onto the analogous claim we are assuming can be made for science. Suppose then that coherence constraints in wide equilibrium turn out to be consensus producing. Then, since these constraints are similar to their analogues in science in other respects, they may also be *evidential*. That is, we have some reason to think that wide equilibrium involves methods that will lead us to objective moral truths *if there are any*. Notice that this conclusion does not presuppose there are such moral truths, nor does it give an account of what kind of truth such a truth would be.

My suggestion is obviously a highly tentative and programmatic route to an account of objectivity in ethics. Nor can I really defend it here. Some qualifying remarks are definitely in order, however.

(A) Developed versions of the arguments for scientific realism do not simply talk about "convergence," but point to a variety of effects indicative of the cumulative nature or progress of scientific knowledge. For example, they may try to account for "take-off" effects indicative of the maturation of an area of inquiry, or they may point to the absence of "schools" or "sects." My supposition that convergence may emerge in wide equilibrium falls far short of specifying this sort of evidence for growth in moral knowledge. There is a related point: I am not sure we know what to count as evidence for convergence in ethics. For example, we do have moral disagreement on numerous issues; but is the level of disagreement compatible with enough other agreement for it to count as convergence, or not? Does existing disagreement merely represent hard or novel problems at the "frontier"? Or is it the result of special social forces which systematically distort our views in areas of political or religious sensitivity? Some of the difficulty may stem from paucity of work in the history of ethics and in moral anthropology adequate to informing us whether we have experienced moral progress.

(B) The piggyback argument seems to rest on the assumption that, if a feature of method (a coherence constraint) is similar in one respect (it produces consensus) in two areas of inquiry, then it holds in both areas for the same reason (it leads to relevant truths). I do not think the assumption is obviously or even generally true; that is why my suggestion is only programmatic.

(C) The arguments for scientific realism depend on some causal account of knowledge – e.g., perceptual knowledge depends on reliable detection mechanisms. We are reminded, therefore, of the burden of proof assumed in section III to provide *some* reliability account of moral judgments (at some level). Suppose we could provide no analogue in the moral case to the causal story we may be persuaded of for perceptual knowledge. If we still wanted to talk about "objective moral truths," we might *retreat* to the view that the objects of moral knowledge were "abstract," that is, more like mathematical objects than the things we can know about through the natural sciences. But our moral realism, then, is open to the worry I earlier expressed about mathematical platonism.[34] To be sure, if our causal accounts of knowledge turn out to be unpersuasive, then the argument for scientific realism may be no better off than this in any case.

(D) My account of wide reflective equilibrium has not provided (not explicitly at least) an obvious analogue to the role of experimentation in science. Some story about moral *practice* and what we can learn from it, and not just about moral thought experiments, seems to be needed. That is, we would need to examine the sense in which moral theories guide moral practice and result in social experimentation. But this account must be left for another project.[35]

A final remark is directed not just at my suggestion about the implications of wide equilibrium for objectivity in ethics, but at my account of wide equilibrium itself. The account I have sketched defines a wide equilibrium for a given individual at a given time. The "convergence" I have been discussing is the (at least approximate) sharing of the same wide equilibrium by different persons; the ordered triples of sets of beliefs are the same for these persons. But there would seem to be another approach.

Suppose we begin by admitting into the set of initial considered moral judgments only those judgments on which there is substantial consensus.[36] There seem to be two immediate advantages. First, ethics looks more like science in that the initial considered moral judgments share with observation reports the fact that there is substantial initial agreement on them. The starting point is more "objective," at least in the sense of intersubjective agreement. One *may* gain a slight edge in respect to the problem of initial credibility discussed earlier. (Revisability is, nevertheless, presumed.) Second, the approach makes the wide equilibrium that emerges (if one does) much more a collective or social product from the start than does my approach, which is a quite unnatural idealization in this regard.

Though I think this alternative merits further examination, which I cannot undertake here, I am not persuaded that it offers real advantages. For one thing, it builds into its procedure the assumption that considered judgments *ought* to function like observation reports in science, a question, I have argued, there is good reason to leave open. Its apparent advantage in making ultimate convergence seem more likely might, consequently, be based on the assumption that we ought to have *initial* convergence where there is no good reason to expect it (given all the things that make *initial* considered moral judgments *un*reliable). For another thing, I have assumed that extensive consideration of alternative background theories and sets of principles will produce reasonable pressures to revise and eliminate divergent considered judgments that there are good reasons to eliminate. The alternative method may shift, in too crude a fashion (losing too many possibilities), the intermediate conclusions of my procedure into the position of methodologically warranted starting points. A less important consideration is historical: reflective equilibrium is advanced by Rawls as a model for the process of justification in ethics. Part of what he wanted to capture is a model for how we may make progress in moral argument – where we have to accommodate initial disagreement on some moral judgments. My approach retains this attractive feature, though it sheds some of the other motivations for Rawls' version.[37]

My remarks on objectivity are admittedly quite speculative; indeed, I think it a virtue of the method of reflective equilibrium that it leaves open metaethical considerations of this kind. Still, I think enough has been said about wide equilibrium, these speculations aside, to make its implications for theory acceptance in ethics worthy of closer study.

NOTES

I am indebted to Richard Boyd, Arthur Caplan, Christopher Cherniak, C. A. J. Coady, Josh Cohen, Daniel Dennett, Jane English, Paul Horwich, Allan

Wide reflective equilibrium and theory acceptance in ethics

Garfinkel, William Lycan, Miles Morgan, John Rawls, Amélie Rorty, George Smith, and M. B. E. Smith for helpful comments on ideas contained in this paper. The research was supported by an NEH Fellowship for 1977/78.

1 Since the notion of justification is broadly used in philosophy, it is worth forestalling a confusion right at the outset. The problem I address in this paper is strictly analogous to the general and abstract problem of theory acceptance or justification posed in the philosophy of science with regard to nonmoral theories. I am not directly concerned with explaining when a particular individual is justified in, or can be held accountable for, holding a particular moral belief or performing a particular action. So, too, the philosopher of science, interested in how theory acceptance depends on the relation of one theory to another, is not directly concerned to determine whether or not a given individual is justified in believing some feature of one of the theories. Just how relevant my account of theory acceptance is to the question, Is so-and-so justified in believing *P* or in doing *A* on evidence *E* in conditions *C* (vary *P, A, E*)? would require a detailed examination of particular cases. I am indebted to Miles Morgan and John Rawls for discussion of this point.

2 The distinction between narrow and wide reflective equilibria is implicit in *A Theory of Justice* (Cambridge, Mass.: Harvard, 1971), p. 49, and is explicit in "The Independence of Moral Theory," *Proceedings and Addresses of the American Philosophical Association*, XLVII (1974/75): 5–22, p. 8.

3 Though Rawls' earlier formulations of the notion [in his "Outline for a Decision Procedure for Ethics," *Philosophical Review*, LX, 2 (April 1951): 177–197, esp. pp. 182/3] restricts considered judgments to moral judgments about particular cases, his later formulations drop the restriction, so they can be of any level of generality. Cf. Rawls, "Independence of Moral Theory," p. 8. These "ideal" conditions may have drawbacks, as Allan Garfinkel has pointed out to me. Sometimes anger or (moral) indignation may lead to morally better actions and judgments than "calm"; also, the formulation fails to correct for divergence between stated beliefs and beliefs revealed in action.

4 Narrow reflective equilibrium might be construed as the moral analogue of solving the projection problem for syntactic competence: the principles are the moral analogue of a grammar. This analogy is not extendable to wide equilibrium, as I show in "On Some Methods of Ethics and Linguistics," *Philosophical Studies* 37 (1980): 21–36. Narrow equilibrium leaves us with the traditional two-tiered view of moral theories and is particularly ill-suited to provide a basis for a justificational argument. It does not offer a special epistemological claim about the considered moral judgments (other than the rather weak claim that they are filtered to avoid some obvious sources of error), nor are there constraints on the acceptability of moral principles beyond their good "fit" with the initial considered judgments. If we have reason to suspect that the initial judgments are the product of bias, historical accident, or ideology, then these elementary coherence considerations alone give us little basis for comfort, since they

provide inadequate pressure to correct for them. Cf. Rawls, *A Theory of Justice*, p. 49.

5   The fact that I describe wide equilibrium as being built up out of judgments, principles, and relevant background theories does not mean that this represents an order of epistemic priority or a natural sequence in the genesis of theories. Arthur Caplan reminded me of this point.

6   My formulation is not adequate as it stands, since there will even be trivial truth-functional counterexamples to it unless some specification of "interesting" and "nontrivial" is given, to say nothing of providing a measure for the "scope" of a theory. This is a standing problem in philosophy of science [cf. Michael Friedman's attempt to handle the related question of unifying theories in "Explanation and Scientific Understanding," *Journal of Philosophy*, LXXI 1 (Jan. 17, 1974): 5–19, esp. pp. 15ff]. I will assume that this difficulty can be overcome, though doing so might require dropping the loose talk about theories. I am indebted to George Smith for helpful discussion of this point.

7   I draw here on my "Reflective Equilibrium and Archimedean Points," *Canadian Journal of Philosophy* 10, 1(1980): 83–103.

8   In particular, Rawls' level III theories rest on no considered moral judgments about rights and entitlements: all such considered judgments are segregated into level I, so that level III theories provide a foundation for our notions of rights and entitlements without themselves appealing to such notions (though they appeal to other moral notions, such as fairness and various claims about persons). Rawls seems attracted to this view of his project [cf. his "Reply to Alexander and Musgrave," *Quarterly Journal of Economics*, LXXXCII, 4 (November 1974), p. 634]. In contrast, Ronald Dworkin argues that a background right to equal respect is needed at what I call "level III." [Cf. his "The Original Position," *University of Chicago Law Review* XL, 3 (Spring 1973): 500–33; reprinted in my anthology, *Reading Rawls* (New York: Basic Books, 1975), pp. 16–53, esp. pp. 45, 50ff.] For an argument that Dworkin is wrong to posit such a level III right, see my "Reflective Equilibrium and Archimedean Points."

9   Rawls leaves himself open to the accusation of "rigging" when he says, e.g., "We want to define the original position so that we get the desired solution" (*A Theory of Justice*, p. 141). Critics have had a field day using this and similar remarks to show that the contract can have no justificational role.

10   We know relatively little about these features of theory acceptance in either domain, a fact traceable to the same empiricist and positivist legacy: too narrow an account of the relation between theory and "data," be it laws-plus-observation or principles-plus-judgments.

11   Compare Derek Parfit, "Later Selves and Moral Principles," in Alan Montefiore, ed., *Philosophy and Personal Relations* (London: Routledge & Kegan Paul, 1973), pp. 149–60. See Rawls' reply in "Independence of Moral Theory," p. 17ff. The degree to which a theory of the person constrains moral-theory acceptance, and conversely, the degree to which moral theory constrains theories of the person are discussed in my "Moral Theory and the Plasticity of Persons," *The Monist*, 62 (1979): 3:267–87. The

Marxist worry that there is no non-class-relative notion of the person substantial enough to found a moral theory on this appears as an argument about level III theory acceptability.

12   "Utilitarianism and Moral Self-Indulgence" in H. D. Lewis, *Contemporary British Philosophy*, IVth Series (New York: Humanities, 1976), pp. 306–21.

13   The charge is made by R. M. Hare ("Rawls' Theory of Justice," in *Reading Rawls*, p. 82ff), by Peter Singer ["Sidgwick and Reflective Equilibrium," *Monist*, LVIII, 3 (July 1974): 490–517, p. 494], and by Richard Brandt (*A Theory of the Good and the Right*, Oxford: Oxford University Press 1979, Ch. I).

14   My characterization of intuitionism emphasizes its foundationalism. For an account that de-emphasizes its foundationalism, see M. B. E. Smith's excellent "Rawls and Intuitionism," in Kai Nielsen and Roger Shiner, eds., *New Essays on Contract Theory, Canadian Journal of Philosophy*, suppl. vol. III: 163–78. Smith agrees that Rawls' "revisionism" in wide equilibrium is contrary to the spirit of intuitionism. Still, he thinks the intuitionist can accept Rawls' method as a "check" on his own, *provided* it does not lead to strongly counterintuitive revisions. It is unclear to me how much of a "check" one has if such a proviso is imposed. Smith also argues that Rawls' method of wide equilibrium cannot yield principles, such as the principle governing the duty of beneficence. If he is right, then the method not only is not acceptable to the intuitionist who wants "definitive" answers, but also does not meet Rawls' requirements. Though he does not note the point, Smith's argument turns on features of the *contract* and *not* on features of *wide reflective equilibrium* as a method.

15   The fact that these sources of error have been minimized does give considered judgments *some* modest degree of epistemic priority, as William Lycan has reminded me.

16   C. F. Delaney suggests quite plausibly that the greater revisability of considered moral judgments in reflective equilibrium in *A Theory of Justice* as compared to "Outline of a Decision Procedure" corresponds to the shift from a more positivist view of the relation between facts and theory to a more coherentist, Quinean view. Cf. Delaney's "Rawls on Method," in Nielsen and Shiner, *op. cit.*, pp. 153–61. The assumption of some critics that Rawls' approach to wide equilibrium is intuitionist may itself derive from their own latent positivism.

17   One reason philosophers have thought reflective equilibrium "intuitionist" is a failure to distinguish narrow and wide equilibria. A more obvious source lies in Rawls' remark, cited by nearly everyone who makes the charge of intuitionism, that "There is a definite if limited class of facts against which conjectured principles can be checked, namely our considered judgments in reflective equilibrium" (*A Theory of Justice*, p. 51). It is tempting to read the remark as follows: "to arrive at a reflective equilibrium, treat considered judgments as a 'definite if limited class of facts' which is to determine the shape and content of the rest of the theory." R. M. Hare ("Rawls' Theory of Justice," in *Reading Rawls*, p. 83) and Peter Singer (*op. cit.*, p. 493) read Rawls' remark this way. But the remark can and should be taken to mean that "the small but definite class" emerges *only*

when reflective equilibrium is reached, and still is revisable in the light of further theory change.

18 Presumably, we could use fairly standard treatments of degree of belief, rooted in probability theory, to formalize what is sketched here. This formalization might give particular content to the assumption that persons are rational, imposing certain constraints on revisability and acceptability. I am indebted to Paul Horwich for discussion of this point.

19 *Loc. cit.* Brandt's discussion draws on early characterizations of justification by Nelson Goodman ["Sense and Certainty," *Philosophical Review*, LXI, 2 (April 1952): 160–7] and Israel Scheffler ["Justification and Commitment," (*Journal of Philosophy*), LI, 6 (March 18, 1954): 180–90]. In Scheffler's discussion, the method is described using the notion of "initial credibility," which is not explicated for us. Later in the article we are told that initial credibility is only an indication of our "initial commitment to . . . acceptance" (187). Perhaps Brandt's argument should be construed as the objection to assuming, as Scheffler is willing to do, that initial credibility and initial commitment to acceptance (Brandt's "credence level") correspond in the moral case the way they do in the nonmoral case.

20 Hare's and Singer's complaints have a similar ring to them, once purged of the mistaken view they share about the unrevisability of considered judgments (see n. 17 above).

21 Cf. Kai Nielsen, "Our Considered Judgments," *Ratio*, XIX, 1 (June 1977): 39–46.

22 A stronger version can be formulated. It would treat some class of observation reports as self-warranting or even incorrigible. I consider only the more plausible, weaker version above. On the strong version, the criticism of reflective equilibrium is just a foundationalist attack. On the weak version, it is an attempt to show that, foundationalism aside, coherence theories of moral justification face special problems not faced by coherence theories of nonmoral justification.

23 The contrast is hardly complete, since observation reports may also be affected by various aspects of a person's "set."

24 Gilbert Harman makes a similar point when he claims that p's obtaining plays no role in explaining my making the moral judgment that p, but q's obtaining does play a role in explaining my nonmoral observation that q. Cf. *The Nature of Morality* (New York: Oxford, 1977), pp. 7ff. I think Harman overdraws the contrast here, but that is a matter for another discussion.

25 Even the access to theoretical considerations generally found in mature and sophisticated adult moral reasoning will not, of course, be as extensive and developed as what I suggest is involved in wide equilibrium, despite my earlier remark that much more structure may be present than we have recognized. Moreover, how much we expect theory to play a role in adult moral reasoning will depend on our purpose in seeking the particular moral justification. These factors affect the degree to which a coherence theory of justification based on wide equilibrium carries over into a theory of individual justification; see n. 1 above.

26 Peter Singer argues that the proponent of reflective equilibrium leaves no room for a notion of the "validity" of moral principles that goes beyond intersubjective agreement. Consequently, the "validity" of moral principles will have to be relativized: it depends on whose considered judgments they are tested against (cf. *op. cit.*, pp. 439ff). I do not see why he thinks so, except that it may be connected to his underestimate of the revisability of considered moral judgments (cf. sec. II above). In any case, Rawls is quite right to deny any straightforward connection between convergence in wide equilibrium and the knowledge of objective moral truths. Cf. Rawls, "Independence of Moral Theory," p. 9.

27 I think the account is implausible, but cf. Gordon W. Allport, *The Nature of Prejudice* (New York: Addison-Wesley, 1954), chs. III, IV.

28 As Singer seems to think it does; cf. *op. cit.*, pp. 494/5; but see also his n. 5, p. 494.

29 If we construe wide reflective equilibrium as providing us with the basis for a full-blown coherence theory of moral justification, then my argument suggests that it faces the same difficulties and advantages as coherence theories of nonmoral justification. I cannot here defend my view that a coherence theory of justification can be made compatible with a non-coherence account of truth.

30 There is some evidence that Rawls is attracted to a view resembling the eliminative view in his portrayal of wide equilibrium as a "constructive" method. Cf. "The Independence of Moral Theory," *op. cit.*, and also a recent unpublished lecture with the same title as the Presidential Address.

31 Cf. Hilary Putnam, *Meaning and the Moral Sciences* (London: Routledge & Kegan Paul, 1978), part IV.

32 I am grateful to Richard Boyd and George Smith for discussion of this argument and of section IV in general.

33 The most persuasive versions of the argument are found in Boyd, "Determinism, Laws and Predictability in Principle," *Philosophy of Science* XXXIX, 4 (December 1972): 431–450; "Realism, Underdetermination and a Causal Theory of Evidence," *Nous*, VII, 1 (1973): 1–12; *Realism and Scientific Epistemology* unpublished ms.; "Materialism without Reductionism: What Physicalism Does Not Entail," in Ned Block, ed., *Readings in Philosophy of Psychology* (Vol. 1. Cambridge: Harvard University Press, 1980); and "Metaphor and Theory Change," in A. Ortony, ed., *Metaphor and Thought*. (Cambridge: Cambridge University Press, 1979). See also H. C. Byerly and V. A. Luzara, "Realist Foundations of Measurement," *Philosophy of Science* XL, 1 (1973): 1–27; and the classic K. MacCorquodale and P. E. Meehl, "On a Distinction between Hypothetical Constructs and Intervening Variables," *Psychological Review*, CLV (1948): 95–107.

34 For a similar suggestion, see Jane English, "Ethics and Science," *Proceedings of the XVI Congress of Philosophy*. For some remarks on the analogy between choosing among alternative logics and choosing among moral theories, see my "On Some Methods of Ethics and Linguistics," *Philosophical Studies*, 37 (1980): 21–36.

35 There are some interesting suggestions along these lines in Ruth Anna Putnam, "Rights of Persons and the Liberal Tradition," in Ted

Honderich, *Social Ends and Political Means* (London: Routledge & Kegan Paul, 1976).

36 Just before her tragic death, Jane English reminded me of the importance of this alternative in comments on an earlier draft of this paper. She argues that ethics should be constructed on such a basis in a brilliant short paper, cited above.

37 In particular, the analogy to descriptive syntactics (see n. 5).

Chapter 3

Reflective equilibrium and Archimedean points

1. THE CONTRACT AND JUSTIFICATION

In *A Theory of Justice*, John Rawls defines a hypothetical contract situation and argues rational people will agree on reflection that it is fair to contractors. He solves the rational choice problem it poses by deriving two lexically ordered principles of justice and suggests the derivation justifies the principles.[1] Its soundness aside, just what justificatory force does such a derivation have?

On one view, there is no justificatory force because the contract is *rigged* specifically to yield principles which match our precontract moral judgments. Rawls provides ammunition for this claim: "By going back and forth, sometimes altering the conditions of the contractual circumstances, at others withdrawing our judgments [about what is just] and conforming them to principle, I assume that eventually we shall find a description of the initial situation that both expresses reasonable conditions and yields principles which match our considered judgments duly pruned and adjusted."[2] Similarly, "We want to define the original position so that we get the desired solution."[3] But if the contract is thus rigged, we gain nothing over "testing" the principles directly by matching them to our considered moral judgments in reflective equilibrium. A rigged contract is redundant. What is worse, such matching of principles to judgments, some argue, tells us only that *we happen* to think the principles acceptable; it is a result in moral anthropology, not moral philosophy. When we add this repudiation of reflective equilibrium to the conclusion the contract is rigged, the wheels of the contract spin freely, providing no justificatory traction.[4]

A second line of argument is that Rawls' hypothetical contract lacks the force of a real contract and cannot stand by itself as a justificatory device.[5] Rather, it is an intermediate step – or vehicle – through which an argument from a "deeper theory" is run. Thus Ronald Dworkin argues that the required deep theory involves a fundamental right of persons to "equal respect and consideration in the design" of the institutions that govern them. The job of the contractors is to narrow down the general right to form a particular concept of justice. Still, the contract has no justificatory force independent of this deep theory, which motivates the contract as "an 'intuitive notion' for developing and testing theories of justice."[6] T. M. Scanlon claims that a social ideal of the person as an autonomous chooser is the central feature of the deep theory.[7] And David Lyons suggests the contract may only be a "special branch" of a coherence argument in which unargued for "presuppositions" about fairness and impartiality play a role. Since Lyons thinks coherence arguments are of dubious value, the justificatory power of the contract, even as an intermediate device, is again challenged.[8]

I shall argue the contract is indeed a special feature of a particular wide reflective equilibrium which contains component theories of the person, of the role of morality in society, and of procedural justice, among others (section 2). These constitute the sought-after "deep theory." Moreover, if they satisfy an "independence constraint" I propose, the contract avoids the rigging charge and the possibility remains open that the derivation has justificatory force (section 3). Still, the acceptability of the contract as a justificatory device depends critically on the acceptability of this "deep theory," so those who find the latter unacceptable "will be unmoved by justice as fairness even granting the validity of its arguments."[9] Rawls' Archimedean point is fixed, but only against components of that wide equilibrium. This observation will suggest an answer to our main question, how choosing principles in the original position can justify them (section 4). My construction draws heavily on Rawls' post–*A Theory of Justice* writings. Still, it does not mark a radical break with, only a shift in emphasis from, the original justificatory argument.

2. WIDE EQUILIBRIUM, THE INDEPENDENCE CONSTRAINT, AND THE CONTRACT

A wide reflective equilibrium is a coherent ordered triple of sets of beliefs held by a particular person, namely, a set of considered moral judgments, (a); a set of moral principles, (b); and a set of relevant background theories, (c). We collect the person's initial moral judgments and filter them to include only those of which he is relatively confident and which have been made under conditions generally conducive to avoiding errors of judgment.[10] We propose alternative sets of moral principles which have varying degrees of "fit" with the moral judgments. Rather than settling immediately for the "best fit" of principles with judgments, which would give us only a *narrow* equilibrium,[11] we advance philosophical arguments which reveal the strengths and weaknesses of the competing sets of principles (i.e., competing moral conceptions). I construe these arguments as inferences from relevant background *theories* (I use the term loosely). Assume that some particular set of arguments wins and the moral agent is thus persuaded one set of principles is more acceptable than the others (and perhaps than the conception that might have emerged in narrow equilibrium). The agent may work back and forth, revising his initial considered judgments, moral principles, and background theories, to arrive at an equilibrium point which consists of the triple, (a), (b), and (c).

There must be more structure here. The theories in (c) must show the principles in (b) are more acceptable than alternatives on grounds to some degree independent of (b)'s match with relevant considered moral judgments in (a). Without such independent support, the principles have no support they would not already have had in a corresponding narrow equilibrium where no appeal to (c) is made. I can raise this point another way: how can we be sure that the moral principles that systematize considered moral judgments are not just "accidental generalizations" of the "moral facts," analogous to accidental generalizations we want to avoid confusing with real scientific laws? In the scientific case, we have evidence we are not stuck with accidental generalizations if we can derive the purported laws from a body of interconnected theories, provided these theories reach beyond the "facts" the laws generalize in a diverse and interesting way.

The analogy suggests one way to ensure independent support for the principles in (b) and to rule out their being mere accidental generalizations of the considered judgments in (a). We should require that the theories in (c) not just be reformulations of the set of considered moral judgments (a) to which we seek to "fit" the principles in (b). The background theories should have a scope reaching beyond the range of the judgments in (a). Suppose some set of considered *moral* judgments, (a'), plays a role in constraining the background theories in (c). Then we are asking that some interesting, nontrivial portion of (a') should be disjoint from the set (a) that constrains the principles in (b). Our *independence constraint* is the requirement that (a') and (a) be to some significant degree disjoint.[12]

It is important to note the acceptability of the theories in (c) may thus in part depend on some *moral* judgments. We are not in general assuming that (c) constitutes a reduction of the moral [in (b) and (a)] to the nonmoral. For example, we might find such a situation if the background theories in (c) incorporate different moral notions (say, fairness and certain claims about the person) from those (say, rights and entitlements) employed by the principles in (b) and judgments in (a).

We can now see that Rawls' contract argument is a feature of a particular wide equilibrium. The contract apparatus (*Level II*, see diagram [Figure 3.1]) is not self-evidently acceptable. Indeed, it contains complex "formal" (publicity, etc.), motivational (mutual disinterest, primary goods), and knowledge (the "thick" veil) constraints on contractors and principles. Rather, philosophical argument must persuade us it is a reasonable device for selecting between competing conceptions of justice (or right). These arguments are inferences from a number of (*Level III*) background theories – of the person, of procedural justice, of the role of morality in society (including the ideal of the well-ordered society). Principles chosen at Level II are subject to two constraints: (i) they must match a relevant set of our considered moral judgments in what I call *partial (Level I)* reflective equilibrium; (ii) they must yield a feasible, stable well-ordered society. *Level IV* contains the body of social theory relevant to testing Level II principles (and Level III) theories for "feasibility."[13]

The independence constraint previously defined for wide equilibrium in general applies in this way: *If* there are any considered moral judgments (a′) which may constrain Level III theory acceptability, they must to a significant extent be disjoint from the considered moral judgments (a) which constrain Level I partial equilibrium. Notice that both (a) and (a′) are in *the same* wide equilibrium with the principles, but they constrain their acceptability in different ways.

I shall now argue that the Level III theories of the person and the role of morality (if not procedural justice) that Rawls uses to argue for key features of the contract (e.g., the publicity and unanimity constraints, the thick veil, the focus on basic structure) do not obviously violate the independence constraint.

3. DEEP THEORY AND THE INDEPENDENCE CONSTRAINT

A. Procedural justice

Rawls elaborates no "theory" of procedural justice as such, only some distinctions between types of procedural justice. He suggests the contract situation is itself an instance of pure procedural justice: if it is *fair* to agents in it, the justice of its procedure will transfer to the principles chosen and, in turn, to whatever entitlements emerge when the principles govern basic social institutions. Thus, "justice as fairness."

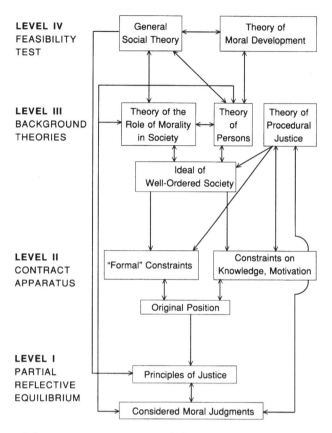

LEVEL IV
FEASIBILITY
TEST

LEVEL III
BACKGROUND
THEORIES

LEVEL II
CONTRACT
APPARATUS

LEVEL I
PARTIAL
REFLECTIVE
EQUILIBRIUM

Figure 3.1. Schematic representation of the wide reflective equilibrium that contains justice as fairness. Arrows indicate that contents of one box are viewed as more plausible in light of contents of a connected box.

Even if we had a general theory of procedural justice, however, it would not by itself resolve how to make the original position fair. Thus the thick veil of ignorance is intended to guarantee fairness by denying agents information that confers unfair advantage. But no theory of procedural justice alone can determine the required thickness of the veil. We must know which facts about individuals are morally relevant or central. Similarly, no such general theory alone suffices to establish Rawls' unanimity condition. Some procedures are fair only if people have proportional voting powers (e.g., a stockholders meeting). Again we need more information to see why unanimity is fair given the task. To get such information, we might turn directly to particular considered judgments about what is fair in these cases, but

Rawls turns instead to other Level III theories, notably of the person (section 3C–D).

Despite these qualifications, two points are worth noting about the nature and role of the theory of procedural justice. First, though some might object that "fairness" is not a *moral* notion, fewer questions are begged if we take the theory to be a *moral* one containing general principles about fair procedures. Consequently, in moving upwards from the moral output of Level II to the Level III theoretical input, we at most "reduce" some moral notions to others, not to the nonmoral.

Second, though the evidence is not conclusive, there is reason to think the theory of procedural justice violates the independence constraint. Some considered judgments about fairness in certain cases ("Such and such an outcome is just because the procedure is fair") appear to constrain both the acceptability of Level III general principles of procedural fairness ("For tasks of a certain kind, if the procedure is fair, the outcome is just") and the acceptability of Level II principles of justice. The problem arises because not all considered judgments about distributions are relevant to Level I equilibrium, but only those that concern outcomes of basic institutions governed by the principles in question. Accepting this restriction to the consequences of basic institutions involves accepting a considered judgment about procedural justice of just the sort employed at Level III to constrain the design of the contract.[14]

B. The well-ordered society and publicity

In contrast, neither the theory of the person nor the theory of the role of morality in society appears to be just a reformulation of Level I considered judgments. In part, these theories overlap to form the ideal of a well-ordered society. Roughly speaking, this ideal specifies the form and function of a conception of justice but omits reference to its content. In this way the ideal shapes many features of the contract, whose task is to supply appropriate content to flesh out the bones of the well-ordered society.[15]

In his recent writings, Rawls lists twelve conditions satisfied by well-ordered societies.[16] Three specify the sense in which the society is regulated by a *public* conception of justice:

(1) Everyone accepts, and knows that others accept, the same principles (the same conception) of justice.
(2) Basic social institutions and their arrangement into one scheme (the basic structure of society) satisfy, and are with reason believed by everyone to satisfy, these principles.
(3) The public conception of justice is founded on reasonable beliefs

that have been established by generally accepted methods of inquiry.

Three further conditions specify that society members are "free, equal and moral persons":

(4) They each have, and view themselves as having, a sense of justice (the content of which is defined by the principles of the public conception) that is normally effective (the desire to act on this conception determines their conduct for the most part).
(5) They each have, and view themselves as having, fundamental aims and interests (a conception of their good) in the name of which it is legitimate to make claims on one another in the design of their institutions.
(6) They each have, and view themselves as having, a right to equal respect and consideration in determining the principles by which the basic structure of their society is to be regulated.

Further conditions specify that such a society is stable (7), operates under the circumstances of justice (moderate scarcity, etc., 8–10), and takes the basic structure to be the primary subject of justice (11–12).

Two points about the notion of publicity used in (1–3) are important to the justificatory structure of Rawls' overall argument. First, though he calls the publicity constraint "formal," it is not a priori. At least conceptual analysis and the theory of meaning alone will not determine just how *strong* a notion of publicity should be incorporated at Level III.[17] Second, though the strong publicity condition affects the acceptability of principles in the contract position, this is not the reason given to justify it. Thus, if egoism cannot be coherently accepted as a public moral conception, as some have argued, then the formal notion turns out to have moral force. Similarly, Rawls uses the strong publicity condition in his argument that justice as fairness is more stable than utilitarianism.[18] A weaker publicity condition would weaken this argument. But Rawls nowhere cites these consequences of the publicity condition as reasons for choosing *it*. Nor is there *specific* evidence these consequences motivated its selection, only Rawls' general remarks that conditions defining the contract may be adjusted to give the desired result.

Why does Rawls think we should accept the strong publicity constraint? One overly vague suggestion is that we adopt it because of the way in which it "fits" or coheres with overall theoretical considerations. A bit less vague is the suggestion in *A Theory of Justice*: "The publicity condition is clearly implicit in Kant's doctrine of the categorical imperative insofar as it requires us to act in accordance with principles that one would be willing as a rational being to enact as law for a kingdom of ends."[19] Though not itself an argument, this appeal to Kant might be converted into one. Still, it is not clear that just the strong publicity condition would follow; a weaker one might suffice.

A more specific suggestion is that a strong publicity constraint fits best with the theory of the person thought most acceptable at Level III. Since persons are dependent on social institutions which shape them in particular ways, certain conceptions of a person may not be realizable unless the publicity condition is strong rather than weak. Rawls suggests, but does not argue,[20] that a Kantian conception of the person as a law-making member of a kingdom of ends requires a fairly strong publicity constraint. But he does not show that other plausible conceptions of the person are not also tied to the same condition. Suppose, however, that some other theory of the person fits best with a weak constraint. Then if Rawls' adoption of the strong constraint is based on its fit with the Kantian theory, the arguments for that Kantian view of the person assume key importance. The theory of the person thus takes priority in the selection of this "formal" constraint,[21] which is clearly no longer just formal. Though we have not yet found an argument incompatible with the independence constraint, it remains to be seen how the theory of the person itself fares.

C. The theory of the person

A numer of high-level generalizations about the nature and interests of persons form the core of what I am loosely calling a "theory." Among them are the following:

(a) "Each person has, and views himself as having, fundamental aims and higher-order interests (a conception of their good)."[22]
(b) Persons do not "think of themselves as inevitably bound to, or as identical with, the pursuit of any particular array of fundamental interests they have at a given time." Rather, "they think of themselves as capable of revising and altering these final ends" and "they have an interest in protecting that capability."[23]
(c) Social institutions, including social attitudes of encouragement, support, and training, shape the desires, aspirations, and abilities of their members and determine, in large part, the kind of persons they want to be as well as the kind of persons they are.[24]
(d) Persons have a highest order interest, and are aware they do, in how all their other interests, including their fundamental ones, are shaped and regulated by social institutions. Consequently, they have an interest, and are aware they do, in determining the principles that govern their institutions.[25]

(e) Persons have, and are aware they have, a realized sense of justice at the age of reason which informs their conduct for the most part.[26]

(f) Persons are rational.[27]

What type of theory is this? Rawls says he wants to "reinterpret" traditional Kantian notions "within the scope of an empirical theory."[28] Unfortunately, this remark leaves the status of these generalizations unclear. If we take them to be straightforward empirical generalizations about past and present (human) persons, they are probably false. We might construe them as an *idealized model* of the human person, one that merely abstracts from certain distorting contexts in which humans have lived. But (a), (b), and (e) may not even be idealizations generally true of human persons throughout history.[29] A yet weaker construal of the idealization distinguishes the theory of persons from a theory of human nature. The former is a more general, but still empirical theory: not every person may be a human. But not every human may actually be a person either: social contexts and facts of human psychology and sociology may sometimes (or often) prevent humans from being persons. But on the Kantian view Rawls is developing, what is relevant about humans for the purposes of moral and political theory is that they *can* be persons, not the facts (of interest to philosophical anthropology) about normal human motives, interests, and emotions.[30]

Features (a–f) may form an *ideal* in a different sense: they may be statements about how "we" *want* persons to be constituted in a well-ordered society. The ideal has empirical constraints: *desired* properties must also be *feasible* ones, but "feasible" here may mean realizable under conditions that have not actually obtained. This ideal person is not simply an empirical idealization of the standard or undistorted human case. Rawls seems to have an ideal and not an idealization in mind when he says, "Let us begin, then, by trying to describe the kind of person we might want to be and the form of society we might wish to live in and to shape our interests and character. In this way we arrive at the notion of a well-ordered society."[31]

Whether we construe these claims about persons as a desirable ideal or as an empirical idealization may have epistemological import. If our Level III theory of the person were just an empirical idealization, its support and acceptability would derive from factors quite independent of Level I considered moral judgments, thus satisfying our independence constraint. If, however, the theory of the person is a desirable ideal, the issue is more complex. Whether or not there is a violation of the independence constraint will depend on *which* considered moral judgments support the ideal. We might, for example, want persons to satisfy feature (d) ("be aware of their interests in determining the principles that govern their institutions") because we consider it unjust when social institutions are designed so that some persons have only "false consciousness" of their interests. If the ideal of the person depends primarily on such Level I moral judgments, then it probably violates the independence constraint. But the ideal need not depend in this way on Level I moral judgments. Other considered moral judgments may be involved, leaving room for the independence constraint to be satisfied.[32] This outcome seems more probable if prominent Level I moral notions like "just" and "unjust" or "rights" and "entitlements" are not found in the Level III ideal or theory of the person.

At just this point a serious question arises. In feature (d), I deliberately use the word "interest," not "right," to refer to the interest persons have in determining the principles that govern their institutions. Yet, in Rawls' condition (6) on well-ordered societies, persons are ascribed a *right* to equal respect and consideration in determining such principles. Positing rights at Level III makes it more likely that the same types of considered judgments found at Level I are also constraining the Level III ideal, significantly reducing the chances that the ideal satisfies the independence constraint. I cannot establish that the theory of the person does satisfy the independence constraint, but I would like to see if its chance of doing so can be enhanced by avoiding rights at Level III.

D. *"Deep theory" rights*

Is Rawls' reference to rights at Level III eliminable?[33] Ronald Dworkin offers the only argument I know which says it is not. Dworkin asks what deep theory can make sense out of the features of the original position, especially its unanimity or veto constraint? Positing a deep "goal-based" theory (e.g., maximize total or average goodness) would not allow us to make sense of a veto based on contractor self-interest. Nor would positing a deep duty (e.g., to perform only certain sorts of acts). By elimination, the only remaining type of deep theory is one that posits a general and abstract right (to equal respect and consideration in the design of social institutions). The veto exercises and protects the right.[34]

On Dworkin's view, the task of the contractors is to refine this vague right into specific rights and entitlements determined by the principles of justice. No doubt this task is an important one. But it is far less bold and profound than the reductive task Rawls appears to undertake, namely to derive those rights and entitlements from an entirely different set of moral notions having to do with fairness, the nature of persons, and the role of morality in society.[35] In my view this provides another reason, in addition to satisfying the independence constraint, to want to eliminate, if possible, such Level III rights.

Fortunately, there is a problem with Dworkin's argument. Suppose we posit Dworkin's deep right. Why think it justifies or makes sense of the *veto* provision? After all, a person's right to equal respect and consideration is respected when his arguments are given a fair hearing and his vote counted, even if he is required to abide by some form of majority rule. A right to equal respect and consideration does not by itself *imply* veto powers. Indeed, it seems *ad hoc* to assume that showing equal consideration to persons requires granting them veto powers. Consequently, positing such a deep right, though *compatible* with the veto *in some circumstances*, gives no special support to it.[36]

Rawls' own arguments for the veto, whatever their problems, do not seem to depend on appeals to hidden rights. Sometimes Rawls treats the unanimity constraint as a mere consequence of the thick veil of ignorance: behind the veil all persons would *have* to arrive at the same principles.[37] Since there seem to be no ineliminable appeals to Level III rights in arguments for the veil (see section 3E), on this account the veto would not need them. Elsewhere Rawls suggests the unanimity condition has a separate basis from the veil, though it is the veil that permits contractors to achieve unanimity.[38] Indeed, he suggests that other devices (the impartial spectator) may also permit rational persons to achieve unanimity and that "the idea of unanimity among rational persons is implicit throughout the tradition of moral philosophy."[39] Rawls' direct justification for the unanimity constraint appeals to his Kantian notions of the person and the kingdom of ends. The argument seems to be: (1) "All [persons] are similarly free and rational"; therefore (2) "each must have an equal say in adopting the public principles of the ethical commonwealth."[40] On the face of it, (2) does not entail a veto even if the argument is sound. But Rawls attempts an explication: "The force of the self's being equal is that the principles chosen must be acceptable to other selves ... This means that as noumenal selves, everyone is to consent to these principles."[41]

I confess to not understanding Rawls' explication, nor to seeing how it saves the argument. (Nor am I convinced there is an available sound argument.) But it does seem Rawls *intends* here no appeal to deep rights but rather an argument rooted in a view of the (transcendental?) nature of persons.[42] The best reply to Dworkin would have been to point to a successful, non-right-based argument for the veto[43] to supplement my claim that Dworkin's right-based theory does not require the very unanimity condition it is invoked to explain. Instead I can only point to an *intent* to avoid an appeal to rights. Given the scope of my inquiry, I can therefore draw only a modest conclusion: the case for deep rights is not established; moreover, since we have no good reason to posit such rights and some good reasons to avoid them, Level III theories of the type I have been discussing remain a plausible alternative to Dworkin's proposal.

E. *The basic structure and the thick veil*

Rawlsian contractors seek principles to govern the basic structure of their society, a constraint that derives from the Level III theory of the role of morality. One argument for this constraint, a reply to Robert Nozick's criticisms in *Anarchy, State, and Utopia*,[44] seems to violate the independence constraint. Though it is initially attractive to think "society should develop over time in accordance with free agreements fairly arrived at and fully honored,"[45] we still must acknowledge that such markets accumulate inequities over time. As a result, individual transactions that seem fair and free may not really be so because of these background inequities. Therefore, some principles regulating the basic structure must be provided if the conditions required for fair and free individual action are to be maintained. The contract seeks just such principles. Rawls' argument here turns on considered moral judgments that cumulative inequities undermine freedom and fairness in individual transactions. But these judgments constraining the theory of the role of morality in society – however plausible they seem – are just the type that also play a role in Level I partial equilibrium. This suggests a violation of the independence constraint.

Rawls sketches a different argument which may avoid this difficulty by drawing on his theory of the person. Social institutions affect not only the manner in which we realize our desires but also what our desires, ambitions, and hopes are. They affect not just the kind of persons we are, but the kind we want to be.[46] After all, our abilities and talents are not fixed natural gifts: they are shaped by social attitudes of encouragement and support and by social institutions governing their training and use. Rawls does not quite complete the argument; to do so he might plausibly invoke feature (d) of the theory of the person, namely, persons have a highest-order interest in how social institutions shape their abilities, talents, desires, and selves. Then he might claim that only principles directly applicable to the basic structure can properly protect this highest-order interest. So, if we agree to these facts about the nature of persons, we should agree to make the basic structure the subject of justice.

A variant, actually an extension, of the same argument is used to support the thick, rather than thin, veil of ignorance. Suppose we agree that the basic structure shapes persons in various important ways and should itself be the subject of justice. Then we should also agree the thick veil is needed. A very thin veil that gives us a glimpse of ourselves, or a thin one that lets us see main features of our society though not ourselves, introduces information already affected by the workings of *some* basic structure. The chance thus arises we will select particular principles because we are directly or indirectly *causally* influenced by a basic structure not regulated by principles of justice we otherwise would rationally select. This danger should incline us to choose the thicker veil.[47] In any case, this argument clearly counters the view that Rawls overtly rigs a thick, rather than thin, veil *just because* it then implies a maximin strategy rather than average utilitarianism.[48]

Considered moral judgments appropriate to Level I seem to play no overt role in this second argument for the basic structure and its extension, as they seem to in the reply to Nozick. But, as we have already seen, we are far short of showing conclusively that the theory of the person to which the argument appeals instead is itself free from violations of the independence constraint. For example, at the heart of that theory there seems to lurk a Kantian distinction between what properties are central and what peripheral to the notion of a moral person. Such a distinction *may* not rest on particular considered moral judgments relevant to Level I partial equilibrium. But the suspicion remains that considered moral judgments about moral relevance that may enter at Level I may also underlie the Kantian distinction. In my own view, such a violation of the independence constraint would not be as serious or damaging as one that involved Level III moral judgments about entitlements and rights, though my defense against Dworkin has not conclusively ruled out even the latter. I have only shown that if there are violations, they are not glaring, overt ones. Rather, they lie deep in the theory of the person, which indicates an important subject for some future inquiry.

4. WIDE EQUILIBRIUM AND JUSTIFICATION

If I am right, key features of Rawls' contract are defended by appeal to deep theories which do not obviously violate the independence constraint. Consequently, there is (at least) no overt rigging of the contract.[49] Set in a wide equilibrium, the contract derivation draws on a circle of justificatory support wider than the simple matching of moral principles to considered judgments in partial equilibrium. This suggests we should answer our original question about the intended justificatory force of the contract as follows:

(i) principles chosen in the original position are justified not (just) because they match relevant considered judgments in partial equilibrium, but because the original position is an acceptable justificatory (or principle-selection) device;

(ii) the original position is an acceptable justificatory device because
the relevant deep theory is acceptable, as are inferences from it to
the features of the contract.

In short, the principles contractors choose are justified because we have
adequate reason to treat the contract as justificatory.

But there is a price to be paid for so freeing the contract from the
rigging charge: the acceptability of the contract now depends on the
acceptability of the deep theory against which the Archimedean point
is fixed. The contract is not automatically acceptable to all rational
persons "on reflection," but only if particular component theories are
also accepted. Consequently, rejection of features of that deep theory
may lead to rejection of the contract device.[50] For example, it has been
suggested that the utilitarian and the Kantian (like Rawls) are committed to different conceptions of the person, specifically to different
criteria for personal identity.[51] Such differences might lead utilitarians
to reject a contract and select something else as a justificatory device,
rendering academic debates about which view follows from the contract. Clearly more has to be said about the method of seeking wide
equilibrium, for the articulation and testing of these deep theories
assumes priority over the contract argument itself and looms as the
more fundamental contribution to method in ethics.

Two roles can be ascribed to the method of seeking wide reflective
equilibrium, a modest and a daring one. In its modest role, the method
is primarily analytic and explicative. It forces us to see that moral
theories have a more complex structure than the traditional two-tiered
view of principles plus judgments. Understanding this structure may
help explain central features of our moral reasoning not usually discussed by philosophers. For example, our judgments about what is
problematic, plausible, and relevant in moral argument may well be
determined by the content and structure of relevant background theories, as their analogues in science are. Clarity about this structure may
help us locate more effectively sources of moral agreement and disagreement. We may even be able to reduce disagreements that seem
intractable at the level of moral judgments and principles to more
tractable disagreements about deep theory. Of course, how much
convergence will result, especially if some component theories are
themselves constrained by considered moral judgments, remains an
empirical question.[52]

In its daring role, which it has in Rawls' work, wide equilibrium
also serves as the basis for a coherence account of moral justification.
Several properties of wide equilibria are suggestive of this role:

(1) No considered moral judgments at any level are taken to be
unrevisable, that is, *strongly foundational*; moreover, they are

subject to revisionary pressures from considerations at all levels.[53]

(2) Nonmoral deep theories (Levels III and IV) in general under-determine moral theory selection; for example, Rawls' feasibility constraints at best narrow down the field.[54]

(3) Important deep theories (e.g., of the person, of the role of morality) are in general constrained by (revisable) considered moral judgments.

Suppose we ask what justifies us in accepting (if we do) the particular Level III theories that are contained in the Rawlsian wide equilibrium. The answer is, of course, many different things, since these theories are constrained by numerous moral and nonmoral factors. But most generally what justifies us is the coherence of those theories with the other beliefs we think justified in wide equilibrium (including some account of how we have acquired them). This suggests we complete our account of the justificatory force of the contract by adding:

(iii) the deep theory is acceptable because it coheres best with the rest of our beliefs at all levels in wide equilibrium.

The juxtaposition of (3) and (iii) raises an important question, which is at least worth noting here. Included among the beliefs with which the deep theories must cohere are some (Level III) considered moral judgments. These are not [by (1)] strongly foundational and do not function like intuitions in traditional moral intuitionism. That is, they are not a "given" which our theories must accommodate but are open to revision in light of theoretical considerations at all levels. Despite this revisability, some will still balk at just this point. They will object to the fact that such *moral judgments* play any role at all in moral theory acceptance. After all, such judgments are still "our" judgments and therefore are open to standard objections, for example, that they only reflect what we *think* is right, not reliably what *is* right, or that they are subject to standard forms of bias. Consequently, we have no reason to think coherence among such judgments – even a fancy one with levels – should count as justificatory. Elsewhere I argue against this complaint and its implied contrast with the scientific case. Specifically I argue that coherence considerations in the moral case may be *evidential* in just the way they are in the sciences, though to make the case persuasively, some account of the initial credibility of moral judgments is owed. I cannot pursue these matters here.[55]

Instead I shall conclude by considering another question raised by my inclusion of (iii). On such a coherence view of justification, someone might argue, it does not matter if the contract is rigged: "let's rig it, see what we get by way of conditions, and if we like them, if they 'fit' with our wide equilibrium, then so be they." This objection misses the point of the independence constraint, which is intended to make sure support for the moral principles is brought from as wide a justificatory circle as possible. Moreover, insisting on its satisfaction has another benefit: it may force revision of considered moral judgments that otherwise would have gone unchallenged. The more casual approach behind the "rigging does not matter" objection forces no such widening of the justificatory network and provides no such revisionary pressure. My insistence that the contract argument has justificatory force only if the independence constraint is satisfied is thus not incompatible with the coherence account of justification contained in (i–iii).[56]

NOTES

1 Cf. John Rawls, *A Theory of Justice* (Cambridge, Mass.: Harvard, 1971), pp. 17, 21, 577–87.

2 Rawls, *A Theory of Justice*, p. 20.

3 Rawls, *A Theory of Justice*, p. 141.

4 Cf. R. M. Hare, "Rawls' Theory of Justice," *Philosophical Quarterly* 23 (1973), pp. 144–55, 241–51; reprinted in Norman Daniels, ed., *Reading Rawls* (New York: Basic, 1975), esp. pp. 82ff. Hare cites (p. 84) the Rawls passages quoted above (cf. n. 2 and n. 3 supra).

5 We are not bound to principles to which we did not actually agree. Nor, merely because we would have agreed to them had we agreed to make the contract (they would have been in our *antecedent* interest) must we now accept them (they may not be in our *actual* interst). Cf. Ronald Dworkin, "The Original Position," *University of Chicago Law Review* 40 (1973), pp. 500–33; reprinted in Daniels, *Reading Rawls*, pp. 16–53.

6 Dworkin, "The Original Position," in *Reading Rawls*, p. 51.

7 T. M. Scanlon, "Rawls' Theory of Justice," *University of Pennsylvania Law Review* 121 (1973), pp. 1010–69; reprinted in part in Daniels, *Reading Rawls*, pp. 169–205, cf. p. 178; Scanlon's view has important similarities to mine.

8 Cf. David Lyons' interesting argument in "Nature and Soundness of Contract and Coherence Arguments," in Daniels, *Reading Rawls*, pp. 141–67, esp. 159–60.

9 John Rawls, "Reply to Alexander and Musgrave," *Quarterly Journal of Economics* 88 (1974), p. 637.

10 E.g., the person is calm and has adequate information about the cases being judged. Considered moral judgments may be of any level of generality, a shift from earlier characterizations. Cf. Rawls, "The Independence of Moral Theory," *Proceedings and Addresses of the American Philosophical Association* 48 (1974–75), p. 8.

11 The distinction between narrow and wide reflective equilibria is implicit in *A Theory of Justice*, p. 49, and explicit in "The Independence of Moral Theory," p. 8. Rawls has compared the search for moral principles in reflective equilibrium to the search for a grammar in descriptive syntactics: each captures a relevant "sense" or competence. But the analogy at best

holds for narrow, not wide equilibria; cf. my "On Some Methods of Ethics and Linguistics" *Philosophical Studies*, 37 (1980), pp. 21–36. More importantly, narrow equilibrium is particularly ill suited as a basis for a justificational argument: its elementary coherence constraints provide inadequate pressure to revise considered moral judgments, which have no special epistemological status and are open to many charges about bias, historical accident, and ideology. Cf. Rawls, *A Theory of Justice*, p. 49.

12 My formulation is not adequate as it stands since there will even be trivial truth-functional counterexamples to it unless some specification of "interesting" and "nontrivial" is given. I also say nothing about how to measure the scope of a theory. The problem is a standing one in philosophy of science (cf. Michael Friedman's attempt to handle the related question of unifying theories in "Explanation and Scientific Understanding," *Journal of Philosophy* 71 (1974), pp. 5–14, esp. 15ff.). I assume this difficulty can be overcome, though doing so might require dropping the loose talk about theories. I am indebted to George Smith for helpful discussion of this point.

13 General social theory, which is used to test the feasibility of Level II principles (from behind the veil of ignorance) and Level III theories (from outside the veil), is presumably independent of Level I considered moral judgments. How much the feasibility test narrows the field is an open question.

14 This point only suggests, but fails to prove, a violation of the independence constraint. Little hangs on the conclusion in what follows.

15 "The aim of the description of the original position is to put together in one conception the idea of fairness with the *formal* conditions expressed by the notion of a well-ordered society, and then to use this conception to help us select between alternative principles of justice." (Rawls, "Reply to Alexander and Musgrave," p. 638, italics added.) Many features of the well-ordered society are not just formal, since they draw directly for support on the theory of the person.

16 All conditions are taken from "Reply to Alexander and Musgrave," pp. 634–5.

17 Definitions, for example, would still have to be assessed in light of a well worked out theory. A *weak* publicity condition might drop (3), for example.

18 Cf. *A Theory of Justice*, pp. 177–9. Similarly, a strong publicity condition imposes broad limits on the allowable complexity of principles and on the amount of information needed to apply them. But Rawls does not argue for the strong publicity condition because of its connection with these effects nor because these effects might favor his principles over others. Cf. "Independence of Moral Theory," p. 14.

19 Rawls, *A Theory of Justice*, p. 133.

20 Rawls, "Independence of Moral Theory," p. 13.

21 The situation is more complex. See my "Moral Theory and the Plasticity of Persons," *Monist* 62:3 (1979), pp. 265–87.

22 Rawls, "A Kantian Conception of Equality," *Cambridge Review* (February, 1975), p. 94. The wording also appears in condition (4) of well-ordered societies; see above.

23 Rawls, "A Kantian Conception of Equality," p. 94.
24 Cf. Rawls, "A Kantian Conception of Equality," p. 95; also, John Rawls, "The Basic Structure as Subject," *American Philosophical Quarterly* 14 (1977), p. 160.
25 Rawls, "A Kantian Conception of Equality," p. 94.
26 Cf. Rawls, "A Kantian Conception of Equality," p. 94.
27 Cf. Rawls, *A Theory of Justice*, section 25.
28 Cf. Rawls, *A Theory of Justice*, pp. 256ff.; also, Rawls, "Kantian Conception of Equality," p. 98.
29 Rawls treats some of these as straightforward empirical claims about humans. Thus he thinks that (e) is true except for pathological cases, and he therefore treats "having a capacity to form a conception of the good and to develop a sense of justice" as a natural (range) property. Since this range property is equal in all persons, he infers it is a relevant basis on which to view persons as equal. Cf. *A Theory of Justice*, pp. 505–8.
30 I am indebted to Josh Cohen for discussion of this point.
31 "A Kantian Conception of Equality," p. 94.
32 Rawls thinks philosophy of mind and general social theory underdetermine even such a central feature of persons as the criterion of personal identity: its selection depends on coherence of the theory of the person with the rest of moral theory in wide equilibrium. This view raises many of the same questions about the independence constraint. In any case, Rawls' view of the "plasticity" of the person suggests he treats the theory of the person as an ideal, not an idealization. Cf. my "Moral Theory and the Plasticity of Persons," section V.
33 There is only one reference to rights in Level III arguments in *A Theory of Justice*: In section 77 Rawls discusses the equality of moral personhood as a basis for determining to whom justice is owed, and he remarks in a note that "This fact can be used to interpret the concept of natural rights" (p. 505, n. 30). But here the talk of rights can be viewed as (misleading) shorthand for the underlying theory of the person. References to Level III rights enter Rawls' writings more freely after Ronald Dworkin's "The Original Position" appeared (e.g., "The Kantian Conception of Equality," p. 94); moreover, Rawls cites Dworkin in a relevant context, while discussing the role of the well-ordered society (cf. "Reply to Alexander and Musgrave," p. 634, n. 1). The real issue is not, of course, whether Rawls accepts Dworkin's view (I think he does not), but whether we are compelled to accept it.
34 Cf. Dworkin's more detailed argument, "The Original Position," pp. 42–53.
35 Cf. Rawls, "Reply to Alexander and Musgrave," p. 638.
36 I am indebted to Miles Morgan for discussion of this point.
37 Rawls, *A Theory of Justice*, pp. 140, 564–5.
38 Rawls, *A Theory of Justice*, pp. 141–2.
39 Rawls, *A Theory of Justice*, p. 264.
40 Rawls, *A Theory of Justice*, p. 257.
41 Rawls, *A Theory of Justice*, p. 257.
42 Cf. Rawls, *A Theory of Justice*, pp. 564–5.

43 It should be remembered I am nowhere assessing the soundness, only the structure, of Rawls' justificatory argument.

44 Robert Nozick, *Anarchy, State, and Utopia* (New York: Basic Books, 1974), pp. 204ff.

45 Rawls, "The Basic Structure as Subject," p. 159.

46 Rawls, "The Basic Structure as Subject," p. 160.

47 Rawls, "The Basic Structure as Subject," p. 161.

48 Cf. Hare's criticism in "Rawls' Theory of Justice," pp. 89–94, 101–7.

49 What still needs explanation are Rawls' remarks suggestive of such rigging. The key lies in the heuristic role of the contract idea. Imagine asking, "can we work backwards from the contractarian task of choosing principles to figure out what conditions on choice will yield the preferred principles?" We can, and we may suppose Rawls did. But after such heuristics, we still have to show why the conditions are acceptable.

50 Rawls, "Reply to Alexander and Musgrave," p. 637; cf. G. E. Pence, "Fair Contracts and Beautiful Intuitions," in Kai Nielsen and Roger Shiner, eds., *Canadian Journal of Philosophy*, Supplementary vol. 3, Guelph: Canadian Association for Publishing in Philosophy, 1977, p. 143.

51 Cf. Derek Parfit, "Later Selves and Moral Principles," in Alan Montefiore, ed., *Philosophy and Personal Relations* (London: Routledge and Kegan Paul, 1973), esp. pp. 149–60; and Rawls, "Independence of Moral Theory," pp. 17ff.; and my "Moral Theory and the Plasticity of Persons."

52 These and some of the following points are pursued further in my "Wide Reflective Equilibrium and Theory Acceptance in Ethics," *Journal of Philosophy* 76 (1979), pp. 255–82.

53 Confusion on this point leads some to construe reflective equilibrium as a form of intuitionism. Cf. Hare, "Rawls' Theory of Justice," p. 83, and Peter Singer, "Sidgwick and Reflective Equilibrium," *Monist* 58 (1974), pp. 493–4.

54 Points (2) and (3) are clearly stated in Rawls' "Independence of Moral Theory." Cf. n. 32 above.

55 Cf. my "Wide Reflective Equilibrium & Theory Acceptance in Ethics," sections IV and V.

56 The National Endowment for the Humanities Fellowship program funded this and related research. I am grateful to Josh Cohen, Miles Morgan, John Rawls, and George Smith for helpful discussion.

Chapter 4

On some methods of ethics and linguistics

I

Characterizing a person's syntactic competency by formulating a grammar that accounts for it may be the main task of descriptive syntactic theory, but determining that a person's moral competency is characterized by a particular set of principles is not the main task of moral philosophy. To be sure, moral philosophy must formulate precise statements of different moral conceptions. But it also must face the task of choosing between competing moral conceptions, of solving the problems of justification and theory acceptance in the moral domain. Because I believe the method of wide reflective equilibrium reveals a complexity in the structure of ethical theories that makes the problem of theory acceptance more tractable than it is on other approaches, I would like to free wide equilibrium from an unnecessary or, at least, overstated analogy to linguistic method. That analogy, first proposed in Rawls' *A Theory of Justice*,[1] only reinforces the erroneous view that the moral philosopher interested in reflective equilibrium has confused moral anthropology with moral philosophy.[2]

I shall first distinguish narrow and wide reflective equilibria, showing in the process that narrow equilibrium has a strong similarity to methods in syntactic theory. It is wide equilibrium, however, not narrow, that is of interest to the moral philosopher – and for just the features which distinguish it from certain features of syntactics. As we shall see, because of these features choosing between competing moral conceptions in wide equilibrium has a close analogy to the problem of choosing between alternative deductive logics. I shall conclude by arguing that the disanalogy to certain features of syntactic theory does not imply a disanalogy to other scientific methods.

II

Characterized in its most abstract form, a *narrow* reflective equilibrium consists of an ordered pair of (a) a set of considered moral judgments acceptable to a given person P at a given time, and (b) a set of general moral principles that economically systematizes (a). The set of considered judgments (a) is pared down from a set of initial moral judgments in two stages. First it is pruned to eliminate judgments that P is not confident of, has made without adequate information about the situation, or has made in a state of mind conducive to moral error. Second, the resulting considered judgments are further adjusted to eliminate irregularities that may block their fit with the most desired set of principles. Such principles not only must economically systematize the considered judgments that result from the first stage of pruning, but if possible should somewhat extend the set of acceptable considered judgments to include some about which the person was not so confident or found indeterminate. The resulting set (b) might then be taken to characterize the moral views held by P.

This abstract characterization of narrow equilibrium shows its amenability to a linguistic analogy. Suppose we view a person as having a moral "sensibility,"[3] a competency which should be investigated like other competencies, in particular, syntactic competency. The competency is manifested in the indeterminately large range of moral judgments people feel competent to make about a wide variety of cases, including judgments about the rightness and wrongness, justice and injustice of acts, policies, and institutions, as well as about the moral status of agents involved in such acts. To be sure, there will be many cases about which people feel unable to make any judgment at all. But this incompleteness in the moral capacity to make judgments does not detract from its remarkable scope and power. Nor need the moral theorist think there is some special or privileged epistemological status adhering to such judgments in order to think it an interesting task to explicate the content and structure of such competency.

I believe Rawls, in introducing this analogy, intends us to see a similarity to the "projection problem"[4] in syntactic theory. People who have encountered only finitely many sentences can make judgments of grammaticality (actually, of acceptability) about indeterminately many sentences, which suggests we should look for general principles or rules when we seek to characterize their syntactic competency. Similarly, people who have encountered only finitely many moral situations can make indeterminately many judgments. In both cases people may cite principles which they appeal to in forming judgments of grammaticality (acceptability) or rightness or justice, but such principles may not, in fact, be the principles which would be needed to explain their linguistic or moral competency.[5] Of course, we are some-what more tolerant of someone who says that his linguistic intuition tells him some string is grammatical (acceptable), but who can cite no principle to explain why, than we are of people who claim confident moral judgments, but can give no reason based on principle or theory to defend their view.[6] Still, we should not expect the set of principles (b) to be read off ready-made by our "moral informant" *P*.

Critical to making the analogy to syntactics work, however, is the need to provide a moral version of the distinction between perform-ance and competence so important to the syntactic case. Not all initial judgments of grammaticality need be accepted into the set of judg-ments we take to reveal syntactic competence and for which we try to provide a grammar. Rather, some such judgments – perhaps many – can be discounted as performance-based errors or distortions. There are at least two categories of such performance errors. The first is, intuitively speaking, nonlinguistic and includes the conditions that affect the subject's state of mind: inebriation, inattention, fatigue, and so on. We saw a rough analogy to some of these conditions in the moral case: initial moral judgments are filtered to include only those made when the informant is in a state of mind conducive to making error-free moral judgments.

The second type of performance-based error or deviation from com-petency is more properly seen as linguistic. Suppose we assume the person making the judgments contains an "on-line processor," that is, actual computational hardware and software whose heuristics, shortcuts, and approximations may deviate in many ways from what might be computationally pure or ideal procedure. (Such deviations reflect the design limits of the system and may make it more efficient.) Then some performance problems will be attributable to limitations of the processor, such as short-term memory limits, or to the fact that the on-line processor contains only heuristic devices for accomplishing some tasks that are called for by the underlying competency. Such heuristic procedures may yield different results from what a more straightforward programming (on a processor of different design) of the underlying competency would yield. For example, suppose we hear a string that reads: "buffalo buffalo buffalo." We might well judge it to be unacceptable or ungrammatical. Then our friendly linguist says, "Think of it on the model, 'Men admire women.'" We probably can then see that the original string is grammatical. We might explain our failure to hear its grammaticality as a failure of heuristic procedures of our on-line processor and we are no longer forced to view the initial judgment of ungrammaticality as part of the data that needs explicat-ing by the grammar.[7]

It is important to note that the performance–competence distinction

is heavily theory dependent.[8] Various theoretical considerations enter
to determine how this distinction is to be drawn. For example, suppose
our theory of language-acquisition gives us good reason to believe we
share a common genetic endowment which helps explain the presence
of certain universal features of grammar. We might then learn from the
study of Italian that it can only develop the way it does if a particular
principle of universal grammar is assumed. In turn, we might be compelled to revise our theory of English, redrawing the line we might
have originally drawn between performance and competence in English. But this sensitivity of the performance–competence distinction to
various theoretical considerations, leading as it does to the revisability
of initial judgments of acceptability or grammaticality, does not undermine the fact that we take the grammar to be a theory of syntactic
competency.[9] This holds even if we take the "hardness" of the data for
that grammar to depend on our confidence in the theoretical support
for the performance–competence distinction as drawn.

With some exercise of fancy, we may find a parallel between the
appeal to the performance–competence distinction in syntactics and an
analogous distinction we might draw for the moral case. Consider, for
example, cases in which we are led to revise moral judgments because
we realize they are incompatible with other judgments we hold, contrary to what we had been able to see at first.[10] A specially constructed
moral dilemma, for instance, might convince us we had "overlooked"
relevant features in judging the original case. Or a number of related
cases might be shown to us, on the basis of which we see similarities we had not seen before. We might then say that our on-line
moral processor erred and failed to match our real moral competency.[11]
Here we can suppose our moral performance–competence distinction
may be theory dependent in ways analogous to the theory dependency
of the syntactic version (for example, psychological theories of attention or reasoning ability may affect how the moral version might be
drawn).

The fact that narrow equilibrium stops at the point at which it
characterizes a person's moral competency, which is what supports the
analogy to syntactics, shows that it is not of central interest to moral
philosophy. In moral philosophy we are interested in understanding
how to justify moral principles and choose between competing sets of
such principles. When the linguist produces a grammar which seems to
characterize a syntactic competency, given his best version of the performance–competence distinction, his descriptive task, at least, is done.
Moreover, he has no further *justificatory* and *prescriptive* task of trying
to show why one descriptively (and, we may suppose, explanatorily)
adequate grammar is to be preferred over another.[12] Narrow equilibrium leaves us in the position of the descriptive linguist (though we

should keep in mind that worries about explanatory considerations help determine what counts as adequate description for the linguist).[13]

The situation is different with wide reflective equilibrium. Suppose we collect, as with narrow equilibrium, a set of initial considered moral judgments. Instead of immediately settling for a "best fit" set of principles, however, we now propose alternative sets, some obviously being better fits than others. The task for the person seeking wide equilibrium is to choose between such alternatives on the basis of philosophical arguments which reveal the strengths and weaknesses of the competing moral conceptions. Such arguments may be viewed as inferences from a body of relevant theories. They may include, for example, a theory of the person, a theory of the role of morality in society, a body of general social theory, and so on. Suppose some set of arguments "wins" and the person adopts a particular set of moral principles. To establish wide equilibrium, of course, he must adjust his set of initial considered judgments and, in turn, make further adjustments in his set of principles or even in the relevant theories. The wide equilibrium can now be characterized as an ordered triple of (a) the considered moral judgments, (b) the moral principles, and (c) the set of relevant theories invoked or presupposed by the winning arguments for (b), all duly "adjusted" to be compatible with each other.

A number of qualifying remarks are in order. First, there is no assumption that the set (c) of relevant theories is a set of nonmoral theories, which thus constitutes a reduction of the moral [sets (a) and (b)] to the nonmoral. The theories in (c) may themselves be constrained by a set (a') of considered moral judgments. Second, if the theories in (c) are to provide support for (b) that is in any way independent of the support for (b) provided by its fit with (a), then some significant portion of (a) and (a') must be disjoint. Otherwise, the theories in (c) might simply be recharacterizations of the considered judgments in (a). Then, we would have no greater justificatory gain in accepting (b) on the basis of (c) than we would have were we simply to establish a partial equilibrium directly between (b) and (a) without any appeal to the arguments derived from (c).[14] Third, the method assumes that persons are rational and will be persuaded by sound arguments; they will not, for example, simply believe every third argument they hear. Fourth, there is no assumption that all persons will converge on a unique equilibrium.[15]

One central feature of wide equilibrium requires special note. It permits, indeed requires, that considered moral judgments be held revisable on far wider grounds than is the case with narrow equilibrium. The acceptability of deep theories in (c) can force the revision of initial considered judgments in (a). Considered moral judgments (a') that constrain the acceptability of theories in (c) are also revisable in light of many considerations that affect the acceptability of the theories in (c) and their equilibrium with principles in (b) and other judgments in (a). No considered judgments are foundational in any sense; all are subjected to great pressures for revision and are accordingly revised. To the extent that we "firm up" a set (a) of considered judgments in wide equilibrium, it is held firm only relative to the rest of the equilibrium, and is in any case revisable if anything destabilizes the equilibrium.

This revisability of considered judgments in (a) points to a disanalogy between wide equilibrium and syntactics. In the linguistic case, we allow revision – even extensive revision – of initial judgments of grammaticality (acceptability), but we do so subject to an important constraint. We revise or discard initial judgments only if we can pass them off as performance-based errors. To be sure, the performance–competence distinction is itself revisable in the light of theory, as noted earlier. But the task of (at least descriptive) syntactics is to produce a grammar for the set of competency-revealing judgments, as best our theory allows us to pick out that set. In wide equilibrium, however, theories act in a far more varied way to force revisions of considered moral judgments. Their main effect is not at all to constrain a performance–competence distinction by reference to which we can in turn discard certain considered judgments (even though they may, among other things, help us develop a theory of moral "performance" errors). Instead, the theories force us to choose, as it were, which among alternative competencies we want to see realized in persons.

A second disanalogy follows from the first. Whereas in the linguistic case we are interested in a person's *actual* syntactic competency, and in narrow equilibrium we are interested in his *actual* moral competency, in wide equilibrium we may not be seeking to characterize a competency at all. At best, we might describe our goal as seeking a hypothetical competency: the one a person would have were he to be persuaded by such and such arguments and revise the components of his system of beliefs accordingly. In linguistics, we pursue no such hypothetical competencies, except, perhaps, for very special purposes (see n. 12).

It might be objected that such a nonactual competency is not the target of wide equilibrium. Rather, the process of philosophical argument in wide equilibrium is intended to get a person to make explicit his actual underlying conception, not to revise an existing one. The philosophical argument is needed because the conception is quite deep, like certain transformational features in grammatical theory, and therefore not consciously accessible (without theory) to the person seeking wide equilibrium. The philosophical argument allows us to explicate the deep structure by getting the person to see what he is really committed to believing true and right.

This objection does not capture the full force of what is involved in achieving wide equilibrium. To be sure, there may well be features of a person's moral conception of which he is not aware and of which argument may make him aware. Thus someone may not be aware that in advancing a particular moral principle or judgment he is really committed to – and "drawing on" – some theory of the nature of the person. Philosophical argument might bring this fact out. But it is also clear that philosophical argument changes peoples' moral beliefs. It would seem perverse to insist that all such changes and revisions are just part of the process of explicating beliefs that are already implicitly there though hidden.[16]

If the revisability of considered moral judgments in wide equilibrium does not hinge on the formulation of an appropriate performance–competence distinction, and if the target of such equilibrium is not just the explication of a person's actual moral competency, then the heart of the analogy to the case of descriptive syntactics is gone.[17] Nor is the search for a moral conception in wide equilibrium like the search for a characterization of English grammar abstracted from idiosyncratic differences in English competency. Nor is it like the search for a theory of universals incorporating features all grammars have, whatever their differences in other ways. I turn, then, to what I believe may be a more convincing analogue to the justificatory task of wide reflective equilibrium: the justification of alternative logics.

III

The analogy to the problem of characterizing and justifying alternative inductive and deductive logics is suggested in passing by Rawls.[18] We might pursue the analogy for the case of induction as follows. There are judgments we all make about what count as reasonable or acceptable patterns of inductive inference. We might try to characterize this practice by formulating a set of principles of induction that can account for these inductive practices. Suppose, however, that our task is not simply to formulate principles that capture a particular person's practice at a given moment. Rather, we formulate alternative inductive logics and bring philosophical argument to bear to persuade ourselves to adopt one alternative rather than another. Doing so might require us to modify our inductive practice. The resulting wide reflective equilbrium would include not only sets of inductive principles and sets of judgments about acceptable inference patterns, but also would include whatever relevant theories were either invoked or implicit in the winning arguments.

A more developed analogy can be found in the literature on alternative deductive logics, well illustrated, I believe, by Michael Dummett's recent arguments about the basis for choosing between classical and intuitionist logics.[19] Suppose we view formalizations of both classical and intuitionist logics as sytematizations of different sets of judgments about acceptable inference patterns, say those of the classical and intuitionist mathematicians. How are we to choose between the two logics? The choice of either will involve revising someone's intuitions.

Dummett's answer is that we must look at the theories of meaning which are presupposed by the two logics. In general we might agree that one "test" of the adequacy of such a theory of meaning is that it provides us, through semantic completeness and soundness proofs, with an account of the forms of inference which we generally employ in our linguistic practice. Thus, we might have an initial prejudice in favor of a theory of meaning that can account for our use of indirect proof (or double negation elimination), since it is part of nearly everyone's (except intuitionists') linguistic practice. The realist or platonist theory of meaning, which posits bivalency with regard to truth for all sentences, regardless of our ability to come to recognize their truth, here seems to have the edge. It seems to explain classical, that is, general, practice.

Suppose, however, we find that the semantics employed in such a realist theory violates certain conditions of adequacy for a theory of meaning (say conditions rooted in certain views about language learning). Then we have some basis for saying that the realist semantics "fails the test" of justifying our practice. There may then be reason to reject features of that practice, if the only way to account for them required such a semantics. In the case at hand it would mean rejecting the assumption of bivalency imported to account for indirect proof. Thus, we may be led to see good reason to reject even widespread linguistic practices, here certain deductive inference patterns, since we cannot give adequate justification for them. We can, however, give adequate justification for an alternative logic not containing them. That is, a different semantic theory, one that bases its notion of truth on constructive provability, or verifiability, can account for all linguistic practices except the ones we now find problematic in classical theory.

I am not concerned here with the soundness of Dummett's complex argument, which I have here only sketched. Instead, I cite it to point out a general structural feature it shares with the method of wide reflective equilibrium. Dummett uses philosophical argument to persuade us of what he hopes we will agree is an acceptable and relevant theory, in this case a verificationist semantics and certain views on language learning. His goal is to resolve a choice between competing "conceptions" of logic held by classical and intuitionist mathematicians.[20] His strategy shares with wide reflective equilibrium the appeal to theory to force a revision in our considered judgments, in this case about the acceptability of an inference pattern rather than the rightness of an action. There is no mediating appeal to a performance–competence distinction (however theory dependent), as in the case of (descriptive) syntactics, for our very task is to determine which competency is superior. Despite this analogy, however, there remains an important difference, at least in the case of Dummett. Dummett views the theory of meaning as foundational in a way that is not true of the theories relevant to constraining the choice of moral principles.[21]

Although I have argued that the way in which relevant theories can compel revision of considered moral judgments is different from the way in which similar revision is compelled in syntactic theory, I do not mean to suggest that wide reflective equilibrium thereby deviates from scientific procedure. Indeed, the kind of revisability it permits is quite consistent with scientific practice in other domains. I turn to consider an opposing view in the next section.

IV

Ronald Dworkin argues that the extensive revisability of considered moral judgments in (wide) reflective equilibrium implies we should interpret the process in terms of a legal model (the "constructive model") rather than a scientific model which fits laws to data (the "natural model").[22] Both models emphasize the consistency between initial judgments and principles, but for different reasons. The natural model interprets the moral principles as "laws" which articulate the natural order among the phenomena accurately described in the set of judgments. The constructive model values consistency for what might be called moral and political reasons: consistency in the public advocacy of principles, as a basis for social action, is a desideratum of a conception of justice.

We get a clearer view of the way the two models are supposed to work by considering some examples Dworkin offers. He asks us to consider an official who has conflicting "intuitions" and who can think of no set of principles capable of reconciling them. For example, he might feel it is wrong to punish an attempted murderer as severely as a successful one, but also feel that what counts in the case is the intention to murder. Similarly, he might feel that special consideration is due a minority group which has been discriminated against, but also feel that any discriminations on the basis of race are wrong.[23]

Suppose the official were guided by the "natural model." Dworkin argues he would then have to abide by the troublesome intuition, "submerging the apparent contradiction, in the faith that a more sophisticated set of principles, which reconciles that intuition, does in fact exist though it has not yet been discovered."[24] One point is immediately unclear: how can the official follow *both* intuitions? Dworkin seems to label only the feeling that attempted murder is less serious as an "intuition." But what, then, is the "sense" the person has that intention ought to count? Let us set this problem aside. Dworkin believes the official would have to stick with his intuitions because the case is, on the "natural model," analogous to one in science in which clear, hard data "outstrips the explanatory powers of those who observe."[25] Here the datum we are stuck with is the intuition to punish less severely. Dworkin's argument turns, I believe, on comparing considered moral judgments (Dworkin calls them "intuitions" or "convictions") to direct perception reports of a relatively privileged sort.

Now suppose the official is guided by the "constructive model." Rather than holding firm to his intuitions, the official would have to give up his conflicting intuitions and work out a principled policy. This constructive course leaves open the possibility that later some principles may be found to reconcile the conflict. But meantime, the pressure of the need to act and the overriding commitment to consistency force the official to reject one of the intuitions on the basis of principles he is willing to stand by and be criticized by.

I believe the contrast is overdrawn. Consider the very example Dworkin appeals to as a model for the scientific case, that of an astronomer with a set of measurements ("clear observational data") for which he can give no account, for example, by fitting them into a theory of the origin of the solar system. Suppose the scientist has no reason to reject any of his data: it depends on reliable theories of instrumentation, and he can be sure there has been no instrument malfunction. Need the scientist stick to his data as Dworkin insists? I think not. He may instead try to build a theory incorporating some of the data. The rest he may leave aside in the hope that further development of the interim theory will allow him to account for it later on, or at least will later allow him to explain it away. To be sure, he is not in this process rejecting as erroneous or unfounded the data that is set aside, however anomalous it may seem to him from the point of view of the interim theory.

But so far, my account of the astronomer makes him sound very much like the "constructive" official trying to formulate a consistent policy in the context of conflicting moral intuitions. There are two possibilities. The official may just arbitrarily set aside one intuition and rely on principles invoked to support the other. Alternatively, he may think there is some reason to give more weight to the principles supporting the preferred intuition. The first alternative sounds neither like the astronomer just described, who has some reason (a more promising line of theory construction) for setting aside the data, nor like what goes on in seeking reflective equilibrium (where relevant theories provide reasons for revision). Suppose, however, we have an instance of the second alternative: the constructive official rejects one of the intuitions because he thinks the principles supporting the other one are better supported by some acceptable theory. Perhaps the principles cohere better with other accepted principles in a theory of punishment or are supported by a theory of effective administration. Then what he is doing in modifying his intuitions in the way I suggested earlier characterizes wide reflective equilibrium.

I conclude Dworkin's contrast is overdrawn. The scientist, even one working with "hard" data, may act more like Dworkin's "constructive" official than like the "natural model" official. Still, there is an important point behind Dworkin's discussion: the extensive revisability of considered moral judgments does count against construing them as hard or privileged (I only mean completely reliable) observation reports.[26] But this point does not count against applying the "natural model" to wide equilibrium any more than it counts against applying it to much of science. For very little of scientific theory construction is directly built on a foundation of privileged observation reports – and in any case, on none held unrevisable.

Dworkin offers several other arguments to show that the natural model should be rejected in favor of the constructive one, but they can be considered more briefly. First, Dworkin argues that in seeking reflective equilibrium, we are allowed to modify proposed principles to allow for the fact that they serve as the basis for a public conception of morality. We might, for example, select principles which are easier to understand. Such considerations do not, however, rule out the natural model. After all, simplification or idealization of models in science is a common phenomenon. The fact that we view such models as "not strictly speaking true" does not mean we are not better off for adopting them as roughly true. Similarly, in the interest of the clear administration of justice, we might select principles we know are only roughly true without compromising the belief we may hold that they purport to be objective moral truths.

A second argument rests on the fact that the end point of a wide equilibrium depends on its starting point. Which principles we settle on in wide equilibrium is "relative" to what alternative sets of principles have been proposed. Dworkin argues that the natural model does not allow us to give any authority to principles so chosen if we think there may be better principles that have not been considered. But this objection is not persuasive. Most scientists would probably agree that some other theories, unknown to us right now, are more likely to be true than the ones we now accept. Indeed, were they now presented, they might be accepted in preference to our current favorites. But such an admission does not diminish our confidence that we have the best theory possible under current circumstances. Any form of scientific realism, such as underlies Dworkin's natural model, must be able to accommodate the possible revision of our laws when alternative theories are considered. Providing a precise formulation of such a position is notoriously difficult, but that is not sufficient support for Dworkin's objection which, after all, supposes the natural model is a good one for science.

Finally, Dworkin argues that we cannot reach a reflective equilibrium in the case where different persons disagree on some initial judgments unless we include in the set of considered judgments only those on which there is consensus. But, he urges, an adherent of the natural model cannot accept the exclusion of such disputed data – *some* of it may be sound. Here too the argument fails. In some scientific contexts, it is necessary to construct a theory using only undisputed data. Disputed data is set aside in the hope that further theory development and resulting improvements in experimental method will allow eventual resolution of the disputes. In short, then, none of Dworkin's arguments against the "natural model" are effective.

My motive for countering Dworkin's attack on the "natural model" for wide equilibrium is not that I am already convinced that general moral principles are of the same ilk as scientific laws. I am not sure how they should be treated. Moreover, I think I shall not be sure until I understand more about the structure and content of theories I think acceptable in wide equilibrium. Still, I think it important not to rule out the possibility too quickly, especially on inadequate descriptions of science. But more important, I think that the method of wide equilibrium, with its emphasis on theory construction as the basis for evaluating considered judgments, functions much like the process of theory acceptance in other areas of science.[27] This contention has greater plausibility, and I hope greater acceptability to moral philosophers, once the misanalogy to syntactics is dispelled.[28]

NOTES

1 Cf. John Rawls, *A Theory of Justice* (Harvard, Cambridge, 1971), p. 46ff. The distinction between narrow and wide reflective equilibria is implicit in: *A Theory of Justice*, p. 49, and explicit in his "The Independence of Moral Theory," *Proceedings and Addresses of the American Philosophical Association* XLVIII (1974–75), p. 8.
2 Such is the force of R. M. Hare's criticism in "Rawls' Theory of Justice," *Philosophical Quarterly* 23 (1973), pp. 144–55, 241–51; reprinted in Norman Daniels (ed.), *Reading Rawls* (Basic, New York, 1975), esp. p. 86. See also Thomas Nagel, "Rawls on Justice," Daniels, *Reading Rawls*, p. 2, n. 2.
3 The term is Rawls'; cf. *A Theory of Justice*, p. 46ff.

4 Cf. Jerrold J. Katz and Jerry A. Fodor, "Structure of a Semantic Theory," in the same authors' *Structure of Language* (Prentice Hall, New Jersey, 1964), p. 482.

5 Cf. Rawls, *A Theory of Justice*, p. 47.

6 Though we do sometimes tolerate such pronouncements, and do not press the matter further, especially if they are declared "matters of conscience."

7 Some examples, such as multiple embeddings, may produce judgments of ungrammaticality (unacceptability) or judgments of unknown grammaticality which our systematic grammar could not accommodate without becoming unduly complex. Such judgments may just be discounted. R. M. Hare's remark that "people's *linguistic* 'intuitions' are indeed, in the end, authoritative for what is correct in their language" ("Rawls' Theory of Justice," in my *Reading Rawls*, p. 86), must be revised relative to a performance–competence distinction. So, too, for Nagel's remark, "Rawls on Justice," p. 2, n. 2.

8 I am indebted to Noam Chomsky for emphasizing this point to me, including the example.

9 Nor do I mean to suggest that the descriptive task of producing a comprehensive grammar for a language is the main or most interesting task of syntactics; the descriptive task is likely to be of considerably less importance than, and as suggested above, dependent on, the explanatory task of showing how the language capacity works and grows.

10 On the view that all we are doing is capturing a moral competency, it can hardly be a requirement that the competency be characterizable by a consistent set of moral principles, since the moral judgments may be inconsistent. Similarly, if a person's linguistic practice was inconsistent (the same string is sometimes held acceptable and sometimes not), the grammar that accurately captured it might have to be inconsistent.

11 As I understand it, the competency that is attributed to the speaker of a language by Chomskyan theory may never – as a whole – have been possessed by the speaker at a given time. It may have existed only in bits and pieces prior to the acquisition of the program for the speaker's on-line processor. Still, the theory is needed to explain what enabled the programming of the on-line processor to take place in the bits and pieces manner that characterizes its evolution. Notice that a moral "grammar" that in this same way accounted for or explained moral competency might be of questionable relevance to what we usually take to be the task of a moral theory, namely, to publicly guide our behavior.

12 For special purposes, such as constructing a speaker–hearer machine, choosing between grammars may have a point. There is another phenomenon worth noting because it suggests that theory may lead to revisions of intuition. The linguist sometimes "loses his ear" and seems unable to give "intuitive" judgments of grammaticality in certain cases. The phenomenon may have an explanation at the performance level. But it may also reflect an incomplete revision of the linguist's competency, not unlike what happens when people deliberately adjust their syntax to bring it into line with what they take to be publicly acceptable.

13 William Lycan has pointed out to me that some "value clarification" advo-

cates in the field of moral education act as if achieving narrow equilibrium is of supreme importance.

14   A partial equilibrium is part of a wide equilibrium; it holds between a component theory or set of principles and some set of considered judgments. A fuller discussion of this independence constraint can be found in my "Reflective Equilibrium and Archimedean Points," *Canadian Journal of Philosophy* 10 (1980): 1:83–107.

15   The implications of this assumption are discussed in my "Reflective equilibrium and theory acceptance in ethics," *Journal of Philosophy* LXXVI (1979), pp. 256–82, esp. Section IV.

16   A qualification is needed here. Some moral intuitionists may, in fact, want to construe all such choices between competing moral conceptions – or competencies – as revelatory of the one, underlying moral competency they believe is there to be made explicit. I do not think wide equilibrium requires such a strong view. In any case, Rawls clearly rejects such a view, when he says narrow equilibrium characterizes a person's sense of justice "pretty much as it is although allowing for the smoothing out of certain irregularities," whereas in wide equilibrium a person's sense of justice "may or may not undergo a radical shift" (*A Theory of Justice*, p. 49). Nevertheless, see M. B. E. Smith, "Ethical Intuitionism and Naturalism: A Reconciliation," *Canadian Journal of Philosophy* 9 (1979): 609–29, and "Rawls and Intuitionism" in: *New Essays in Contract Theory*, Kai Nielsen and Roger Shiner (eds.), *Canadian Journal of Philosophy*, Supplementary Volume III, Guelf: Canadian Association for Publishing in Philosophy, 1977, pp. 163–78.

17   Actually, my point may be too strong as it stands since my discussion has been restricted to approaches to syntactics that view it as a branch of psychology, broadly construed. These are the approaches Rawls has in mind in proposing the analogy, but alternative approaches, such as the one indicated in Jerrold Katz's recent work, reject the psychologizing of linguistics.

18   He cites Nelson Goodman's discussion in: *Fact, Fiction and Forecast* (Cambridge, Mass.: Harvard University Press, 1955), pp. 65–8. Cf. *A Theory of Justice*, p. 20, n. 7.

19   Cf. Michael Dummett, "The Justification of Deduction," Hertz Lecture, *Proceedings of the British Academy* (Oxford University Press, London, 1974), pp. 3–34; also "Philosophical Basis of Intuitionist Logic," in: *Logic Colloquium '73*, H. E. Rose et al. (eds.), (Amsterdam, 1975), pp. 5–40.

20   A standard position, however, is to deny that there is a problem of choosing between alternative logics. It holds that different logics formalize different notions of truth, and there is no problem of choice between them. Dummett's strategy is to suggest that we can find out which is the correct notion of truth by taking the matter outside the court of logic and even mathematics and into the field of semantics and the theory of language acquisition. I suspect that even if one took alternative logics to be formalizations of different notions of "consequence" rather than of "truth," a similar strategy of moving to a broader field of relevant theories would seem equally appealing (or unappealing).

21 I discuss the sense in which wide reflective equilibrium supports a coherence theory of justification or theory acceptance in my "Reflective Equilibrium and Theory Acceptance in Ethics," Section IV.

22 Ronald Dworkin, "The Original Position," *University of Chicago Law Review* 40 (1973), pp. 500–33; reprinted in my *Reading Rawls*, esp. pp. 27–37; quotations will be from latter source. The same material also appears in Chapter 6 of Dworkin's *Taking Rights Seriously* (Harvard, Cambridge, Mass., 1977).

23 Cf. Dworkin, "The Original Position," p. 29.

24 Dworkin, "The Original Position," p. 29.

25 Dworkin, "The Original Position," p. 29.

26 I argue against the analogy to observation reports in another context in my "Reflective Equilibrium and Theory Acceptance in Ethics," pp. 270–1.

27 This is the main contention of my "Reflective Equilibrium and Theory Acceptance in Ethics."

28 I am deeply indebted to my colleague George Smith for discussion of material in Sections II and III; my understanding of the competence-performance distinction and the problems posed by alternative logics and Dummett's arguments would have been far less were it not for his help. I would also like to thank Ned Block, Art Caplan, Noam Chomsky, Josh Cohen, William Lycan, Hilary Putnam, and M. B. E. Smith for many helpful suggestions and comments on earlier drafts. This work has been supported by a National Endowment for the Humanities Fellowship.

Chapter 5

Two approaches to theory acceptance in ethics[1]

1. "INTUITIONISM" VS. "MORAL EMPIRICISM"[2]

Just what role should be assigned to moral judgments or moral intuitions in the process of selecting among or justifying moral theories is a matter of ancient controversy. Egoists and utilitarians, for example, have always had to do battle with those who urge a tribunal in which a moral theory must match commonly held moral judgments. Proponents of such tribunals have been hard pressed, in turn, to provide credentials for these judgments. This old debate has taken on a modern form in the contrast between two recent proposals for solving the problem of theory acceptance or justification in ethics, the method of wide reflective equilibrium, which derives from Rawls, and the moral empiricism advocated by Brandt. My intention is to contrast these methods to see what lessons we may draw about the role of moral judgments in theory acceptance.

It is fair to construe these two recent proposals as major alternatives. Indeed, Brandt elaborates his own view in response to the "intuitionism" he thinks undermines the method of wide reflective equilibrium and, specifically, Rawls' use of the method in constructing his contractarian approach to the problem of choosing among competing moral conceptions. I shall concentrate on Brandt's methodological proposals, both because of their intrinsic interest and because I have discussed the strengths and weaknesses of wide reflective equilibrium in detail elsewhere (1979a, 1979b, 1980a, 1980b). I will, however, offer a brief sketch of the method of wide reflective equilibrium so that some points of contrast with Brandt's approach will be clear.

I shall argue that Brandt's strategy is an attempt to comply with two main methodological constraints, which he views as conditions of adequacy on any account of justification in ethics. Both of these constraints, an *empiricist constraint* and a *disalienation constraint*, are advanced by Brandt to correct what he takes to be fatal flaws in Rawlsian "intuitionism." The fact that Brandt's own proposal runs afoul of his own constraints points to some serious questions both about the plausibility of the constraints themselves and the adequacy of Brandt's proposal, viewed as an alternative to wide reflective equilibrium.

2. WIDE REFLECTIVE EQUILIBRIUM[3]

A wide reflective equilibrium is a coherent triple of sets of beliefs held by a particular person; namely (a) a set of considered moral judgments; (b) a set of moral principles; and (c) a set of relevant background theories, which may include both moral and nonmoral theories. We collect the person's initial moral judgments, which may be particular or general, and filter them to include only those of which he is relatively confident and which have been made under conditions generally conducive to avoiding errors of judgment. We propose alternative sets of moral principles which have varying degrees of "fit" with the moral judgments. Rather than settling immediately for the "best fit" of principles with judgments, which would give us only a narrow equilibrium, we advance philosophical arguments that reveal the strengths and weaknesses of the competing sets of principles (that is, competing moral conceptions). I construe these arguments as inferences from relevant background theories (I use the term loosely). Assume that some particular set of arguments wins and the moral agent is thus persuaded that one set of principles is more acceptable than the others (and perhaps than the conception that might have emerged in narrow equilibrium). The agent may work back and forth, revising his initial considered judgments, moral principles, and background theories, to arrive at an equilibrium point that consists of the triple – (a), (b), and (c).

There must be more structure here. The theories in (c) must show that the principles in (b) are more acceptable than alternatives on grounds to some degree independent of (b)'s match with relevant considered moral judgments in (a). Without such independent support, the principles have no support which they would not already have had in a corresponding narrow equilibrium where no special appeal to (c) is made. I can raise this point another way: How can we be sure that the moral principles that systematize considered moral judgments are not just "accidental generalizations" of the "moral facts," analogous to accidental generalizations we want to avoid confusing with real scientific laws? In the scientific case, we have evidence that we are not stuck with accidental generalizations if we can derive the purported laws from a body of interconnected theories, provided these theories reach beyond the "facts" the laws generalize in a diverse and interesting way.

The analogy suggests one way to ensure independent support for the principles in (b) and to rule out their being mere accidental generalizations of the considered judgments in (a). We should require that the theories in (c) not just be reformulations of the set of considered moral judgments (a) to which we seek to "fit" the principles in (b). The background theories should have a scope reaching beyond the range of the judgments in (a). Suppose some set of considered moral judgments, (a'), plays a role in constraining the background theories in (c). Then we are asking that some interesting, nontrivial portion of (a') should be disjoint from the set (a) that constrains the principles in (b). The *independence constraint* is the requirement that (a') and (a) be to some significant degree disjoint.[4]

It is important to note that the acceptability of the theories in (c) may thus in part depend on some moral judgments. We are not in general assuming that (c) constitutes a reduction of the moral in (b) and (a) to the nonmoral. Thus the independence constraint may be satisfied if the background theories in (c) incorporate different moral notions (say, fairness and certain claims about the nature of persons) from those (say, rights and entitlements) employed by the principles in (b) and judgments in (a).[5]

Wide reflective equilibrium as I have described it is not a standard form of moral intuitionism because it is not foundationalist. Despite the care taken to filter initial judgments to avoid obvious sources of error, no special epistemological priority is granted to considered moral judgments. We are missing the little story that intuitionist theories usually provide, explaining why we should pay homage to those judgments and indirectly to the principles that systematize them. Without such a story, we have no foundationalism and so no standard form of moral intuitionism.

Nevertheless, it might be thought that reflective equilibrium involves an attempt to give us the effect of intuitionism without any fairy tales about epistemic priority. The effect is that a set of principles gets "tested" against a determinate and relatively fixed set of moral judgments. We have, as it were, foundationalism without foundations. Once the foundational claim about moral judgments is removed, however, we have nothing more than a person's moral opinion, however considered. Since such opinions are often the result of self-interest, self-deception, historical and cultural accident, hidden class bias, and so on, just systematizing some of them hardly seems a promising way to provide justification for them or for the principles that order them.

This objection rests on two distinct complaints: (1) that reflective equilibrium merely systematizes some relatively determinate set of moral judgments; and (2) that the considered moral judgments are not a proper foundation for an ethical theory. The first complaint is unfounded. Wide reflective equilibrium does not merely systematize some determinate set of judgments. Rather, it permits extensive revision of these moral judgments. There is no set of judgments that is held more or less fixed as there would be on a foundationalist approach, even one without foundations.[6] In seeking wide reflective equilibrium, we are constantly making plausibility judgments about which of our considered judgments we should revise in light of theoretical considered judgments at all levels. Wide reflective equilibrium keeps us from taking considered moral judgments at face value, however much they may be treated as starting points in our theory construction.

The second complaint, that considered moral judgments are an inappropriate foundation for moral theory, brings us to the heart of Brandt's rejection of wide reflective equilibrium as a form of intuitionism. In seeking reflective equilibrium, Brandt argues, we begin with a set of moral judgments or intuitions to which we assign an *initial credence level* (say from 0 to 1 on a scale from things we believe very little to things we confidently believe). We filter out judgments with low initial credence levels to form our set of considered judgments. Then we propose principles and attempt to bring the system of principles plus judgments into equilibrium, allowing modifications wherever they are necessary to produce the system with the highest overall credence level.

But why, asks Brandt, should we be impressed with the results of such a process? We should not, he argues, unless we have some way to show that "some of the beliefs are initially *credible* – and not merely initially believed – for some reason other than their coherence" (1979, p. 20, emphasis added) in the set of beliefs we believe the most. For example, in the nonmoral case, Brandt suggests that an initially believed judgment is also an initially credible judgment when it states (or purports to state) a fact of observation. "In the case of normative beliefs, no reason has been offered why we should think that initial credence levels for a person correspond to *credibilities*" (p. 20).[7] The result is that we have no reason to think that increasing the credence level for the system as a whole moves us closer to moral truth rather than away from it. Coherent fictions are still fictions, and we may only be reshuffling our prejudices.

I believe some of the force of Brandt's argument derives from an inappropriate analogy between considered moral judgments and observation reports in science. But since I have responded to Brandt's argument in some detail elsewhere, and since David Copp has discussed my arguments in Copp and Zimmerman (1985), I shall not defend wide reflective equilibrium directly here. Rather, I shall turn to the alternative methodology Brandt proposes to see if it really does avoid problems facing reflective equilibrium.

3. BRANDT'S METHODOLOGICAL CONSTRAINTS

Brandt insists that moral intuitionism, even in its more sophisticated Rawlsian version, wide reflective equilibrium, is worse than hopeless: "We must avoid intuitionism even if this were to mean (as it does not) that we must end up as complete skeptics in the area of practice" (p. 3). The problem, as we have seen, is that we have no positive account of why we should grant initial credibility to these data, and we have excellent reason to be skeptical of moral intuitions, influenced as they often are by cultural tradition, social class, and other sources of bias. Consequently, Brandt argues, appeals to intuitions prevent our adopting an adequately objective critical perspective. "What we should aim to do is *step outside our own tradition* somehow, see it from the outside, and evaluate it, separating what is only the vestige of a possibly once useful moral tradition from what is justifiable at the present" (pp. 21–22, emphasis added).

Anti-intuitionism is not surprising coming from a utilitarian like Brandt. But if we must not appeal to moral judgments in answering the fundamental questions of moral theory – like "What is good?" and "What is right?" – then where are we to turn? Brandt answers that we must see "how far facts and logic alone carry us in criticism of a moral system: this is the question my conceptual framework has been designed to answer" (p. 244; cf. p. 10). To make facts and logic maximally relevant, these fundamental questions must be reformulated so that they are "sufficiently clear and precise for one to answer them by some mode of scientific or observational procedure" (p. 2). Such reformulation must not be based on mere appeals to linguistic intuitions, since ordinary usage is vague and conflates important distinctions.

Brandt argues that we must adopt a method of "reforming definitions." These do not mean the same as the expressions they replace, but they let us address more effectively the central issues raised by the original questions. Specifically, Brandt proposes that the term "rational" be taken to "refer to actions, desires, or moral systems which survive maximal criticism and corrections by facts and logic" (p. 10).[8] He then replaces "What is the best thing (for a given agent) to do?" with the reforming question, "What is the fully rational thing to do?" (pp. 14–16). Finally, he replaces "good" by "rationally desired" (pp. 126–129) and "morally wrong" by the following: "would be prohibited by any moral code which all fully rational persons would tend to support, in preference to all others or to none at all, for the society of the agent if they intended to spend a life-time in that society" (p. 194).

Two constraints emerge as central in Brandt's repudiation of intuitionism and his advocacy of reforming definitions. Brandt believes
that if justification in ethics is to be possible, it must rest on facts and
logic alone. Call this requirement the *empiricist constraint*. As we shall
see, we may need to distinguish weak and strong versions of the
empiricist constraint, governing explicit and implicit moral influences,
respectively, but for now it will suffice to refer to the exclusion of moral
judgments or intuitions from the process of justification as the empiricist constraint. Brandt insists on a second constraint as well. He wants
to close the gap between justifying a moral theory or code and motivating someone to accept its requirements. For him, no justification will be
significant if it is not also motivating. Consequently, a moral code must
appeal to the agent's actual desires or to his rational desires (in a sense
of "rational" to be explained). This is the *disalienation constraint* (pp.
186–187).

These two constraints are viewed by Brandt as conditions of adequacy on a successful theory of justification in ethics. They are clearly
violated by the method of wide reflective equilibrium as it is used in
Rawls' hands to construct his contractarian argument for justice as
fairness. The appeal to considered moral judgments, both in the design
of the Original Position and in the constraint on principles selected
there, violates the empiricist constraint. For example, it is a moral ideal
of persons as free and equal that underlies the design of the constraints
on choice in the Original Position. Moreover, since the selection of a
moral conception in the contract situation depends on the *hypothetical*
interests of agents in it, then there appears to be a straightforward
violation of the disalienation constraint. Indeed, Rawls' arguments
about the "reasonable" vs. the "rational," and his solution to the problem of moral motivation by positing a "sense of justice" as a fundamental moral power of persons, constitute an alternative to the
disalienation constraint only at the cost of directly violating the empiricist constraint.

That wide reflective equilibrium violates both constraints when used
by Rawls is a problem only if the constraints are themselves really
conditions of adequacy on methods of theory acceptance in ethics. I
think they are not, but I shall try to raise problems for these constraints
not by direct argument, but by examination of the way in which
Brandt's own method is forced to violate them. Specifically, I shall
argue that Brandt fails to justify his reforming definition of "the good,"
since he simply substitutes the new problem, "Why should I be rational?" for the traditional problem, "Why should I be moral?" This
means that he cannot guarantee that the disalienation constraint will be
satisfied when we pursue his method for choosing moral codes. Second, the rational desires that provide the bedrock facts motivating the

choice of moral codes do not in any way let us "step outside our own tradition" and achieve the "objective" stance Brandt promises. This violates at least some form of the empiricist constraint. The combined force of these criticisms is to suggest that a more enlightened approach to theory acceptance in ethics may result if we abandon these methodological constraints.

Before it is possible to take up these criticisms, we must discuss Brandt's treatment of rational choice. His method of theory selection in ethics depends critically on the details of his account of rational choice, and some of my criticisms will therefore turn on these details. Still, certain general features of the approach underlie other criticisms, which bodes ill for attempts to improve on Brandt's approach by modifications of its details.

4. RATIONAL DESIRE AND COGNITIVE PSYCHOTHERAPY

The boldest feature of Brandt's discussion of rational action and rational agents is his attempt (p. 110) to supplant the Humean view that reason cannot criticize desire. Brandt offers an account of rational desire, and indeed an operational definition of rational desire. He argues that "cognitive psychotherapy" is the appropriate operation to use in such a definition. This is the process of "confronting desires with relevant information by repeatedly representing it, in an ideally vivid way, and at an appropriate time. . . . The process relies simply upon reflection on available information, without influence by prestige of someone, use of evaluative language, extrinsic reward or punishment, or use of artificially induced feeling – states like relaxation" (p. 113). Accordingly, desires that result from or survive cognitive psychotherapy are rational; those that are extinguished are irrational.

What motivates Brandt to go beyond Hume's purely instrumental view of rationality is that he does not want what is good and what is right to be held hostage by what are intuitively bizarre or crazy desires. However, his reforming definitions of "good" and "right," which turn on what is best for a rational agent to choose, risk just such moral terrorism. If we search for a way to sort the acceptable desires from the unacceptable, we face serious problems. Had we an acceptable teleological theory of the ultimate function or ends of man, we might be able to derive constraints on the set of desires that can be counted as rational. But without this account, any other such "theory" is really a value-laden ideal,[9] an appeal to which would violate Brandt's restriction that we rely on facts and logic alone in the justification of moral beliefs.

Brandt's appeal to cognitive psychotherapy is an attempt to meet just this constraint: "It is," he suggests, *"value-free reflection"* (p. 113).

His underlying idea is that many of the desires we think irrational are not consonant with important facts about the world and ourselves. These desires are "mistaken" not because it is a mistake to think we can act on them, but because we have such desires via beliefs about the world and ourselves that are mistaken. Hume viewed a passion, such as hope or fear, grief or joy, as "unreasonable" when it is "founded on the supposition of the existence of objects which really do not exist."[10] Brandt extends this view to desires. He suggests that someone may have an aversion to a certain food because he mistakenly believes it will make him ill (p. 115); he may desire that blacks be denied prestigious jobs because he believes they are less intelligent. A related group of mistaken desires or aversions is based not on false beliefs, but on generalizations from untypical examples: aversion to eating all fish after not liking cod (p. 120) or aversion to all on welfare because some are "cheaters." Another category of example seems to depend on a different relation to "the facts": I may desire something (food, money, attention) "too strongly" because I am overcompensating for an earlier deprivation (p. 133). Brandt's "artificial" desires are even more complex: I may have an aversion to entering a nonprestigious occupation or interracial marriage (p. 117) because I have acquired my parents' negative attitudes, although I might otherwise find the occupation or marriage satisfying.[11]

Brandt's central idea, then, is that we are generally reliable desire-acquisition devices. We tend to acquire nonmistaken desires and to shed mistaken ones when we are suffused with adequate representations of relevant truths. We have, in short, an account of rational desire "naturalized." Brandt's proposal can be summarized as follows: (1) the "mistaken" desires are a significant portion of the desires we intuitively or pretheoretically view as irrational; moreover, it is the only category of intuitively irrational desires we can pick out by reference to facts and logic alone; (2) cognitive psychotherapy is a value-free procedure for eliminating most of these mistaken desires; (3) the operational definition that involves cognitive psychotherapy is a reasonable refinement of the intuitive notion of irrational desires. We may now ask, are the mistaken desires an adequate refinement of the intuitively irrational ones? And is cognitive psychotherapy adequate to the task Brandt sets it?

The category of mistaken desires seems too narrow. Some desires we intuitively consider irrational are not clearly based on false beliefs. Certain obsessive or fetishist desires may not rest on false beliefs or on false estimates of the happiness produced by satisfying them. The Humean example Brandt cites (p. 110) when he promises to go beyond Hume ("It is not contrary to reason to prefer the destruction of the whole world to the scratching of my finger") may also not be mistaken in Brandt's sense, although some would view it as irrational. (Of course, the irrationality here cannot turn on some notion of gross evil without violating Brandt's methodological constraints.)

The category of mistaken desires is too broad, including desires that are not intuitively irrational. In Brandt's view, a desire is mistaken if it is based on beliefs that it would be unjustified to hold in light of all relevant information available to society (pp. 12, 70, 113); it is then a legitimate target for cognitive psychotherapy. But I may lack some of that information and still be justified in holding certain false beliefs. Desires based on these beliefs will then be mistaken, but they are not (at least intuitively) irrational. Brandt is led to this counterintuitive result because he wants our choices of what is good and what is right to be as informed as possible, without requiring the impossible, that we be omniscient – thus the "all relevant information available" criterion.[12] But by defining the category of mistaken desires through reference to such a strong criterion, Brandt idealizes the concept of rationality in a way that invites trouble.

The situation is even worse for Brandt. We are likely to call a mistaken desire irrational only if someone clings to it despite becoming aware that there is information that falsifies its underlying beliefs. Astonishingly, it is just when such a mistaken desire resists cognitive psychotherapy that Brandt calls it rational! Because of the disalienation constraint, Brandt wants actual outcomes of the therapeutic process to determine what is rational, not outcomes that "ought to" take place. So, if I am so "hung up" on a mistaken desire that it survives cognitive psychotherapy, it counts as rational. Now, I may fail to extinguish a mistaken desire if I cannot draw all the relevant inferences from the information presented in therapy, or if I am in some other way very stupid. But then, the more dense I am, the more my mistaken desires will count as rational, given Brandt's operational definition.[13]

This point brings us to the question whether cognitive psychotherapy is the appropriate technique for ridding ourselves of mistaken desires. Brandt admits that it will fail to extinguish some mistaken desires, such as those acquired in early childhood. Incidentally, Brandt does not consider the opposite problem: I might extinguish desires that are not mistaken (such as the desire to make love or to complete this essay) if I vividly repeat to myself all relevant information at the appropriate time, say at the occurrence of the desire. The price of letting mistaken desires slip through is high, for we fail to dispel our worry that the good and the right will be hostage to irrational desires. Yet Brandt does not strengthen cognitive psychotherapy so that the purification process brings more powerful techniques to bear. We cannot resort to psychotherapy by an expert, or to drugs, or to behavior modification techniques involving reward or punishment (cf. p. 113). All we may do is vividly and repeatedly represent the relevant truths to ourselves.[14]

The unrestricted use of more powerful techniques, like behavior modification, is presumably barred on two counts. Not only might they smuggle in the therapist's prior values, but also, they are powerful enough to extinguish both mistaken and nonmistaken desires and so cannot be used to sort them from each other. Yet if some mistaken desires are unconscious, they will surely escape detection without expert help.[15] Brandt may fear that we will err in identifying a given belief as mistaken, but if we do not supplement cognitive psychotherapy with more powerful techniques, too many mistaken desires will slip through. An intermediary approach would use more powerful techniques on clearly mistaken desires. These points about the adequacy of cognitive psychotherapy are connected to deeper worries: The classical learning theory underlying Brandt's account may be only a fragment of an adequate learning theory.[16]

5. WHY SHOULD I BE RATIONAL?

If Brandt's reforming definition for "good" is to work, then he must show that there is recommendatory force to my knowing that some of my desires or actions are (or would be) rational and others irrational. Such a demonstration is both a condition of adequacy on the reforming definition (pp. 14–15, 151–152) and an important step toward satisfying the disalienation constraint. If knowing that a certain choice would be the rational one for me does not recommend it to me, then there is little hope that I can be disalienated from (what would be) my rational choice of a moral code.

Brandt's argument that there is recommendatory force rests on claiming that people have certain second-order aversions and desires. Specifically, he suggests that we are made uncomfortable by the awareness that we have irrational desires and aversions (p. 157). These desires, moreover, are inefficient sources of happiness: Satisfying them is likely to make us less happy than we would be made by satisfying rational desires (p. 157). Since "probably everyone with an adequate conceptual scheme (with the concept of long-range happiness) will take a positive interest in his net happiness over a lifetime" (p. 158), people will disfavor such inefficient desires and aversions. As Brandt points out, however, "if you are uninterested in happiness or avoiding dissonance, the 'argument' does not work" (p. 159).[17]

Brandt's argument proves too much. Suppose my initial desires include some irrational desires and aversions. Brandt wants to show that, if I know some of my desires are irrational, I have a reason or motivation to want to acquire the rational set by undergoing cognitive psychotherapy. But suppose someone shows me that there is another, superior set of desires, one which would be an even more efficient source of happiness than my rational set. This superior set might even contain some irrational desires. Now I have a reason or motivation to seek the superior set over the rational set – the very same motivation that leads me to prefer the rational set to my initial set. The rational set is at best only one among many sets of desires that commend themselves to me, once I let my hedonistic desire to maximize happiness carry the weight that it does in Brandt's argument.[18]

There may be a way around this problem for Brandt. After all, we often think there is a point to modifying our desires to make ourselves happier, but this modest fact does not compel us to strive to be, or to become, whatever person is constituted by a superior happiness-producing set of desires.[19] We hold some things more dear than that. Specifically, we tend to define ourselves through the systems of long-term desires that form our life plans. Accordingly, Brandt might suggest that abandoning initial desires in favor of rational desires does not threaten our sense of self or integrity, whereas abandoning original desires for the superior set might.

Unfortunately, even if this appeal to integrity is on the right track, it is unclear how far it carries us. I might now *resist* the suggestion that I undergo cognitive psychotherapy and give up my quirky and irrational desires because I view them as part of what makes me quirky old *me*. My integrity in this case prevents me from becoming rational, and Brandt's argument proves too little. A middle course for Brandt's argument must tell us just when and how the concern for integrity modifies the desire to maximize happiness. Since Brandt does not address this issue, I do not know which, if any, of my rationalized desires are recommended to me.

If the argument about recommendatory force fails, there is little hope of meeting the disalienation constraint. Knowing that a moral code would be the best one for me to choose were I rational (were I to undergo cognitive psychotherapy) is irrelevant if I have prevailing irrational desires that lead me to choose a different code. The fully rational me might just as well be another person for all the grip *his* motives have on me.

6. CAN A FULLY RATIONAL AGENT STEP OUTSIDE HIS TRADITION?

I have suggested that Brandt adopts an empiricist constraint on justification in ethics: No appeal to moral intuitions or judgments may play a role in the justification of moral principles or codes. Does Brandt's own procedure for selecting moral codes respect the spirit or just the letter of that constraint? To answer this question and the one raised in the next section about the role of consensus, we must be clear about the procedure for selecting among alternative moral codes.[20]

The rational agents in Brandt's choice problem are intended to contrast sharply with both the traditional "ideal observer" and Rawls' hypothetical contractors. Brandt's fully rational agents know less than omniscient observers, but they know far more than Rawlsian contractors, who operate behind a veil of ignorance. In the process of becoming fully rational agents by undergoing cognitive psychotherapy, they appeal to all relevant information available in the society. They have all relevant information about themselves – their skills, talents, abilities, social position, sex, and so on – and all available information about the society they will live in. No special assumptions are made about their degree of benevolence or selfishness. Their rational desires, whatever they are, all play a role, with the important exception: Explicitly moral desires and aversions are not to play a role in the choice. Including these would violate the empiricist constraint.[21] Each rational agent is then asked to consider which social moral code he would choose to govern the society he will live in. Finally, the area of convergence, if any, among codes chosen by all fully rational agents gives us the content of the notions of "the right" (p. 194).

Brandt suggests that his code-selection procedure offers an important advantage lacking in such alternatives as Rawls'. A central constraint on the outcome of Rawls' contract procedure is that principles have to match "our" considered moral judgments in reflective equilibrium. This constraint, Brandt argues, traps us in our own tradition (pp. 21–22, 186, 236). It takes the perspective of our own tradition as the ultimate one for critical purposes. Yet once we realize that there is diversity among moral codes, we are led to inquire "which of these codes is 'correct' – that is, criticized by facts and logic as far as possible. We do not like to think that our moral thinking is confined to making our intuitions coherent; we should like to step outside our tradition, look at it from the outside, and see where more basic kinds of criticism would lead. Now identifying the moral code that a fully rational person would support does just this" (p. 185; see also pp. 186–187).

Does Brandt's version of the choice problem allow us to step outside our tradition in the ways these passages suggest? Brandt believes that cognitive psychotherapy allows the fully rational agent to do so because value judgments have played no role in purifying his desires. Moreover, all of the actual results of cognitive psychotherapy play a role in the choice: There is no value-laden filter screening out some of them (in the manner of Rawls' veil of ignorance) and there are no special assumptions about the degree of benevolence moral agents ought to exhibit (p. 138). Rather, the desires that emerge after cognitive psychotherapy are among the "facts" that must be reconciled with the choice of a moral theory. Here Brandt's goal of disalienating people from morality reinforces his qualms about letting prior moral judgments influence the justificatory process. But has the purified, fully rational agent been lifted outside his own tradition merely by avoiding such value-laden filters? Pretty definitely not. The agent is still the product of his culture and the social institutions in it. Consequently, he is a product of its implicit and explicit social moral code, for this code presumably shapes the basic institutions that in turn shape the desires individuals acquire. Merely excluding the desires that are explicitly moral from the deliberation, as Brandt does (p. 203), does not remove the imprint of the social setting upon desires.

Consider an example. Suppose that the society from which one comes is highly benevolent and pays considerable attention to inculcating benevolent attitudes in children from an early age. It reinforces these attitudes with highly egalitarian distributions and tends to play down competitive individualism. Such societies may produce more persons approximating Brandt's perfectly benevolent agents than would societies like ours, which have highly inegalitarian distributions along class, race, and sex lines. Toleration for these unequal distributions and nonbenevolent attitudes is greatly enhanced by an ideology and accompanying emotional structure that glorifies competitive individualism. At the extreme, we find societies with highly entrenched – even stable – race or caste structures. The rational desires, in Brandt's account, of superior caste persons from such societies may well include desires to be treated better than members of the inferior race or caste. Such desires may be inculcated in the early phases of childhood and be reinforced throughout youth. Brandt might object that any ideology that justifies such practices is likely to rest on false beliefs about the inferiority of the low-caste group, and so the corresponding desires should be extinguished with cognitive psychotherapy. But such ideologies are highly resistant to extinction merely through exposure to "all the relevant facts." Witness the difficulty in eradicating the "blaming the victim" ideologies that help "justify" American racism (Ryan 1976).

This sketch suggests that the likelihood of producing persons who are highly benevolent, rather than benevolent only toward an "in" or preferred group, depends very much on prior moral judgments – specifically on those operating as the social moral code in the society that produced the rational agent. The desires that play a role in theory (code) selection thus bear the imprint of such prior moral judgments. Brandt operates under an illusion: He believes that, since moral desires do not explicitly play a role in the selection of the code, only "facts and logic" do. Brandt's apparent lack of concern for the social structuring of desires in a morally laden way is indeed surprising; my complaint is but a version of the traditional criticism that utilitarianism is biased toward the status quo. This complaint points to a deep tension between the empiricist and disalienation constraints.

There is also a deep irony here. Brandt argues that the imposition of Rawls' thick veil of ignorance is equivalent to making special assumptions about benevolence (p. 244) and thus violates the empiricist constraint. But a central justification that Rawls gives for the thick veil is that it corrects for the way in which existing basic social institutions shape the desires of moral agents. Its intended effect is to eliminate the hidden influences of prior moral values that are embedded in the social structures that shape the chooser. Brandt's fear of allowing moral judgments to play any role in the justificatory process, his empiricist constraint, may thus make his procedure more subject to the charge of failure to step outside of tradition than Rawls' is. That is, the known moral influence may be less dangerous than the unknown one.

Given Brandt's concern for stepping outside tradition, it is surprising to discover that we must rely on tradition to construct the pluralist ideal moral code (pp. 289–290). Brandt urges us to take existing legal and moral rules as our starting point. We then modify them according to their ability to maximize happiness. Strictly speaking, Brandt is not committing the same error as the one that he ascribes to Rawls. For the process of constructing – or discovering – the ideal code is not itself a justificatory process. Thus he is not relying on accepted moral judgments to justify other moral judgments. Even if Brandt restricts his empiricist constraint to "contexts of justification," not "contexts of discovery," two problems arise. First, the ultimate structure of the moral code will probably be affected by the fact that the existing code is taken as a starting point (p. 293 not withstanding). This parallels the objection to reflective equilibrium; that even if considered moral judgments are revisable, the equilibrium is going to be a function of the starting point. We need some account of why the starting point is a plausible one. Yet Brandt seems to believe that the existing moral and legal code is a good place to start. It reflects society's experience in regulating certain kinds of behavior and conflict. It is a heritage we dare not ignore. But this very respect for the existing social moral code is quite out of keeping with the near contempt Brandt expresses when he worries about the problem of choosing a general moral position. Why give credibility to the code for one task but not the other?

7. WHERE DOES BRANDT'S METHODOLOGY TAKE US?

Is there any moral code that all fully rational agents would prefer for the society in which they live? If there are such codes, "is morally wrong" should be replaced by "would be prohibited by any such code," which fixed its descriptive meaning. However, if there is no such code, then we need a relativized definition for "is morally wrong," one that fixes its descriptive meaning for each agent. To determine whether "wrong" has the force of "wrong according to everyone" or just "wrong according to me," we must know what moral codes rational agents will choose.

Brandt seems undecided among three possible outcomes of such choices, which yield strong, modest, and minimal conclusions, respectively. The *strong* conclusion is that "roughly, and in the long run, rational selfish persons will support a happiness-maximizing moral system, not intentionally, but inadvertently, since of course each rational selfish person will support his best – his expectable welfare-maximizing – option among the viable ones open to him" (p. 220). The strong conclusion immediately follows Brandt's argument that "the moral principles which will be most viable will be those which arouse least total resentment, counting both numbers and intensity; and hence equalitarian principles will tend to be more viable" (p. 219). Brandt implies that even selfish, fully rational persons would choose a comprehensive, relatively egalitarian moral code and not just the minimal self-protections of what Brandt calls the "Hobbesian core." If this conclusion could be sustained, "is morally wrong" would presumably have the content "is prohibited by the egalitarian code."

But Brandt backs away from the strong conclusion because selfish persons enjoying advantageous social positions might not accept a happiness-maximizing egalitarian code (p. 221). He retreats to the *modest* conclusion that a "central [Hobbesian] core – the protective system roughly supportive of the criminal law – can be justified to all selfish persons alike, and indeed to persons of any degree of benevolence; but various possible additions to this might not, any of them, be justifiable to all selfish persons" (p. 221). Indeed, if anything is "wrong according to everyone," it is only what falls in this core.

Brandt hints at the need to retreat still further. After his discussion of egoism, he remarks, "neither will a selfish person want an egoist moral system, unless he is in a special position of power, in which case he may not care about a moral system at all" (p. 270). This admission, nowhere else remarked on, suggests the *minimal* conclusion, that some fully rational moral agents, who are both selfish and especially well situated, may not even find that the Hobbesian core is in their long-run interests. Perhaps the lackluster selfish person will support the Hobbesian core, but the bold and powerful will not.

Brandt may feel justified in ignoring the minimal conclusion because of the rarity of such fortunate, selfish people. But it is important to see that, if we do not ignore it, and if we also insist that the replacement expressions refer to a code that all rational persons prefer, then we are left with vacuous definitions of "morally right" and "morally obligatory." Brandt's mention of the relativized reforming definition ("wrong according to my code") thus implies that we may not be moved beyond the minimal conclusion. Definitions aside, there is another problem: The function of a moral code – to serve as a public and final court of appeal in resolving a broad range of conflicting claims – is undermined if the core is very thin. Even the modest Hobbesian core may not provide enough of a basis of agreement to sustain real cooperative social effort. Brandt seems unworried about such lack of consensus (p. 242), but it may be more than the social fabric can bear.

Just what is the importance of agreement on a code? Suppose I have undergone cognitive psychotherapy and my irrational desires have been eliminated. Suppose further that I am benevolent and am concerned as much about the happiness of persons in other groups, say blacks, as I am about my own happiness. Unfortunately, the society in which I am to live has a long tradition of racial discrimination, on the model of the Jim Crow laws of the South. Unlike the case of the South, however, the black population is quite small. Nevertheless, the racist expectations and desires of the white population are deep and strong, and not everyone in the society is likely to shed them even with cognitive psychotherapy. So it is reasonable to anticipate the instability of any social moral code that does not cater to these desires and expectations.[22] Even allowing for some black noncompliance with a Jim Crow code, we would expect it to be far more stable. It is even possible that such a code would in fact maximize happiness, given the respective population sizes. Consequently, the Jim Crow code might be the best one for me to support, given my high level of benevolence.

Of course, this code may not be chosen by everyone. At the risk of appearing selfish, fully rational blacks might not choose it. But, *ex hypothesi*, this lack of support does not make the code unstable, so Brandt cannot insist on unanimity on these grounds. Nor can Brandt insist on unanimity in the way Rawls does, through the veto available to agents in his Original Position. Indeed, Brandt is quite disparaging about this unanimity requirement (pp. 242–243), which in any case needs a justification. For Rawls, the justification depends on moral assumptions about free and equal moral agents.[23] But Brandt's empiricist constraint bars any such justification, and he insists that the appropriateness of the reforming definition of "morally right" should depend on the actual outcomes of the justificatory choice procedure. So Brandt is left with the problem of assigning a status to the Jim Crow code given that it meets these conditions: (1) it is stable compared to alternatives; (2) it would be chosen by enough of the population (say 90 percent) to make it generally current; and (3) it is happiness maximizing. Should we now say that this code gives us the content of "it is morally right and wrong" because the overwhelming majority would choose it, were they rational? Or do we retreat to the relativistic "right according to the majority" but "wrong according to the minority?" Brandt insists that "we let the chips fall where they will" (p. 3) but either result seems unacceptable to me.

Indeed, Brandt's problem here (if it is a problem) brings to mind a criticism that David Lyons has made of Rawlsian contractarianism: We have no reason to think the outcome of such a rational choice procedure determines what is *moral* rather than merely what is *prudential* (Lyons 1975). Of course, the outcome of the Rawlsian choice procedure is also constrained by the requirement that the preferred principles match considered moral judgments in reflective equilibrium. This constraint gives some assurance that the outcome is moral. But Brandt rejects any such constraint: It would be completely counter to his empiricist constraint. So if it is prudent for the majority of fully rational agents to choose the Jim Crow code, there is no further requirement that the outcome match moral judgments. Thus Lyons' criticism has a far greater bite when directed against Brandt than against Rawls.

8. SOME LESSONS

The question was asked, in Section 6, whether Brandt's own procedure for selecting moral codes respects the spirit, and not just the letter, of the empiricist constraint. We may now clarify that question in light of the problems raised for Brandt's methodology in the last two sections. Brandt's method, it appears, at best conforms to a *weak* version of the empiricist constraint: No *explicit* appeal to moral intuitions or judgments may play a role in the process of justifying a moral code. But conformity with the weak empiricist constraint is compatible with the presence of at least two types of moral influence on the justificatory process.

First, it is possible that explicit moral beliefs or desires can act causally, but in undetected ways, to affect our other desires. Merely ruling out appeal to such explicit desires will not then eliminate their other effects on our desires and choices (see notes 15 and 21). Second, our desires, even after cognitive psychotherapy, are a product of the social structures in which we are raised. Consequently, moral codes that influence the design of those social structures will leave their imprint – overt or covert – on our rational desires. As a result, Brandt's method is likely not to conform to a *strong* version of the empiricist constraint: Prior moral judgments or intuitions may play neither an explicit nor implicit role, inferential or causal, in influencing the outcome of the justificatory process.

The failure of Brandt's method to conform to the strong empiricist constraint, even if it complies with the weak one, violates the spirit in which the empiricist constraint is advocated by him. The point behind Brandt's repudiation of intuitionism was (1) that appeals to such moral judgments trapped us in our tradition and lacked objectivity, and (2) that they lacked "credibility" as a basis for moral-theory construction or justification. In contrast, Brandt sought a method that relied on facts and logic alone. But now we see that the desires that survive cognitive psychotherapy are not free from important moral influences. They are not "just facts," but facts that reflect the influence of prior moral choices. These desires, too, trap us in our own traditions. And their "credibility" as bases for moral-theory construction or justification will be neither greater nor less than the credibility of the moral judgments that are embodied in the moral codes that have causally influenced their content and structure.

It might be argued that there is some advantage to conforming to the weak empiricist constraint even if the strong one is violated. At least one source of bias, one source of skeptical objection, is removed. But if we are in a rowboat, the unseen leaks will wet our feet as thoroughly as the visible ones, and at least we can patch the ones we see. Brandt seems to be in basically the same leaky boat as Rawls, although at least Rawls is clear that we must do some bailing.

Even if Brandt is in the same boat as Rawls, perhaps some modest modification of his strategy would permit us to find a way to purify desires of moral influences. This suggestion brings us to a point noted in Section 6 – that there is a tension between the empiricist and disalienation constraints. The disalienation constraint requires that, in the procedure for choosing moral codes, we employ only those desires we *actually* have, or at least those it is "recommendatory" for us to have. This constraint imposes severe limits on the degree to which we can "purify" our desires. But the stricter our compliance with the disalienation constraint, the more likely our violation of the strong empiricist constraint. Suppose, for example, we could correct, at least hypothetically, for the influence of prior moral codes on our desire sets by determining just which desires are morally influenced. We could make these corrections in "our" choice of an ideal moral code only if we resorted to hypothetical choices, which would violate the disalienation constraint, or if we could show that each correction can be "recommended" to us, which seems totally implausible. So any strategy for conforming to the strong empiricist constraint would probably have to abandon the disalienation constraint. This is no minor concession for Brandt.

There is another constraint on the ways in which Brandt might try to modify his basic strategy. If conformity to the strong empiricist constraint is to be achieved, it must be complete: *All* moral influences on the desires that play a role in justification must be eliminated. In contrast, if only some such influences are eliminated, and others are viewed as "acceptable," then it begins to look as if we are invoking moral distinctions in another guise. But to seek the elimination of all moral influences on desires may leave us with too small a desire set to permit any "rational" choice of a moral code.

If Brandt is forced to concede violation of the strong empiricist constraint, then the issue between his method and the method of wide reflective equilibrium – for example, in Rawls' use of it – becomes one of degree and not principle. It becomes the issue of how best to correct for the possibility that prior moral judgments that influence moral theory acceptance may be biased or otherwise epistemologically worrisome. What is then needed is a comparison of the resources for criticism and the pressures for revision that are present in both methods. We will have to abandon the illusion that there is a knockdown epistemological objection to one method to which the alternative is immune. Of course, there is another alternative open to Brandt, which is hinted at in his remark quoted earlier: "We must avoid intuitionism even if this were to mean (*as it does not*) that we must end up as complete skeptics in the area of practice" (p. 13, emphasis added).

NOTES

1 This essay, especially sections 4–7, is to a significant extent based on my "Can Cognitive Psychotherapy Reconcile Reason and Desire?" in *Ethics* 93 (1983): 772–85. I wish to thank Hugo Bedau, Charles Beitz, Judith Wagner DeCew, and Susan Wolf for provocative discussion of Brandt's work during the fall of 1979, Richard Brandt for helpful comments on an early draft, and David Copp and David Zimmerman for suggestions about this version. All references to Richard Brandt's *A Theory of the Good and the Right* (1979) will be indicated parenthetically in the text.

2 The term moral empiricism is taken from Nicholas Sturgeon's (1982) review essay.

3 This section is based on material from Daniels (1979b), pp. 265–8, and (1980a), pp. 85–8.

4 My formulation is not adequate as it stands, since there will even be trivial truth-functional counterexamples to it unless some specification of "interesting" and "nontrivial" is given. I also say nothing about how to measure the scope of a theory. The problem is a standing one in the philosophy of science. I am indebted to George Smith for helpful discussion of this point.

5 Rawls' contract argument is a feature of a particular wide reflective equilibrium. The contract apparatus is not self-evidently acceptable. It contains complex "formal" (publicity), motivational, and knowledge constraints on contractors and principles. Philosophical argument must persuade us that

it is a reasonable device for selecting between competing conceptions of justice. These arguments are inferences from a number of background theories – of the person, of procedural justice, of the role of morality in society. Principles chosen must be in a (partial) reflective equilibrium with a relevant set of considered judgments and must yield a feasible, stable, well-ordered society. General social theory tells us what is feasible.

6 I believe that if this point is taken seriously, it undercuts the force of David Copp's claim that wide reflective equilibrium is a "conservative" theory. He argues that if *j* is a considered moral judgment of which a person remains confident, and *j* does not fit with the rest of the otherwise coherent package of beliefs and theories held by the person, then *j* remains justified for the person. I am inclined to say that such a person has not achieved wide reflective equilibrium and *j* is not necessarily justified for the person. See David Copp's essay [in Copp and Zimmerman 1985].

7 Brandt's discussion draws on early characterizations of justification by Nelson Goodman (1952) and Israel Scheffler (1954). In Scheffler's discussion, the method is described using the notion of "initial credibility," which is not explicated for us. Later in the article we are told that initial credibility is only an indication of our "initial commitment to . . . acceptance" (p. 187). Perhaps Brandt's argument should be construed as the objection to assuming, as Scheffler is willing to do, that initial credibility and initial commitment to acceptance (Brandt's "credence level") correspond in the moral case in the way they do in the nonmoral case.

8 More specifically, there are three senses of "rational": (1) an action is rational to the first approximation if and only if, taking desires and aversions as a given, it reflects optimal use of "all relevant available information" concerning means and ends and weighted probabilities of satisfaction; (2) a desire or aversion is rational if and only if "it is what it would have been had the person undergone *cognitive psychotherapy*"; and (3) an action is fully rational if and only if it is based on rational desires and is rational to the first approximation (p. 11). A fully rational agent is one in a position to carry out fully rational actions.

9 Rawls' "model conception" of persons as free and equal moral agents has such a status. Persons are "free" to form and revise conceptions of the good and "equal" in their possession of a sense of justice. Such complexity in the theory or ideal of the person – human nature, if you will – is not only absent in Brandt's account, but it is ruled out by Brandt's methodological constraints. John Rawls (1980); cf. also Daniels (1979a).

10 See Hume (1739), bk. II, sec. 3, and Brandt (1979), pp. 110–11. Brandt, incidentally, credits Rashdall with giving an approximation to cognitive psychotherapy (p. 209). In the passage Brandt cites, however, Rashdall suggests that we can ferret out the truly moral content from our intuitions. These cleansed intuitions then form the foundation of our moral system, contra Brandt. See Hastings Rashdall (1924), vol. I, p. 212.

11 Brandt defines a desire as artificial if it "could not have been brought about by experience with actual situations which the desires are for and the aversions against" (p. 117). The counterfactual is problematic. If it permits major changes in a person's system of desires, then some changes will

make the same test desire natural, whereas others will make it artificial. If it involves only minimal alteration of his desires, changing only the test desire, then artificiality depends on quite incidental facts about him. Some aversions that then intuitively seem artificial will turn out to be natural.

12 Brandt wants "relevance" to be both a *causal* notion (p. 12) and a *content* notion (p. 112). Unfortunately, some information that ought to count as relevant by the content criterion may not count as such because it fails to have the proper causal effect. So although we (in contrast to Brandt) might want to call a desire irrational because it resists extinction when exposed to relevant information, Brandt is free to conclude that the information is not relevant.

13 Brandt's problem here is part of a more general problem with idealized views of rationality. Cf. Cherniak (1986).

14 Paul Meehl has pointed out to me that Brandt's version of cognitive psychotherapy should not be confused with the more aggressive therapist-guided techniques usually known by the same name.

15 Although the problem of unconscious desires is a problem for Brandt's approach, he does not mention it. Instead, he makes an entirely inappropriate criticism of Rawls' veil of ignorance, which, he says, cannot block the operation of unconscious desires (p. 240). Rawls' construction is here an analytic or formal construction, not an empirical process to be foiled in the way Brandt suggests.

16 For example, Brandt makes little effort to connect his account of learning theory to recent work in cognitive psychology, especially the developmental literature.

17 The higher-order desire to maximize happiness is a requirement of the motivational and learning theory Brandt sketches (p. 154). The strong claim on page 154 takes desire as given and does not avoid the argument above.

18 Indeed, if some behavior-modification method much more powerful than cognitive psychotherapy would lead me to the superior set and increased enjoyment, I would be foolish not to try it. For Brandt's considered remarks on hedonism, see pp. 132–8.

19 As part of a general argument that "satisfaction" is an inappropriate criterion for well-being in important moral contexts, Rawls suggests that the deep social-utility functions needed for maximizing satisfaction interpersonally commit us to the view that persons are just containers. See Rawls (1982), especially pp. 173–9.

20 Brandt devotes Chapter IX to "psychologizing" the notion of a moral code, so that a code is not a set of principles, but a set of underlying desires and aversions. Yet the entire argument about choosing moral codes is conducted as if we are talking about principles. I adhere to this "intellectualist" approach throughout, despite its "disastrous problems" (p. 171).

21 Excluding them, however, exposes Brandt to a criticism he raises (implausibly) against Rawls; namely, whether we can simply ignore desires it is posited that we have (p. 240). If so, we may be violating the disalienation constraint (see note 15).

22 Brandt's use of the term "intrinsic" desire or aversion does not exclude us from having a nonmistaken and possibly nonartificial desire to have blacks treated in discriminatory ways. Nor does he turn to a restriction to "self-regarding" desires like Dworkin's. See Ronald Dworkin (1977).

23 See Rawls (1980) for explicit claims about the centrality of the ideal or "model conception" of the person to the design of the Original Position. See also Daniels (1980a).

REFERENCES

Brandt, R. 1979. *A Theory of the Good and the Right*. Oxford: Oxford University Press.

Cherniak, C. 1986. *Minimal Rationality*. Cambridge, MA: MIT Press.

Copp, D., and Zimmerman, D., eds. 1985. *Morality, Reason and Truth*. Totowa, NJ: Rowman & Littlefield.

Daniels, N. 1979a. "Moral Theory and the Plasticity of Persons," *The Monist* 62:265–87.

Daniels, N. 1979b. "Wide Reflective Equilibrium and Theory Acceptance in Ethics," *The Journal of Philosophy* 76:256–82.

Daniels, N. 1980a. "Reflective Equilibrium and Archimedean Points," *Canadian Journal of Philosophy* 10:1:83–103.

Daniels, N. 1980b. "Some Methods of Ethics and Linguistics," *Philosophical Studies* 37:21–36.

Dworkin, R. 1977. *Taking Rights Seriously*. Cambridge, MA: Harvard University Press.

Hume, D. 1739 (1969). *Treatise of Human Nature*. Edited by L. A. Selby-Bigge. Oxford: The Clarendon Press of Oxford University Press.

Goodman, N. 1952. "Sense and Certainty," *The Philosophical Review* 61:160–7.

Lyons, D. 1975. "Nature and Soundness of the Contract and Coherence Arguments." In Norman Daniels, ed., *Reading Rawls*, pp. 141–67. New York: Basic Books.

Rashdall, H. 1924. *The Theory of Good and Evil*. 2nd ed. Oxford: Oxford University Press.

Rawls, J. 1980. "Kantian Constructivism in Moral Theory," *Journal of Philosophy* 77:515–72.

Rawls, J. 1982. "Social Unity and the Primary Goods." In A. K. Sen and B. Williams, eds., *Utilitarianism and Beyond*, pp. 159–85. Cambridge: Cambridge University Press.

Ryan, W. 1976. *Blaming the Victim*. 2nd ed. New York: Vintage.

Scheffler, I. 1954. "Justification and Commitment," *The Journal of Philosophy* 51:180–90.

Sturgeon, N. 1982. "Brandt's Moral Empiricism," *The Philosophical Review* 91:389–422.

Chapter 6

An argument about the relativity of justice

1. IS JUSTICE "LOCAL"?

Recently, many American universities, some local governments, and some major corporations have taken a stand against Apartheid in South Africa by divesting themselves of investments in corporations with major holdings there. There is even a strong movement in Congress supporting economic sanctions against South Africa. Similar – or stronger – stands have been taken around the world. Millions of individuals believe that divestment is a proper action to take in opposition to a system of government which denies fundamental liberties and opportunities to the majority of its population on the basis of race.

Other campuses have taken a stand against complete divestment. Their trustees have decided to pursue selective divestment, abiding by the Sullivan Principles. The intention here is to produce selective pressure to reform Apartheid through corporations which have the economic clout to implement some reforms. Many individuals believe it is better to try to work from within and thus prefer this "hands on" tactic for promoting reform.

Notice that both sides of this *tactical* dispute share some moral assumptions about Apartheid, namely that it is an unjust set of practices and institutions which it is everybody's business, South African or not, to try to change. Of course, some people believe that practices in South Africa are not the proper object of concern for anyone but South Africans. More specifically, some people may believe that practices in South Africa should be judged just or unjust only by reference to principles of justice South Africans affirm.

The view that judgments about justice are "local" judgments, which have truth value – or application – only *within* a society, is a view which runs counter to the moral *practice* of many of us. This does not mean we are justified in our practice. Perhaps we are just moral busybodies. For example, the former Chairman of the Board of Tufts Trustees, Allan Callow, suggested that Tufts students interested in fighting racism should "go to Roxbury," a predominantly black section of Boston, rather than insist on Tufts divestment. But even Callow was not really saying that Tufts students are being moral busybodies, because his remarks imply that injustice exists in both places and that Tufts students can be more effective in Roxbury than by trying to get Tufts to abandon the Sullivan Principles in favor of complete divestment. Still, the metaethical principle that all principles of justice are local principles has normative implications about our – or most of our – practice of being moral busybodies. The principle says the practice is unjustified if it simply rests on our appeal to our own local principles.

Actually, it is not the metaethical principle that justice is local which rules out our practice of taking action against perceived injustice elsewhere. Rather, the metaethical principle is readily coupled with a normative principle prohibiting "intolerance" of the "unjust" practices of another society. The metaethical principle seems to lend support to the normative principle. Both seem to imply that we had better be able to defend our inclination to be moral busybodies. (Actually, the principles are independent: either could be defended while the other is denied.)

One way to defend the inclination to be busybodies is to criticize the metaethical view that justice is always local justice, which is what I propose to do here. Specifically, I will consider one recent argument that justice is relative, namely Michael Walzer's argument in *Spheres of Justice*. Of course, showing that Walzer's claim about local justice is not defensible because it is too strong does not show that other versions of relativism are too; but the "communitarian" view that Walzer defends has become one of the more popular bases for defending a strong form of relativism, and so it is an important position to discuss. Similarly, showing that Walzer's relativism is unfounded does not justify all kinds of moral busybodiness, but that is not my intention either. In what follows I shall have to reconstruct Walzer's position, characterize the form of relativism involved, uncover the argument that underlies it, and criticize the argument.

2. PROBLEMS WITH THE LOCALITY THESIS

The anthropological feast Walzer lays before his reader – as expansive as an Indonesian "rijsttafel" or a Scarsdale Bar Mitvah – is far more inviting and entertaining than the austere rations of social choice theory or the minimal diet of the Kantian rational agent. Indeed, the meal is a rich rebellion against that thin fare. How tasty this tidbit about Athenian metics, and that about German Gastarbeiter! How authethic that saucy snippet about Aztec education, which complements so well the tangy tales about Hillel on the roof of the schul and George Orwell's prep school! The repast Walzer sets out for us is no mere smorgasbord, however. Like a Seder, the ritual Passover feast, it has an agenda and is intended to teach us a moral lesson. Walzer's exotic presentations are intended to make palatable his normative theory of "complex equality" and his metaethical claims about the relativity of justice.

My main concerns will be about the indigestibility of the latter and about Walzer's suspicion about "abstract philosophy" and his view that philosophical inquiry is discontinuous with, and stands apart from, our real moral life – though here Walzer is more concerned to document this view by appeal to moral anthropology than he is to appeal to moral psychology. I will argue that it is Walzer's own "communitarian" stance that is untrue to our real moral life, and that philosophical critique and the search for justification in ethics is continuous with important features of our life as real moral agents. But I shall want to lead up to these concerns by commenting briefly on Walzer's normative theory, for the limitations of that theory will show us why it is so important to consider Walzer's methodological stance.

Walzer's theory of pluralist or complex equality has two central normative claims: (a) The Spheres Thesis is the moral claim that social goods – welfare, office, education, recognition, and others – divide into "spheres" governed by distinct distributive principles; these principles determine allowable inequalities in each sphere. (b) The Non-Domination Thesis is the moral claim that inequalities in one sphere ought not to dominate other spheres, at least in societies which differentiate these spheres. When spheres are kept appropriately distinct, Walzer contends, no "simple egalitarian" formula will capture the kind of complete equality justice requires (pp. 14ff).

By adding further empirical and methodological claims, Walzer's theory takes on a more striking form, as we shall see, but let me begin with this normative core. What exactly is the contrast with "simple egalitarian" theories? Consider Rawls' theory, which Walzer often contrasts with his own.[1] Is it a simple egalitarian theory? Not obviously. Basic rights and liberties are governed by one principle; the distribution of offices and jobs by another; economic welfare by yet another. So Rawls has distinct principles for distinct "spheres" (of course, Rawls' principles govern only basic institutions), though not the same list of spheres or principles advocated by Walzer. Where Walzer distinguishes them, Rawls argues that certain "spheres" – such as offices, jobs, education, and possibly health care – ought to be linked because the same distributive principle governing the primary social good opportunity should encompass them all. Finally, Rawls takes considerable effort to argue that inequalities permitted in one sphere can and should be blocked from dominating other spheres through appropriate design of the basic institutions. Walzer and Rawls may thus disagree about how many distinct principles are needed to distribute social goods in different spheres, and they may disagree about how to keep the spheres distinct (Rawls says more on this subject than Walzer actually does), but their theories do not stand in the relationship of complex to simple theories of equality (at least if we focus on the normative core of Walzer's theory).

Consider the disagreement about which spheres are distinct. Walzer urges that (in our society) medical care should be distributed according to need, but certain jobs or offices according to merit or desert. Are these distinct spheres? I have argued elsewhere for this linkage: meeting health care needs is more important than meeting other preferences because of the impact of disease and disability on equality of opportunity. So too emphasizing individual traits that bear on the performance of jobs or offices, not on irrelevant features of individuals, is what we must do to protect equality of opportunity. A principle guaranteeing fair equality of opportunity ought to govern institutions delivering both kinds of goods.[2]

Walzer says very little against this type of argument. Indeed, we are not told what makes for distinct spheres: a difference in social goods? in principles governing them? both? Nor are we told *in general* what spheres must be kept distinct if complex equality is to be achieved. These are questions which one would expect answered in a philosophical theory about justice. To see why Walzer does not address them, we must look beyond the normative core of his theory to his method. In fact, we shall see that Walzer thinks no general questions as these should even be asked – they are not legitimate subject for philosophical inquiry (pp. 318–9).

To the Spheres and Non-Domination Theses [(a) and (b) above], we must now add an assortment of claims which flesh out Walzer's methodological stance: (c) The Cultural Relativity Thesis is the empirical claim that different cultures give different social meanings to the goods in these spheres. (d) The Moral Anthropology Thesis is the methodological claim that we can discover these meanings only by doing something like moral anthropology, not traditional ethical theory. (e) The Incommensurability Thesis is the methodological claim that there is no acceptable method for ranking the goodness of cultural products, that is, goods with their social meanings are interculturally incommensurable. Finally, (f) the Justification Thesis is the metaethical claim that we cannot justify assigning a distributive principle to a sphere if it does

An argument about the relativity of justice

not fit the social meanings people ascribe to the goods in that sphere, and thus is not acceptable to them. Together, these claims lead Walzer to assert that justice is relative to social meanings: "A given society is just if its substantive life is lived in a certain way – that is, in a way faithful to the shared understandings of the members" (p. 313). That is, we cannot use the theory of complex equality as a normative theory except from *within* the system of social meanings created by a particular culture. (It is striking, incidentally, that Walzer offers his theory while mentioning none of his apparent philosophical predecessors – Westermarck, Winch, Pitkin, and others.)

It is now clear why Walzer does not provide the missing arguments about the nature of the spheres that are needed to flesh out the normative theory of complex equality. The "theory" is at best a *scheme* – and then not a uniform one – for theories of complex equality. ["Every substantive account of distributive justice is a local account" (p. 314).] It does not tell us what the spheres must in general be and what principles must govern them, but only that, if a society attributes certain social meanings to goods, marking off spheres in which distributive principles are to apply, then its spheres must be kept distinct. "We never know exactly where to put the fences [between spheres]; they have no natural location. The good they distinguish are artifacts; as they were made, so they can be remade" (p. 319). The content of this schema can only be provided by finding the principles already embedded in a particular culture, and so *moral theory becomes moral anthropology*.

Despite these passages in which Walzer clearly affirms a commitment to the Cultural Relativity and Moral Anthropology Theses [(c) and (d)], and despite passages which demonstrate differences in the social meaning attributed to certain goods, such as leisure [holidays in some cultures affirm community, vacations in ours affirm our individuality (pp. 190ff)], a serious ambiguity arises. There are many contrasting passages in which a social good is talked about as if it *ought* to be in a distinct sphere whose *internal logic* makes only a particular distributive principle appropriate to it. The claims in these passages do not appear to relativize the "ought" either to the society in question or to ours. For example, Walzer argues that expertise has its limits in political decision making (pp. 285ff), and that "Once we have located ownership, expertise, religious knowledge, and so on in the proper places and established their autonomy, there is no alternative to democracy in the political sphere" (p. 303). Similarly, he says, "'One citizen/one vote' is the functional equivalent, in the sphere of politics, of the rule against exclusion and degradation in the sphere of welfare, of the principle of equal consideration in the sphere of office, and of the guarantee of a school place for every child in the sphere of education" (pp. 305–6). Another example: we are told health-care providers, from ancient Greece to medieval Jewish doctors to our own superspecialists, have had a collective bad conscience about distributing health care on any other basis except need (pp. 86–87).

Perhaps there is an intended relativization here. Walzer may intend us to qualify all these claims by the phrase "from the perspective of our own moral beliefs," as the Cultural Relativity and Moral Anthropology Theses seem to require. But are these conclusions Walzer articulates about merit and office, need and health care really only made *relative* to the shared meanings in our society? It would be difficult to follow his argument in the passages cited if that qualification were made. Yet elsewhere Walzer does insist that his argument that health care should be distributed according to need only holds for our society and turns on the social meaning we attribute to health care. He remarks that a comparably wealthy society might devote its resources to curing souls, not bodies, and philosophy could not show the injustice of that decision.[3]

This ambiguity about the scope of distributive principles aside, there are more serious difficulties facing Walzer's anthropological stance. Ronald Dworkin has already noted one of these: it is difficult to find a unified "social meaning" for important social goods in many cultures.[4] Disputes abound and it may take appeals to "abstract justice" to resolve them. Thus the commitment of public funds to meet some level of medical needs in our society has always been a matter of dispute and that dispute may not merely be about how to interpret the commitments already embedded in shared social meanings. It also remains unclear why the shared meaning – if one does emerge – rules out a principle providing health care for only certain kinds of needs and not others (which is in fact our practice). Why should the spending of public funds to meet *some* health-care needs force the conclusion Walzer draws that we are committed to meeting all health-care needs through public funds? Cannot shared meanings come in all possible variations? Walzer's *method* seems to pull him one way, his own *normative* views another.

Even if active internal disputes do not prevent discovering unified social meanings, there is the serious problem of "authenticity." A culture may reflect a history of class struggle and domination by a ruling class, or domination by external cultures. Nevertheless, the shared social meanings may be ones to which dominant groups acquiesce – over time it may seem like true consent, but it may only be "false consciousness." If the effects and artifacts of such history are now reified into a shared social meaning, we seem to discover *right* where there is only a history of *might*. Walzer's reply is that all cultural products are really "joint" ones (p. 9, note), and that there is no real inauthenticity. But this reply leaves the integrity of social meanings resting on highly controversial empirical claims which Walzer never substantiates.

The problem inauthenticity raises for Walzer is that it challenges his own view that we are all equal in the sense that we are all "culture-producing creatures" (p. 314). This moral principle about transcultural equality (we might call it the Meadean Measure) is a normative reflection of the Incommensurability Thesis (e). If some cultures are in fact inauthentic, then they do not deserve the respect the Meadean Measure requires. We also face the obvious problem: Is the Meadean Measure itself only relative to social meanings? If so, some may be justified in denying it. If not, where did this transcultural moral principle come from?

One possible solution to the inauthenticity problem would be to propose that only shared meanings which result from a democratic process must be treated with the respect demanded by the Meadean Measure.[5] In effect, we give content to the notion of authenticity by appealing to the notion of a morally acceptable democratic procedure for selecting – or consenting to – the cultural product. In this case, consent is to the shared meanings and the distributive principles appropriate to the goods defined by those meanings. Principles that are democratically chosen may be culturally relative, for not all democratic choices will be of the same principle. This strategy carries a high price tag: it makes the appeal to democratic theory itself nonrelative. We would need an account of why this democratic theory, which I would have taken to be part of a general theory of justice, is immune to the relativity that infects the rest of distributive justice. Walzer, as I have suggested, does not pursue any such account, which would seem quite alien to his overall project. I turn instead to a slightly different issue.

The problem of authenticity points to an even deeper issue, which Joshua Cohen has recently discussed.[6] Consider how Walzer, in his role as moral anthropologist, tries to discover the shared meanings of a given society. His working assumption is that we can abstract those meanings by examining the institutions and institutionalized practices which characterize the society. But this assumption ignores the fact that people in a given society comply with those institutions for very different reasons. Some may go along with the practices out of indifference, some despite opposition, and some to promote their own interests. Therefore "commitment" to the values embedded in these institutions may not be a central motivational feature for individuals who are surrounded by them, and there is no plausible inference from the "shared meanings" we abstract from the institutions to the commitment individuals have to them. It thus is not very clear in what sense the meanings are really shared. Of course, this would pose obvious problems for any theory of consent.

Cohen's point has an even deeper implication which I do want to pursue. If we individuals differ in our commitments to the meanings or values which appear to be embodied in our institutions, then we must be equipped with the capacity to detach ourselves in various ways from both our own actual commitments and the alleged shared meanings in our everyday reasoning about what we ought to do. These shared meanings are really only a fragment of each individual's system of beliefs and desires. We are equipped, in fact, with the capacity to search for reasons on the basis of which we assess and criticize and adopt or reject aspects or implications of these "shared" meanings. But if our everyday moral life reflects these capacities for detachment and for "impartial" critical inquiry – that is, if we are practiced in "stepping outside" at least some elements of our tradition – then Walzer's methodological and metaethical theses, and his relativist conclusions, may rest on assumptions which are not true to our actual moral experience. It is to this set of issues I now want to turn.

3. LOCALITY AND STRONG INTERNALISM

We need to understand better the roots of Walzer's relativism. Consider first the Incommensurability Thesis (e) (remember, these are my terms), which says that there is no acceptable method for ranking the goodness of cultural products. The Thesis appears to be a social version of Rawls' claims about the incommensurability of individual conceptions of the good. On Rawls' view, we can have no *social* ranking of conceptions of the good that does not do violence to the very ideal of a person we all share and which would not lead to unacceptable results. For example, such a measure would seem to commit us to wanting to be whichever person has the conception of the good that makes him happiest or best off.[7] Walzer treats social meanings as if they were individual conceptions of the good writ large, and he rejects the possibility of ranking them (p. 314).

Rawls' response to the incommensurability of individual conceptions of the good, which he views as fundamental to the circumstances of justice, is to develop a conception of primary social goods and a hypothetical contract situation in which rational deliberators can respect the importance, if not the content, of their conceptions of the good. These constructs he defends by reference to theories of the person and of the role of morality in society, which he takes to be a part of our overall system of beliefs. (Incidentally, Walzer mistakes the primary social goods for anthropological generalizations on p. 8; cf. Rawls at n. 8 above.) Reasonable persons, he argues, would accept this model for selecting principles of justice, though it abstracts from their actual preferences, because it is procedurally fair to them and because it represents them in a way that preserves the "ideal" of free and equal persons which they share. Walzer, in contrast, is not willing to retreat to any such exercise in abstract philosophy. He thinks no such constructions will adequately respect the social meanings shared by actual persons in actual societies (cf. p. 8). This position points us toward the fundamental importance of his Justification Thesis (f), but before turning to it, I want to make a point about the analogy between individual conceptions of the good and shared social meanings.

Even though individual conceptions of the good may not be ranked on a social scale of happiness or satisfaction which allows us to compare them, in Rawls' view, they are the results of individual rational deliberation about a plan of life. Moreover, conceptions of the good may be revised and rejected, and individuals have a fundamental interest in protecting their liberty to carry out such revisions. But the process of rational deliberation and revision means that individuals will assess *the reasons* they have for their fundamental preferences. Individuals must be able to detach themselves from some of their actual preferences in order to carry out this process of rational deliberation and revision. To some extent, they must be able to adopt an independent or impartial perspective in assessing the reasons for their basic preferences. So, despite the *social* incommensurability of conceptions of the good, there is rational assessment of them by *individuals* who reason about and compare and revise them. The preferences that form such conceptions are not just givens we hold fixed – they are themselves the subject of rational assessment, and it is a fundamental feature of our moral experience that we have the capacity to carry out such assessment.[8] This is not to say that we have the capacity to revise these fundamental preferences all at once, without appeal to other preferences to which we hold firm. But none are values we hold in principle unrevisable, and many people vary in what they revise over a lifetime.

But similar capacities for individual rational assessment must play a role in deliberation about "shared social meanings" – even if we grant, for the sake of argument, that these too are incommensurable because we lack an intersocietal scale of goodness on which to rank them. These shared meanings form components of individual conceptions of the good; they penetrate individual plans of life which together comprise the life plans of the community. As a result, these shared meanings must also be subject to rational assessment and revision, from both individual and social perspectives. We would expect that the moral experience of the individual includes the opportunity and capacity to assess shared meanings by searching out the reasons for accepting them or revising them. The point I made earlier, Cohen's remark about varieties of commitment to shared meanings, is but an implication of the more basic point here. In effect, then, our acceptance of the notion of a rational plan of life presupposes our ability to step outside of parts of our tradition; we must have this ability if we are to assess our reasons for including certain values within our conception of the good. This point raises serious worries about the Justification Thesis Walzer advances, to which I now turn.

What I have called the Justification Thesis is Walzer's metaethical claim that we cannot justify assigning a distributive principle to a sphere if it does not "fit" the social meanings people ascribe to the goods in that sphere, and is thus not acceptable to them. (This needs unpacking, and in view of the lack of explicit unpacking Walzer provides, I clearly risk overattributing.) I believe Walzer is committed to something like the following argument: (1) To justify a moral principle to someone is to give him adequate reasons for accepting or adopting the principle. But (2) something is a reason for a person to perform an act (or to accept a rule or principle) only if consideration of it motivates him to perform the act (or accept the principle). However, (3) consideration of a fact about an act (or rule) will motivate someone to perform the act (or adopt the rule) – that is, the fact will be a reason – only if it is appropriately connected to some desires or "values" or "shared meanings" which the person already (actually or dispositionally) has. Specifically, (4) something will be a reason for us to accept a principle of distributive justice only if it is appropriately connected to the values and shared meanings which motivate us to distribute the good in a particular way. Therefore, (5) philosophical arguments, such as those based on hypothetical contracts (in which we must abstract from our conceptions or the good) will not give us reasons for adopting a distributive principle unless they happen to be appropriately connected to the values or meanings we already share. But, then, (6) we have no philosophical method which provides reasons which will motivate a person to accept a distributive principle regardless of the shared meanings which he already possesses.

If I have not read into Walzer's view too much that is not there, the roots of his relativism reach back to a very strong form of internalism.[9] Walzer – without argument, I might add – has rejected any form of externalism. An externalist is someone who thinks reasons are guides to action – they allow us to judge what action is best – but denies that something can be a guide to action "only if it is capable of motivating the agent."[10] For the sake of argument, I will let that rejection stand. I am more concerned that Walzer has – also without argument – assumed an overly strong version of internalism. Specifically, he has assumed that something will be a reason for an agent to do something only if it motivates him to do it because of its connection to desires (or "values" or "shared meanings," which at least involve preferences ranked in a certain way) that the agent already has (at least dispositionally). Since we cannot justify a distributive principle to someone who lacks the appropriate shared meanings, because we cannot provide him with reasons for adopting the principle, the strong form of internalism leads us rather precipitously into the relativism Walzer espouses.

My main response to this view is that we have little reason to adopt such a strong form of internalism. Certain versions of it have been effectively dealt with by Darwall, but my objection here turns on the degree to which I think the view is untrue to our moral experience. In considering reasons for doing things, we consistently detach ourselves from significant parts of our actual preferences in order to adopt an impartial, rational stance. I have argued that Walzer's anthropological method, which tries to read community values from institutional structures, ignores the various sorts of commitments people actually have to those structures and the implicit values they represent. But these varied commitments presuppose our capacity to detach ourselves from "shared values" in considering reasons. So, too, I argued that rational deliberation about a plan of life presupposes the ability to consider reasons which are not tied to actual desires in the strong way Walzer supposes. If we can rationally deliberate about and revise our conceptions of the good – and we do – then the very strong form of internalism advocated by Walzer is untrue to our moral experience. The parallel point would hold for our ability to deliberate and revise culturally induced values or shared meanings, which, after all, penetrate our life plans and are features of our conceptions of the good which we often want to revise.

If Walzer were right in insisting on the very strong form of internalism he holds, then we could not really have reasons for revising our conceptions of the good, our plans of life, where this means having reasons for thinking some fundamental or intrinsic preferences should be altered in favor of others. Our moral experience would be better described as one in which changes in fundamental features of life plans were all assimilated to inexplicable conversions. Since this is a poor description of our moral experience, Walzer's strong internalism is untrue to it, and I think unsupportable.

Someone may object that the picture I offer of people rationally revising a plan of life – including the shared social meanings that penetrate it – is itself a very particular, "local" cultural product. Even if it is a reasonable description of what deliberation about individual and social values is like in a heterogeneous society such as ours, it is quite inaccurate as a description of moral experience in other societies. But if this moral experience is just a local one, then appeal to it cannot be the basis for criticizing the view that justice is local.

It is certainly possible that the picture of moral experience I paint is more likely to be true of some societies – say heterogeneous ones like ours and most nation-states anywhere in the world – than it is of others – say small, highly homogeneous, perhaps isolated cultures. Now I am not persuaded by Walzer's anthropological evidence that he has described even one context in which moral experience is such that people lack the capacity to criticize their values. But even if there are some cases in which people exhibit no capacity to revise and assess their conceptions of the good, the general range of cases points in the other direction. In general, people can and do detach themselves from actual desires, including shared social meanings, when engaging in moral deliberation. If this is true, then strong internalism is an implausible restriction on the process of justification, including the process of justifying principles of justice. Indeed, in the general range of cases, the problem of justice is the problem of defining institutions that are compatible with diverse conceptions of the good and with individuals' interests in retaining the liberty to reform and revise their plans of life. This is the problem of justice which Rawls treats as central to his construction.

There may be another way to see the relationship between Walzer's strong internalism and the relativism he espouses. Relativists are typically very impressed by disagreements, especially long-standing disagreements that seem immune to easy resolution. Walzer's claim that different cultures disagree about how certain goods should be distributed is a case in point. In a recent article, Sandra Peterson suggests that relativists of various sorts share a common belief.[11] They believe that, if knowledge of moral truths were possible, then the truth would win out, that is, that people would tend to converge – over time, with all the evidence in, with care, etc. – in their beliefs about it. Specifically, they might have an "expectation of the power of belief," that is, they may think this claim is true: "If in the long and careful run we believe that p, then it is true that p." Or they may have an "expectation of the power of truth," that is, they may think this claim is true: "If p is true, then anyone reasonable who reflects on (all) the (relevant) evidence whether p will eventually come to believe p." Since people in different cultures – even when aware of the evidence, in the long run, etc. – may come to believe p and not-p, some cultures one, some the other, then p is not the kind of proposition which can be either true or not true. The appeal to relativism is thus an attempt to save the belief in convergence and the datum of nonconvergence.

We might think of Walzer's strong internalism as an attempt to explain the nonconvergence. People will not be justified in accepting a distributive principle P unless they are motivated to accept it. But they cannot be motivated to accept principles which do not fit with their shared social meanings since strong internalism is true. If we had a philosophical method that could rank alternative social conceptions of the good (or the just), then the evidence available through application of that method could conceivably produce convergence. The problem is that any such method would itself run afoul of the strong internalism Walzer is committed to. Such a method would require that we could get beyond the grip of our own shared social meanings in order to see why one set of such meanings is preferable to another. But strong internalism prevents us from accepting the validity of any such philosophical method. But if convergence is unachievable, then we must make justice relative, or so the argument goes.

My argument that strong internalism is not true to our moral experience turns on the claim that we have a significant capacity to detach ourselves from some of our social attachments and to conduct critical assessment of them. The argument is intended to leave the door open to more possibilities of convergence. It is not an argument which challenges the belief in the relationship between truth and convergence, though I am not committed to any such relationship. For example, someone might simply challenge the premise about convergence, arguing, as Peterson suggests the "umpiricist" would, that the notion of "all relevant evidence" is either trivial or unclarifiable. It is trivial if the evidence includes the explicit answer to the issue in dispute; it is unclarifiable if it does not. For example, there may be a truth of the matter about whether the runner was safe at first, but still no convergence, even when all the evidence is in; that is why we need umpires in baseball.

It is worth noting that attraction to very strong forms of internalism cuts across party lines. For example, Richard Brandt seems to hold a similar view when he insists that justification in ethics must appeal to an agent's actual desires, purified perhaps by cognitive psychotherapy, but actual in any case.[12] In Brandt's case I have labeled the strong internalism "the disalienation constraint," since he wants the justification for a moral position to be directly relevant to answering the question, why should I be moral?[13] I have argued that the disalienation constraint is in tension with his other central methodological constraint, the "empiricist constraint," which prohibits invoking moral intuitions in the process of moral justification. (Walzer clearly does not share the empirical constraint!) My argument against Brandt turns on the fact that the disalienation constraint makes us stay extremely close to our actual desires, which are deeply affected by the moral commitments of our society. But this means we will not be able to "step outside our tradition" to adopt that critical detachment needed in moral deliberation about competing moral conceptions, and this makes us violate the spirit of the empiricist constraint. Rawls, in contrast, rejects any such strong internalism – indeed, he is a target of both Walzer and Brandt because he does. But the method of wide reflective equilibrium, which is central to Rawls' theory of justification, may involve a weak version of internalism and if it does, the concerns driving Walzer may arise at another level.[14]

Walzer could be wrong – as I have argued he is – and Rawls right about our ability to step outside (at least some of) our shared, socially relative motivations. Still, even if we do not keep our anthropological noses as close to the ground as Walzer does, we may still find that Rawlsian wide reflective equilibria will diverge in ways that correspond to certain cross-cultural differences. For example, the Kantian ideal of the person underlying Rawls' contractarian construction may reflect only a certain liberal tradition. It is an Archimedean point only for those who can agree to hold it fixed.[15] Rawls, in his recent writings, makes this feature of his theory explicit.[16] He says that justice as fairness rests on acceptance of a particular ideal of the person and on a conception of the function of justice in a heterogeneous nation-state in which there may be disagreement about conceptions of the good. That is, he intends his theory to be *politically* justifiable to persons operating within a broadly construed democratic liberal tradition. Whether or not justice as fairness would emerge in a wide reflective equilibrium involving people from distinctly different moral and political tradition is not something Rawls is ready to comment on, at least until the ideals of the person and other "background theories" of the other tradition are made explicit. In principle, however, the door is open to some form of relativism with regard to justice, though not to relativism about justice in nation-states in which diverse conceptions of the good may be found and in which people have a fundamental interest in their freedom to pursue and revise those conceptions.

This characterization of Rawls' position may make it seem closer to Walzer's than one might at first have suspected. To be sure, nothing in Walzer's argument shows us that divergence in wide reflective equilibria – and thus relativism – will or must arise. We certainly cannot infer ultimate divergence by merely pointing to some different views currently held by different cultures, for we have to see what would be revised in wide reflective equilibrium. Walzer and Rawls do seem to disagree about the extent to which people can step back from socially dominant motivations and engage in a process of deliberation about the suitability of alternative distributive principles. One way to put the point is that Walzer's strong internalism seems to restrict the process of justification to narrow, rather than wide reflective equilibria. But this fundamental difference between Walzer and Rawls still leaves a nagging worry that relativism will arise even for Rawls, and this may make one sympathetic to Walzer's position even if one is not tempted to hold so strong a form of internalism.

I am not sure this form of relativism can be ruled out by a priori arguments. Perhaps some way of anchoring a notion of practical reason – à la Darwall – might suggest such an argument. It may be that we cannot yet determine whether such relativism is a fact of our political and moral lives, and we will have to do far more work in ethical theory, of the sort Sidgwick began and Rawls has pursued, before we can tell what convergence in wide equilibrium there will be or or even what significance a particular example of divergence has. But I do think we are not driven to the immediate relativism Walzer adopts, because the strong internalism from which it derives is unsupportable.

Let me conclude by returning to the issue with which I began, the inclination many of us have to make judgments about injustice in other societies and to take actions based on those judgments. First, out of fairness to Walzer, it is not clear that in the case of South Africa, we must refrain from such actions because of the need to respect the cultural products of other societies. Internal opposition to Apartheid in South Africa is widespread and long-standing, so there is reason to believe Apartheid is not a "joint" cultural product of whites and blacks. Moreover, even white South Africans espouse some democratic principles with which Apartheid might be thought inconsistent (I recollect Prime Minister Botha saying that the problem with the principle of one man/one vote is that it would lead to majority domination over the minority; presumably whatever is wrong with that would also be wrong with minority domination over the majority.) So it might be acceptable to take actions against the injustice in South Africa because it is up for grabs what should count as justice there.

But I think this will not do. Most of us who oppose racism and Apartheid do not think that such practices and institutions become morally acceptable merely because they are not visibly opposed by their victims, though issues of consent are complex, as I hinted earlier. Greater awareness of the caste system in India, a case Walzer clearly treats as a matter of local justice, would, and I think should, produce external opposition despite (alleged) consent by the lower castes. Here, of course, the difference between Walzer's rapid plunge into relativism and the narrowed range within which relativism can arise in Rawls' account have a definite effect. Nations such as South Africa, where we can expect conceptions of the good to diverge, can be condemned as unjust when they deny liberty and opportunity to all.[17]

Justice and justification

NOTES

1 John Rawls, *A Theory of Justice* (Cambridge, 1971).
2 Norman Daniels, "Health Care Needs and Distributive Justice," *Philosophy and Public Affairs* 10 (1981), 146–79; also see my *Just Health Care* (Cambridge, 1985).
3 See Ronald Dworkin, "To Each His Own," *New York Review of Books* (April 14, 1983), 4–5, and Walzer's reply in " 'Spheres of Justice': An Exchange," *New York Review of Books* (July 21, 1983).
4 Dworkin, "To Each His Own," p. 4.
5 T. M. Scanlon made a suggestion along these lines in his presentation to the Western APA Symposium on *Spheres of Justice*, April 1985.
6 Joshua Cohen, review of *Spheres of Justice*, in *Journal of Philosophy* 83:8 (August 1986), 457–68.
7 John Rawls, "Social Unity and Primary Goods," in Amartya Sen and Bernard Williams, eds., *Utilitarianism and Beyond* (Cambridge, 1982), 159–86.
8 Cf. Darwall's remarks on unified agency in Stephen Darwall, *Impartial Reason* (Cornell, 1983), pp. 102ff.
9 Cf. Gilbert Harman, "Moral Relativism Defended," *The Philosophical Review* 84 (1975), 3–22. Harman, however, restricts his internalism to "inner moral judgments," which assert that an agent ought or ought not to do something; he is not concerned with other normative judgements, such as those which say a certain state of affairs or institutional arrangement is wrong. In contrast, Walzer seems committed to a stronger claim: the judgment that Indian caste society is unjust presupposes that Indians could come to accept certain distributive principles, which their shared social meanings in fact prevent them from accepting.
10 Cf. Darwall, *Impartial Reason*, p. 52.
11 Sandra Peterson, "Remarks on Three Formulations of Ethical Relativism," *Ethics* 95:4,887–908.
12 Cf. Richard Brandt, *A Theory of the Good and the Right* (Oxford, 1979); also see Norman Daniels, "Can Cognitive Psychotherapy Reconcile Reason and Desire?" *Ethics* 93 (1983), 772–85.
13 Cf. Norman Daniels, "Two Approaches to Theory Acceptance in Ethics," in D. Copp and D. Zimmerman, eds., *Morality, Reason, and Truth: New Essays on the Foundations of Ethics* (Rowman and Littlefield, 1984), pp. 120–40.
14 Norman Daniels, "Wide Reflective Equilibrium and Theory Acceptance in Ethics," *Journal of Philosophy* 76 (1979), 256–82.
15 Cf. my "Reflective Equilibrium and Archimedean Points," *Canadian Journal of Philosophy*, 10:1, 83–103.
16 Cf. John Rawls, "Kantian Constructivism in Moral Theory," *Journal of Philosophy*, 77 (September 1980); and "Justice as Fairness: Political Not Metaphysical," *Philosophy and Public Affairs* 14:3, 223–51.
17 I am indebted to Joshua Cohen, C. A. J. Coady, and members of the Tufts Philosophy Department for helpful discussion of these issues. This paper is based on my symposium presentation, "The Roots of Walzer's Relativ-

118

ism," delivered at the Western Division APA Meeting, April 1985; it was also presented at Brooklyn College. In sections I–IV I draw on material from my review of Walzer's *Spheres of Justice* in *Philosophical Review* 94:1(January 1985), 142–8.

Chapter 7

Moral theory and the plasticity of persons[1]

I

There is a hoary tradition in moral philosophy that assumes we cannot determine which moral theory is acceptable or correct unless we have available a correct theory of human nature, or, in its more modern form, of the person.[2] With such a theory of the person, however, we could at least narrow down the choice among competing ethical theories. A more recent tradition, at least in one of its standard interpretations, agrees it would be necessary to have a correct theory of the person before we could determine an acceptable moral theory, but it denies there is a determinate nature of the person to be captured in such a theory. The plasticity of the person, according to this strand of Marxist theory, rules out the possibility of there being universal moral theory at all. In this paper, I would like to explore a view that treads an intermediate path. It agrees with the Marxist denial that there is a determinate nature of the person, a deep fact of the matter, that can be abstracted from the social matrix and made the subject of a (nonmoral) theory of the person. And, it agrees with both traditions that moral theory depends on and embodies a theory of the person. But, by making the problem of arriving at an acceptable view of the person itself something that depends on overall theoretical considerations, including moral ones, the intermediary view may be able to avoid the type of moral relativism associated with the Marxist view.

The immediate source of the view I discuss is an exchange between John Rawls and Derek Parfit[3] on the connection between criteria of personal identity and moral theories. The focus on personal identity is of some interest, because, at least at first sight, it seems to be a less morally loaded notion than other concepts usually dealt with in the theory of the person, such as autonomy and rationality. I will support what I take to be the thrust of Rawls' remarks:[4] even here, in the heart of *echt* philosophy of mind, we find a feature of the concept of the person that is in an important sense indeterminate without input from moral theory. First, however, I will examine Parfit's claims about the connection between two views of personal identity, which he calls the Simple and the Complex, and competing moral theories. I will then look at Rawls' argument that philosophy of mind underdetermines theory selection in ethics. Pursuing the thrust of Rawls' remarks will lead me to the intermediary view just noted and to the connection of this issue to a coherentist or holist view of theory acceptance in ethics.

II

Parfit distinguishes two views of personal identity, the Simple View and the Complex View. The Complex View builds on the important fact that a person's memories and intentions, projects and character, all change over time. Following Parfit, let us call "direct" the psychological relation that holds between a memory and the experience it is a memory of or between an intention and the later act that is intended. Let us say a person's life over a given period of time is "connected" if direct psychological relations hold in that period. Successive periods in a person's life will have "continuity" if they form a chain of connected periods. Suppose on Friday I remember what happened on Thursday, and on Thursday I remember what happened on Wednesday, but on Friday I cannot remember what happened on Wednesday. Then my life has continuity from Wednesday through Friday even if there is no connectedness between Wednesday and Friday.[5]

Continuity can vary in degree, depending on the number and strength of the connections between different parts of a person's life. On the Complex View this fact is taken to imply that personal identity can also vary in degree. The survival of the same person, over time, will be a matter of degree. Successive person-stages or "selves" may not include the survival, to any significant degree, of the person who was ancestor to those "selves." The Simple View rejects this temptation to treat identity or survival of the same person as a matter of degree. It takes the fact of identity or survival of the same person to be "all-or-nothing." A person, in a real or imaginary case (say a Methusela case or a complex fission or fusion case),[6] either is *me* or *someone else*.[7] Given this commitment to an all-or-nothing view of identity and survival, then, since continuities vary in degree, identity cannot consist in these continuities. It must be a special, "further fact" over and above them.

Before turning to the purported implications of these two Views for moral theory, a couple of qualificatory remarks are in order. First, the Complex View is quite compatible with persons having as high a degree of continuity and connectedness as we can imagine. It does not imply that none or many or some of us fail to survive to any significant degree through successive selves. As we shall see this point is of relevance to the argument about the moral implications of scaling identity.

Second, in the normal range of cases – which we can assume is indeed quite wide, especially if we include the pathological, we generally find insufficient variation in the degree of continuity to warrant raising serious questions about the survival of a person. It takes philosophical or science fiction imagination to concoct such cases. Even in the case of significant psychological and character alteration, say that accompanying growth through adolescence, identity crisis, career change, "mid-life" crisis, and old age, we may not be as tempted as Parfit thinks we are to make survival a matter of degree. Indeed, a working assumption of psychologists and sociologists, to say nothing of friends and relatives, is that we can find particular "causal" stories, and perhaps comprehensive theories of personality, that can explain the particular changes the person undergoes.[8] It would take a more detailed discussion than I can undertake here to see what the implications of shifting to talk about sequences of selves are for the possibility of developing such explanations. It is an unexplored empirical question what effect such a conceptual shift would have (it might even lead to improvements). But the question is not just academic: without an ability to explain and understand such changes in persons, we do not know how to relate to, and interact with, people.

Finally, although Parfit indicates there are reasons for thinking the Simple View mistaken, he does not argue the point in the article under discussion. Rather, he treats both Views as if they are involved in some of our usual ways of thinking about personal identity. Parfit is not offering decisive arguments for a particular view of personal identity, showing that view supports a particular moral theory, and thus providing us with decisive arguments for that moral theory.[9]

Parfit claims that the shift from the Simple to the Complex View has two distinct effects on moral principles. The first effect is restricted to cases in which personal identity holds only to a lesser degree: principles that involve our keeping track of personal identity over time, such as principles governing desert and commitment, will be affected in their *scope* and in their *importance*. The second is a general effect that holds regardless of the degree to which identity is diminished in particular cases: personal identity becomes a less deep fact and therefore a less *weighty* moral fact; consequently, moral principles that involve personal identity may be treated as less weighty or important principles. We must consider each of these purported effects in more detail.

Consider first the effect on scope. Suppose there is little continuity between a given criminal and his later self when he is caught and prosecuted for "his" crime. Parfit suggests that our normal principle, which calls for punishing the criminal for his crimes, presupposes the identity of the person being punished and the person who committed the crime. But if identity is here diminished in degree, then the principle may apply to a lesser degree, or not at all if survival of the criminal "self" is minimal. Accordingly, we might punish less severely, or not at all. The scope of a principle of punishment is thus restricted to cases in which it makes sense to claim we are punishing a person who is, to a significant degree, the same person as the criminal. Similarly, suppose a person who makes a promise is only to a small degree the same person who is (if anyone is) obliged to keep that promise. Then principles governing commitment over time, since they presuppose personal identity, may have reduced scope and may apply only to a diminished degree.[10] On the Simple View, however, in both of these cases, if we can ascribe identity to the person over time, then the principles of desert and commitment apply with full force.[11]

Parfit's argument in these cases turns on the assumption that if a "morally important fact holds to a lesser degree, it can be more plausibly claimed to have less importance," or none at all in extreme cases.[12] He does not argue for the assumption except to suggest that we accept instances of it in other cases. For example, he thinks we have "less of a special duty" to help our relatives and friends when they are more distant relatives and friends. Presumably he means we can satisfy our special duty (if there is such) by doing less for distant relatives and friends, and we can be excused from doing anything at all for them by considerations which would not carry as much weight were they closer relatives and friends.

The analogy is not persuasive as a defense of the general assumption, however. More factors affect our acknowledgment of a duty to help our friends and relatives than the degree of closeness of the kinship or friendship relationships. For example, our duty to help our relatives has undergone serious transformations with the erosion of social arrangements that depend on and enhance the extended family as a social unit. At times, or in societies or subcultures, in which the extended family is held more important than it is now, cousins and other more distant relatives might have been beneficiaries of such duties, although they no longer are considered to be. One could try to save Parfit's point by saying that the change reflects an alteration in the *closeness* of the relation – and thus of the degree to which the morally relevant fact of being related holds. But it seems more plausible to conclude that our duties to relatives and friends vary on the basis of many factors other than the degree of kinship. So Parfit's example may not even be an example of our altering the importance of the duty to help relatives and friends depending on the degree of closeness of the relation. But even if it had been, it would show only that we *sometimes* alter the importance of a principle that depends on a particular moral fact when the fact holds to a lesser degree. What is missing is an argument to show that in the case at hand, of personal identity, we should make the analogous dilution. Moreover, it is hard to see how that argument would not itself have to be in large part a moral argument.

Consider next the second effect of the Complex View on moral principles that involve keeping track of personal identity. This effect is general and applies even in cases where psychological connectedness and continuity are strong. The effect, Parfit claims, derives from the fact that on the Complex View, personal identity "is in its nature less deep, or involves less."[13] The effect of this change in the "depth" of the fact of personal identity, Parfit suggests, is that we should change the *weight* (rather than the scope, as with the first effect) we give moral principles that involve, or presuppose claims about, personal identity. "When some morally important fact is seen to be less deep, it can be plausibly claimed to be less important."[14]

This central assumption of Parfit's brilliant article is never argued for.[15] My worry is not simply that there is vague, metaphorical language about the "depth" of certain facts and the "weight" of related principles.[16] Rather, I am worried that there is not a single argument that reducing the (metaphysical?) depth of the fact is sufficient reason to warrant reducing the (moral) weight ascribed to a relevant principle. What we would expect to be in question is the *moral* importance (depth?) of the fact, not its metaphysical depth, if there is to be a relationship of the fact to the weightiness of relevant moral principles. But there is no such argument. To be sure, there is some plausibility, my earlier objections aside, to the claim that if a morally relevant fact (personal identity) does not hold to a sufficient degree, then we should adjust the scope of principles that presuppose the fact obtains to a sufficient degree. But here what is being claimed is that even in cases of strong personal identity, the fact of that identity is "less deep," and "therefore" moral principles that involve personal identity are less weighty. But the argument is missing that personal identity, even when strong, is still not "deep" and therefore is not morally important enough to provide a basis for a weighty moral principle.

Perhaps such an argument could be given. It would require showing that we can characterize a set of "deep" facts independently of moral considerations, by reference, say, only to intuitions about "depth" that derive from philosophy of mind. Then we would have to show that these deep facts are the appropriate set of facts for supporting weighty moral principles. I am suspicious, however, that part of what makes such facts turn out to be "deep" in the first place is that they play a relatively central role in our moral and social theories. We would then need an argument to show that the fact of personal identity *should not* play such a role in our theories and *should not* be viewed as a deep fact. But that is just the *moral* argument missing in Parfit's discussion.

The gap in Parfit's argument for this second effect of the Complex View is serious. I would like, nevertheless, to sketch how Parfit appeals to this effect in his discussion of distributive justice. Parfit wants to show that one might appeal to the Complex View to make more plausible the utilitarian rejection of principles of distributive justice. In particular, utilitarians tend to reject or override principles of fairness which constrain how benefits and burdens are to be balanced between individuals. Instead utilitarians seek to maximize the "net benefits minus burdens"[17] without special regard to how the distribution falls between people.

It is just because utilitarians ignore these fairness principles that some of their critics have charged that either they assume a group of people is like a single person (Gauthier) or that they forget a group is not like a single person (Rawls).[18] Parfit wants to show that utilitarians need not be assumed to believe there is no difference between single persons and groups in order to justify his rejection of the distributive principles. Rather, the utilitarian may appeal to the Complex View, which implies that the differences between persons is a less deep fact, and therefore a less morally important one, than it is taken to be on the Simple View. Because it is less morally important, principles that depend on it, like principles of fairness, may be thought to be less weighty moral principles. In this way, the utilitarian concern for maximization might be thought to outweigh the principles of fairness.

Actually, Parfit's argument is far more complex.[19] To show that what counts here is the pro-utilitarian effect of the Complex View on the *weight* of the principles of fairness, Parfit first shows that the effect of the Complex View on the *scope* of such principles actually runs counter to the utilitarian position. We might think that the relevant effect of the Complex View is to make us treat persons and groups more similarly because personal identity holds to lesser degrees than on the Simple View. But, Parfit points out, we can do that in two ways: (a) we can *reduce the scope* of fairness principles so that they no longer apply to groups; or (b) we can *extend* their scope so that they apply within lives, that is, between successive "selves." If anything, the Complex View seems to favor (b), *extending* their scope, and so its effect on scope is actually counter-utilitarian. That is, we would then not maximize even within a life, as the utilitarian assumes, but we would have to worry that greater benefits to a later "self" may not balance lesser burdens to the earlier self. It is a different view, which Parfit calls "the Reverse View," that seems to favor *reducing* the scope of fairness principles. But the Reverse View involves treating a group as if it were a superperson, a holist view of groups which Parfit rejects as implausible. Yet it is this implausible Reverse View and its effect of reducing scope that would have to be pinned on the utilitarian if Gauthier's or Rawls' accusations were true.

Thus, Parfit concludes, there is a more plausible way to defend the utilitarian: attribute his rejection of the fairness principles to the effect of the Complex View on the *weight*, not the scope, of the distributive principles. The utilitarian does not, as Rawls and others suggest, have an attitude of "conflating all persons into one."[20] Rather, his attitude may derive from treating the unity of each life as less deep in its nature. That is, it may derive from a metaphysical disintegration of the person.[21] The utilitarian is not ignoring the fact that we cannot *compensate* one person's burdens with another's benefits, as the principles of fairness insist. Rather, he is claiming that this fact is outweighed by utilitarian considerations because it is not morally very important that we cannot so compensate persons. In short, the utilitarian position is being defended against the claim that it ignores or forgets an important fact about persons by the claim that it denies the fact is such an important one. Such a denial might rest on the Complex View.

A few qualificatory remarks are in order. First, a reminder: Parfit's argument rests on the unsubstantiated assumption that because the fact of personal identity is "less deep" it is therefore less morally important. Second, another reminder: Parfit does not in the course of this discussion argue that the Complex View is decisively established and the Simple View refuted. Therefore he should not be taken to be arguing that the connection between the Complex View and the utilitarian position amounts to a sufficient defense of utilitarianism. Third, it is not always clear that all utilitarian views are equal beneficiaries of Parfit's arguments. Some of his claims seem most supportive of rather straightforward act utilitarianisms and may not really play much role in defending rule utilitarianisms.[22] Fourth, some deontological theories, and not just utilitarianism, might be thought to be plausibly supported by the Complex View.[23]

One final qualificatory remark. As I have interpreted Parfit's discussion, it contains a rather immodest proposal: that is, the Complex View supports the moral claim that personal identity is not as morally important a notion as some deontological principles make it out to be. Despite what I think is the thrust of Parfit's remarks, some might instead attribute to him only a more modest proposal: the Complex View might be taken to assert that, since persons are "continuous" in varying degrees, then there is no deep or natural fact about their being strongly continuous. Consequently, there is room for claiming that we cannot rule out utilitarianism straightaway on the grounds that it fails to employ a criterion of personal identity as strong as that presupposed by the Simple View. This modest proposal leaves it an *open question* how strong a degree of connectedness one might strive to produce in people and how morally important a fact boundaries between persons should be taken to be. As we shall see, the modest proposal may be compatible with the view advanced by Rawls and to which I now turn.

III

Parfit's discussion, at least if it rests on anything like the "immodest proposal," suggests the following argument.[24] The Complex View supports, or makes more plausible, a utilitarian position on a number of questions, including problems of desert, commitment, and distributive justice. The Simple View supports, or makes plausible, certain deontological positions on the same questions. In particular, a Kantian view, like justice as fairness, seems to require a fairly strong criterion of personal identity in order to keep track of the responsibility and contribution of persons through time so that distributions can be suitably related to them. Similarly, its ideal of an autonomous person responsible for devising and altering a life plan seems to require tracking persons over longer periods of time than are relevant for the utilitarian.[25] The philosophy of mind, however, gives us reason to support the Complex View and reject the Simple View. Therefore, we have reason to support utilitarianism and reject competing moral theories that require the stronger, but false, Simple View of personal identity.

Rawls advances a most interesting reply to arguments of this form. I will paraphrase his argument and then discuss its most important features:[26]

(1) The philosophy of mind provides us with general conditions of adequacy that must be met by any criterion of personal identity; roughly, "persons are mental continuities embodied and expressed in a planned order of conduct through space and time."[27]

(2) These general conditions leave room for a family of possible criteria of personal identity, ranging, among other things, from weaker to stronger, depending on how much they require (or enable) us to keep track of the individual through time.

(3) A moral conception embodies a conception of the person and therefore will involve some particular criterion of personal identity from among the family of possible criteria.

(4) It is plausible to believe that utilitarian and Kantian views (like

127

justice as fairness) require, respectively, weaker and stronger criteria of personal identity.

(5) It is a necessary condition for the acceptability of the particular criterion of personal identity required by a moral conception that it is *feasible*, as determined by general social theory.

(6) The feasibility test is relative to the well-ordered society embodying the relevant conception of the person, not to a society (well-ordered or not), such as our own, which may embody a competing moral theory.

(7) If two particular criteria of personal identity employed by competing moral conceptions are both feasible, then not only does philosophy of mind underdetermine the choice between them, but philosophy of mind *cum* general social theory may underdetermine the choice between them.

(8) We have no reason to think that either the utilitarian or the Kantian theories require criteria of personal identity that fail the feasibility test; indeed, we have some reason to think both criteria pass it.

(9) Therefore, philosophy of mind underdetermines the choice between utilitarianism and a Kantian view such as justice as fairness.

Rawls' sketchy argument clearly needs support for a number of its premises.[28] I will concentrate on what I take to be its central and most interesting contention: that philosophy of mind, even construed in a "broadly empirical" way,[29] can uncover no particular degree of connectedness or continuity within persons that is "natural" or "fixed."[30] Rather, different social institutions, which we may assume reflect different, at least implicit, moral conceptions, can *shape* persons to have different "actual continuities." Call this thesis the Plasticity Thesis. Rawls is saying that philosophy of mind, normally construed, can tell us about the nature of persons, in particular about the criteria of identity for persons, only up to the bounds imposed by the Plasticity Thesis. The task of developing a more complete theory of the person must involve considerations that derive from within moral theory (a broad notion on Rawls' view). Rather than there being some prior, deep and determinate fact of the matter about the nature of persons, it is the task of moral theory to help determine the most acceptable shape or "nature" that we should attempt to have persons realize.[31]

The Plasticity Thesis as stated is limited to the psychological connectedness and continuity of persons. It is in the spirit of Rawls' argument to extend the thesis to cover other important features of the person. Such an extended Plasticity Thesis might claim, for example, that there is no natural or fixed degree to which persons have autonomy, rationality, or a sense of justice. All of these central features of persons, it might be argued, will vary in degree (or within a range of degrees) depending on the features of the basic institutions of the well-ordered (or other) societies in which the persons live. In what follows, I will primarily consider the more limited Plasticity Thesis, the problems facing establishing it, and some of its implications for problems of theory acceptance in ethics.

IV

To establish the Plasticity Thesis would involve at least the following tasks:

(1) characterizing the method of philosophy of mind, at least the part that concerns personal identity, in order to arrive at an acceptable account of just what kind of knowledge it can provide (it would be nice to require agreement of philosophers doing this work, but that seems too strong);

(2) showing that such methods cannot determine a criterion of personal identity but only a family of such criteria;

(3) producing empirical evidence that different criteria of identity are "feasible" for persons living under different social arrangements.

All three steps present problems I am not sure how to resolve. Still, examining them may suffice to establish at least the plausibility of the Plasticity Thesis.

Before considering these difficulties, it is worth noting an obvious objection to the Plasticity Thesis. It might be argued that the thesis confuses variation among persons who share enough of a common nature to still be persons with variation in the nature of persons. The latter might invite the plea that we stop calling entities with such different natures all "persons." Such entities would fail, as it were, to be a natural kind exhibiting mere phenotypic variation. Coupled with such an objection we are likely to find the assumption that philosophy of mind has the task of telling us whether or not there is such a common nature – "it is a conceptual question" – and the social sciences have the task of telling us about the range of variation we can expect among persons shaped by different social settings.

Fortunately, I do not have to turn this paper into a discussion of essence and accident to meet the objection. First, the objection is irrelevant to the Plasticity Thesis in the context of Rawls' argument. Even if the plasticity is only phenotypic variation, it may still warrant Rawls' claim that without specific determination of that phenotype, we cannot decide between competing ethical theories. Even if some discipline, say (a "broadly empirical") philosophy of mind, could still detect a common nature (or essential nature) underlying such variation, it would still underdetermine theory selection in ethics. The common nature would be too sparse or thin a notion to force a choice between traditional moral theories. We would need moral theory itself to help us decide which phenotypic variation we think it is most acceptable to actualize in persons.

Second, the assumption that, were there a nature of persons to be discovered, it would be the task of philosophy of mind, rather than, say, the social sciences, to discover it, presupposes an agreement on features of philosophic method that I find missing in the literature. Seeing what unclarity about method exists here will help us see why tasks (1) and (2) in an argument for (or against!) the Plasticity Thesis are so hard to complete. I will take up two central questions: Can the method of examining puzzle cases in searching for our criteria of personal identity reveal such a common nature of persons as the objection assumes? Can the method extract from our judgments about personal identity some non- or premoral philosophical fact of the matter about the identity of persons?

Consider the first question first. Much work on personal identity consists of probing the limits of "our" concept of it. The method is to construct puzzle cases – transplant and duplication cases, longevity cases, fission and fusion cases – and to examine our inclination to judge the survival or identity of persons through such exotic changes. The cases are intended to test the degree to which we rely on features of bodily or mental continuity in making judgments about the identity of persons through time. But what do we really learn from them?

One problem is that we are never really sure just what the goal of such exploration of our concepts is. Suppose we find that we rely more heavily or decisively on certain features of mental continuity than we do on bodily continuity when asked about a certain kind of transplant case. What does that fact tell us about our concept of personal identity? It might tell us that such reliance is *already* a feature of our concept. Alternatively, it *might* tell us that we are disposed to *extend* our concept in a particular way from its current content, given the particular description of the puzzle case. The puzzle case method seems indeterminate between giving us a synchronic or a diachronic view of our concept. Perhaps either or both could legitimately be viewed as the proper target of the method, but it would be helpful to know which. If we are clear, for example, that we are doing diachronic *descriptive* metaphysics (or *normative* metaphysics, for that matter), we would have to involve ourselves more directly in worrying about the factors which lead us to have the concepts we do and which lead us to change them in the ways we are inclined to.

The uncertainty about the goal of the method shows up in another way. Suppose we are given cases in which we are not sure what we want to say about the survival of a person through an exotic change.

We might be inclined to adopt any of three positions: (a) our existing criteria for personal identity are in the right ballpark but need refinement, say in the weighting and priorities of components, before we can handle these cases; (b) the criteria we have worked out on the basis of previous cases are in fact not the right criteria at all, because they do not allow us to decide what to say in these problem cases; (c) our criteria capture the concept of personal identity for the range in which it is defined, but we need to add to the criteria in order to extend its range to the cases at hand; such extension might be based on good reasons, or it may just have to be an arbitrary decision. Deciding whether the examination of puzzle cases is supposed to yield diachronic or synchronic "descriptive metaphysics" might incline us toward a preference for (a) or (b) or (c). Still, the inclination may not be decisive, and if it is not, we do not know what we are doing.

It may be helpful to speculate about an issue that I think underlies our uncertainty about philosophical method here. Consider two approaches to what is involved in determining the "nature" of persons. One approach (A) operates as if we already have in mind a concept of the nature of persons. That concept of the nature of persons is what allows us to pick out as persons the entities we do, to reidentify them through time, indeed, to refer to them at all. If we can figure out our explicit and implicit necessary and sufficient conditions for referring to and identifying persons, including our criteria for personal identity, then, according to this approach, we will have elucidated whatever constitutes the "nature" of the person. The other approach (B) treats the nature of persons as something we find out about through (broadly speaking) the scientific study of persons. The fact that we can refer to persons and reidentify them through time and change in some range of cases does not mean we can squeeze out of those abilities a correct view of the nature of persons.[32]

My speculation is that something like the approach (A) underlies the vast interest in puzzle cases. Moreover, the approach (A) might incline us to the view that we are primarily interested in synchronic, not diachronic, questions about our concepts. Consequently, it might incline us less toward examining the factors that determine why our concept of the person emphasizes the features of the person it does. Finally, my speculation is that the approach (A) may incline us toward a view of the fixedness of the nature of the person. For example, we might hope to explicate just which particular degree of mental connectedness succeeds in making determinate "our" concept of the person. The risk here is that features of the person found in a certain range of conditions may become, on the approach (A), criteria for the application of the concept person and so part of the "nature" of persons. In contrast, I think approach (B) is neutral with regard to questions about the fixedness of the nature of the person – or indeed about whether there is only one "nature" involved.

My first question was whether the method of puzzle cases can reveal the common nature of persons presupposed by the objection we are considering to the Plasticity Thesis. I have suggested, though hardly proved, that it is unclear what we are intended to derive from the examination of such puzzle cases. Moreover, if my speculation is right that approach (A) underlies the attraction of such cases, then it is unclear what we could learn from this method. But since I do not propose to consider the merits of either approach, I turn to my second question about what we can learn from puzzle cases, which I think can be raised independently of the issues raised so far.

One feature of many of the puzzle cases found in the literature is that they intend to abstract from many features of the social institutions in which we carry on the business of making judgments about personal identity. And, in a sense, this seems like good scientific method, varying as few variables as possible in a situation and thereby hoping to isolate their effect. Thus we might not be told whether a proposed transplant is an isolated phenomenon, funded by the CIA to make some particular deception more likely, or whether it is the first in a projected unlimited number of such transplants, initially funded by the NIH, which are to become a standard feature of health care in the near future. (Or, if we are given such a background story, it is usually fashioned for its entertainment value, not as part of an effort to put the influence of the social forces at work in it to test.)[33] What is not examined, presumably because we are trying to explore a prior question, is whether it makes a difference in our judgment about the typical transplant case if, say, it is seen as a way of ducking obligations incurred prior to the transplant or as a way of providing unhappy, desperate people with a chance at a new life.

Failing to specify the social setting may not be an effective way of abstracting from its effects. Rather, it may be a way of hiding them. Suppose that we take much of the work on personal identity to be an effort to carry on "descriptive metaphysics," leaving aside my earlier worries about just what is thereby described. It is plausible to suggest that such descriptive metaphysics is carried on against a certain background *status quo*, namely the social institutions that surround many of our usual decisions about personal identity and its importance. Within that *status quo* many exotic features of our experience are varied by the puzzle cases. These cases are almost entirely taken to be ways of altering (technologically) the physics, biology, and psychology of our experience. The assumption seems to be that these are the features of our experience of persons which, when varied, will reveal the deep fact of the matter that constitutes the subject matter of descriptive metaphysics. The danger in this assumption is that we will end up having only hidden our *ideology* about the person in the guise of a philosophical fact of the matter about persons (or about our concept of the person).

Let us pursue in a slightly different direction this hypothesis that philosophy of mind may be unwittingly ideological. Many puzzle cases seem to elicit conflicting tendencies we have about how to judge personal identity. We seem pulled in different directions, sometimes with apparently equal force. The response of some philosophers is that we may have to "decide" or "legislate" what we want to say about personal identity for such cases because various theoretical considerations somehow cancel each other out and there may be no clear fact of the matter. That is, the concept seems to be undefined here and we must decide how to define it.

The hypothesis that hidden ideology may be present might throw light on some such cases. Perhaps the conceptual scheme being examined in such cases is really heavily laden with social[34] and moral theory. Moreover, the moral theory may be leading us in conflicting directions; or, there may be fragments of incompatible moral theories which incline us in different directions. What is rarely explored is the possibility that the basis for our indecision in certain cases may be moral, despite the fact that such puzzle cases often explicitly disavow any intention of bringing in such factors and try to abstract from them.

Suppose we are faced with a puzzle case that leaves us undecided about how we want to judge the survival or identity of a person through certain exotic changes. What factors should be thought relevant to "simply deciding" or "legislating" how to handle such cases? The reason such cases often seem so problematic is that we get little help from certain kinds of nonmoral theoretical factors. What is usually not discussed are the social and moral *interests* or *purposes* that might be at stake in deciding the cases one way rather than another. The hope seems to be that we ought to try to solve the problem case by finding a criterion of identity independent of such social and moral considerations. Then we would be able to use the criterion to help us decide the relevant moral questions. There may even be, I think, real resistance to the idea of settling the cases requiring "decision" or "legislation" on moral grounds, as if that would involve putting the cart before the horse. And this even if there is no horse! Or rather, the horse may be one of another color.

My guess is that a fairly deep assumption about a "fact–value" distinction lurks in the background here. Using moral considerations to help decide a criterion of personal identity would be mucking up the "facts of the matter" by bringing values into the question. How much better if we could determine the hard (philosophical) fact of the matter and then use the fact to decide the moral question! One way to put the

Plasticity Thesis is to say that the deep assumption about the fact–value distinction may beg the question about what counts as fact, which is to say, about how sharp the distinction is in at least this critical area.

I believe there is a connection here to a central issue in social theory – the status of methodological individualism. A standard procedure in much social philosophy and social science is to build on the idea that we compose societies out of persons. Persons are the prior fact of the matter. We should examine how societies work on the basis of what we can find out about how persons work. We should propose social reforms and ideals that are realistic in the sense that they reflect what is true about persons. My reservations about the methodological assumptions of philosophy of mind, at least those that run counter to the Plasticity Thesis, may provide a basis for some reservations about methodological individualism in other contexts. But this point cannot be pursued here.

I have given some reasons why it may prove impossible conclusively to establish the first two steps of an argument in favor of the Plasticity Thesis. At the same time, however, I have tried to bring out considerations which leave it an open possibility that the Plasticity Thesis might well be true and which show that little in (some of) the methods of philosophy of mind counts against it. I turn now to a few remarks about the third step that would seem to be needed to defend the Plasticity Thesis, namely, the production of empirical evidence that more than one set of criteria of personal identity are socially realizable or feasible.

I have taken the Plasticity Thesis to be claiming that there is no deep philosophical fact of the matter about persons with regard to their degree of psychological connectedness or continuity. In any case, the exploration of "our" concept of the person through various kinds of puzzle cases may not be capable of uncovering such a fact. In fact, the method may mislead us because it hides the fact that, when using it, we are looking at persons against a particular background of social institutions and moral conceptions. "Facts" so extricated may involve hidden ideology. This difficulty with philosophical method suggests a similar difficulty facing efforts to provide empirical support for the Plasticity Thesis.

Rawls suggests that different well-ordered societies, embodying different moral conceptions and therefore different conceptions of the person, would shape persons in different ways through their different institutions. "I assume that the kind of lives that people can and do lead is importantly affected by the moral conception publicly realized in their society. What sorts of persons we are is shaped by how we think of ourselves and this in turn is influenced by the social forms we live under."[35] Presumably, Rawls has in mind the following sort of mechanism: a society might raise individuals to place great emphasis on the rational planning of their own life plans. It might encourage autonomy, granting individuals great liberty to develop life plans within a framework of principles of justice. It might also provide people with a fair share of the means and opportunities to advance their ends. Not only does such social support for strong connectedness in individual lives derive from the material, educational, and liberty-promoting support of the basic institutions, but people, in their interaction with each other, would presumably place great weight on taking other persons' life plans into account and on advancing their own. Rawls is supposing that these mechanisms would produce people with a greater degree of psychological connectedness than would be produced in societies that encouraged disconnectedness among persons. One might imagine similar "shaping" effects on autonomy and even rationality.

We are required, however, by Rawls' argument to test whether a proposed "criterion of identity" is realizable or feasible. The test does not involve simply examining our society, which may not embody a moral conception containing persons constituted by the relevant criterion. But then what does the test involve? To some extent, it seems to be an exercise in imagination: imagine what the effects on persons might be of the relevant well-ordered society and try to judge if they lead to feasible or unfeasible social systems.

How definitive can such a test be? Some reference to what we know from our own experience in the institutions with which we are familiar must be brought to bear. We might find relevant data for many of the issues we are interested in. In a nonhomogeneous society, such as ours, and through cross-cultural studies, one may find enough diversity to suggest that altering social arrangements might skew the distribution of diverse psychological traits in different ways. There are problems, however. We are constantly at risk of both overestimating and underestimating plasticity. We underestimate it if, as it seems we must, our projection of the possible is based on some estimate of the actual. And we overestimate it if, as it seems we must, we extrapolate from considerable diversity between individuals under some range of conditions to guesses about the plasticity of individuals under some other range of conditions. (As any population geneticist knows, there is great danger in such estimates.)[36]

The philosophical "data" on the concept of personal identity, our judgments about puzzle cases, does not reveal a pure or natural fact of the matter about personal identity, if my earlier discussion is right. It is adulterated by our social and moral interests and beliefs. So too, the empirical data on the range of the feasible is adulterated by the social institutions which shape our lives. Nor do we have available a simple methodology for avoiding either type of confounding factor. This suggests it is of primary importance to learn what we can about how each sort of confounding factor works. We must stop treating them as irrelevant distractions and start treating them as the subject matter of the inquiry.

One final point bears on the empirical evidence for plasticity. I noted in my discussion of Parfit that there might be some difficulties reconciling features of the Complex View with many of our ways of explaining change (causally) in an individual over time. This suggests a possible constraint on the degree of plasticity we might find it reasonable to speculate about. In proposing that certain well-ordered societies might shape persons quite differently from our own, even with regard to the degree of their psychological connectedness, we must keep in mind that in any such society people would have to be able to develop adequate explanatory theories about how people change through time. The holist attitude might be that we could always adjust our explanatory theories to accommodate the "new persons" concerned or sequences of "selves"; and of course, if there are such new persons, we would have to. But it is not clear that we should be willing to allow a significant decrease in the ability to explain psychological growth and change as a "feasible" consequence of altering the social order and persons. Our ability to explain the psychological change in persons through time is not just an abstract academic question but has deep implications for everyday social interaction.

I noted earlier that one might take Parfit to be advancing only a modest proposal, one which in fact sounds like some of Rawls' views. That is, Parfit's claim that the Complex View might support utilitarianism might be reduced only to the more modest claim that, if the Simple View is rejected, the Complex View shows that there is no deep, fixed metaphysical fact about the continuity of persons. This modest claim is compatible with the Plasticity Thesis. It is also compatible with Parfit's goal of showing that the utilitarian may not have forgotten an important fact about the importance of boundaries between persons; he just might not think such boundaries are important. This point of possible agreement between Rawls and Parfit leads us to an important question: if we can suppose that persons can be shaped in different ways by different well-ordered societies, how do we decide which conception of the person is the best one to realize or actualize?

V

I suggested in the opening section of this essay that there is a long tradition in moral philosophy whose proponents want to derive conclusions about which moral conceptions or principles are acceptable from the theory of the person. I have in mind here theorists as diverse as Aristotle, Hobbes, Hume, and even Kant, but I will not defend any of the historical attributions. The Plasticity Thesis, in a manner reminiscent of some strands of Marxist theory, seems to raise questions about the possibility of such a derivation[37] (which, incidentally, need not be an entailment but only an inference to the best account). The Thesis suggests that there are a family of possible theories of the person. Each is associatable with different moral conceptions and, thereby, with different realizations of the conceptions in well-ordered societies (to borrow Rawls' notion). The problem is that it is the preferability of the moral conception embodying a certain ideal of the person that leads us to prefer and to want to realize that conception of the person. Consequently, we cannot appeal to the *prior* acceptability of a particular theory of the person, considered in isolation from its embodiment in a moral theory, in our defense of the preferred moral theory. The acceptability of our moral theory overall, including its component theory of the person, determines the acceptability of the theory of the person.

For the theorist who thinks the derivation has to be from the acceptability of the theory of the person to the acceptability of the moral theory, the Plasticity Thesis seems to threaten the possibility of moral theory resting on a sound, objective foundation. This consequence may be the position of some Marxists, for example, who argue from the historicity of the person (actually, of human nature) to the relativity of moral theory. Does the Plasticity Thesis force such a result? Is there a view of theory acceptance in ethics that may circumvent this difficulty?

The Plasticity Thesis thus raises important general questions about the process of theory acceptance in ethics. To provide a manageable focus, I will consider what issues it raises for Rawls' own methodology of moral theory acceptance.[38] Specifically, the issue arises in this way. Many of Rawls' arguments that the original position is an acceptable device for selecting moral principles depend on a particular theory or ideal of the person he advances, one which presupposes a fairly strong criterion of personal identity. But suppose it turns out that his theory of the person is itself thought acceptable only because it meshes with moral principles and judgments we already hold. Then it is unclear what extra justificational support we get for those principles and judgments from the fact we can also derive them from the contract, for the contract, we just noted, is justifiable only because of the theory of the person. Do we risk a vitiating circle?

To state the problem more precisely, I shall need the notion of a wide reflective equilibrium. A wide reflective equilibrium consists of an ordered triple of sets of beliefs: (a) a set of considered moral judgments; (b) a set of moral principles; and (c) a set of background theories. Initial moral judgments, acceptable to a given person at a given time, are filtered to include only those of which the moral agent is confident and which have been made under conditions conducive to avoiding errors of judgment. Alternative sets of moral principles which have varying degrees of "fit" with the moral judgments are proposed, and philosophical arguments, intended to bring out the relative strengths and weaknesses of the alternative sets of principles, are advanced. These arguments can be construed as inferences from some set of relevant background theories. Assume that some particular set of arguments is persuasive and some set of moral principles is thus found most acceptable. Adjustments may have to be made to the person's considered judgments, preferred principles, and preferred background theories to arrive at an equilibrium of (a), (b), and (c). The theories in (c) may themselves be constrained by a set (a') of considered moral judgments. (There is no assumption that the set (c) is a set of nonmoral theories which constitutes a reduction of the moral, that is, of (a) and (b), to the nonmoral.) But, if the theories in (c) are to provide support for (b) that is in any way independent of the support for (b) provided by its fit with (a), then some significant portion of (a') and (a) must be disjoint. Otherwise the theories in (c) would simply be recharacterizations of the considered judgments in (a) and we would have made no greater justificatory gain in accepting (b) on the basis of (c) than we would have made had we simply established a partial equilibrium[39] directly between (b) and (a) without any appeal to the arguments derived from (c). Let us call the requirement that (a') and (a) be to some significant degree disjoint the independence constraint.[40]

Rawls' contract argument can now be shown to be a feature of a particular wide reflective equilibrium. We are led by philosophical argument, Rawls believes, to accept the contract as an appropriate device for selecting between competing conceptions of justice or right. Just such argument leads us to agree to the various formal and motivational constraints on the original position, and even to viewing the original position as an appropriate theory selection device. These arguments, however, can be viewed as inferences from a number of relevant background theories, in particular, from a theory of the person, a theory of procedural justice, general social theory, and a theory of the role of morality in society (including the ideal of a well-ordered society). Call these the Level III theories. They are what persuade us to adopt the contract apparatus, with all its constraints (call it the Level II apparatus). The principles chosen in the contract situation are subject to two constraints: (i) they must match our considered moral judgments in (partial) reflective equilibrium; and (ii) they must yield a feasible, stable well-ordered society. I will call Level I the partial reflective equilibrium that holds between the moral principles and the relevant set of considered moral judgments. Level IV (which is still behind the veil of ignorance and corresponds to Rawls' second stage of deliberation in the original position) involves testing the resulting principles at Level I for feasibility.

The independence constraint previously defined for wide equilibrium in general applies in this way: the considered moral judgments (a') which may act to constrain Level III theory acceptability must to a significant extent be disjoint from the considered moral judgments (a) which act to constrain Level I partial equilibrium. Our question now is whether the Plasticity Thesis leads to conflict with this independence constraint.[41]

Just how might the Plasticity Thesis lead us to violate the independence constraint? Suppose we are deliberating about which of two views of the person is most acceptable as a Level III theory. One involves a strong, and one a weak, criterion of personal identity. We might be tempted to say the following: "We hold a number of moral judgments and principles about rights and entitlements which match the Kantian view and which fail to match the utilitarian view. Therefore, we should pick the strong criterion of identity and the other features of the theory of the person that fit best with the Kantian moral judgments we hold. Then we can use the resulting ideal of the person to justify the contract apparatus, and, finally, derive our Level I principles from the Level II apparatus." Such an approach allows the considered judgments (a) at Level I to act as the primary constraint on our selection of the Level III theory. This does not by itself show that the whole set of judgments (a') so constraining the Level III theory is not significantly disjoint with (a). But it gives us good reason to be suspicious.

It may well be possible to defend the strong criterion of personal identity without appealing directly to considered judgments in (a). Such a defense would be interesting and important. Perhaps one could make relevant some remarks of Bernard Williams, who suggests that our long-term projects in life are what give meaning to our "going on in life" so that we choose to survive rather than not to survive.[42] Or perhaps a defense lies in Rawls' remarks about the highest-order interests persons have in determining how their fundamental interests are to be ordered. But I will not attempt to defend the strong criterion here. Indeed, demanding a *direct* defense of the strong personal identity criterion over the weak one may be too strong a requirement. It might be enough to show the strong criterion is feasible and that the view of the person as a whole that emerges is preferable to a view that embodies the weaker criterion. The preferability of the "view as a whole," of course, should not depend on Level I considered judgments either; that is only passing the buck. It might even be enough to show that the view of the person as a whole is as good as (or no worse than) any other and that it is feasible and that the moral theory as a whole is better.

Here we face the problem that there are only *vague* constraints on theory acceptance imposed by the holistic view embodied in the notion of wide reflective equilibrium.

I have not provided a clear-cut answer to the question whether the Plasticity Thesis runs afoul of Rawls' general methodological approach, including the independence constraint I have suggested is necessary. There are reasons to be leary of the Plasticity Thesis, but there may well be ways to show that it does not violate the constraint, either by providing a direct defense for it or by defending a more relaxed coherence view that requires no direct defense of the criterion. To be optimistic, at least it is not established that the Plasticity Thesis violates the constraint.

Does the Plasticity Thesis make it more likely that some form of moral relativism will seem true, given wide reflective equilibrium as a method for theory acceptance? Suppose there are no arguments that make a particular criterion of personal identity, and thus some particular view of the person, more acceptable than another, at least not without risking violation of the independence constraint. Suppose further that neither criterion is superior on feasibility considerations. Does this lead us closer to failure of convergence on a wide reflective equilibrium, a failure which might incline us toward the view that a deep relativism underlies moral beliefs?

Here too I can offer nothing decisive. Whether convergence emerges among significantly diverse individuals on a particular wide equilibrium is best left an open empirical question. If we cannot appeal to component theories within that wide equilibrium, such as the theory of the person, as a source of convergence, then intuitively it seems that there will be more leeway for divergence. But the direction of influence can also work the other way: factors which lead to convergence in wide equilibrium as a whole may lead to convergence on the component theory of the person. Again, we cannot give decisive answers.[43] Still, it is worth pointing out that convergence in wide equilibrium is best viewed as neither a necessary nor a sufficient condition for the contained theories to constitute some notion of "objective moral truth." We must attend to explanations of *why* the convergence is attainable. Conversely, divergence is neither a necessary nor sufficient condition for concluding that moral beliefs are ultimately relative and cannot be "objective moral knowledge." These issues require their own full discussion.[44]

NOTES

1 I am indebted to C. A. J. Coady, Josh Cohen, Daniel C. Dennett, Barbara Herman, Miles Morgan, and Amélie Rorty for helpful suggestions about

the ideas contained in this paper, and to The National Endowment for the Humanities, which funded my research on this and related papers cited herein.

2 I do not mean to suggest these are the same, for it will be a contingent question whether every human is a person and every person a human. In general, persons can be thought of as a broader class, with humans a particular instantiation. On the Kantian view under discussion here, what is relevant about humans for the purposes of moral and political theory is that they *can* be persons, not the facts, of interest to philosophical anthropology, about special human motives, interests, and emotions.

3 See Derek Parfit, "Later Selves and Moral Principles," in *Philosophy and Personal Relations*, Alan Montefiore, ed. (London: Routledge and Kegan Paul, 1973), pp. 137–69; and John Rawls, "Independence of Moral Theory," *Proceedings and Addresses of the American Philosophical Association* 48 (1974–75): 5–22.

4 The title of Rawls' paper, and some of his remarks, suggest he is arguing for the independence of moral theory and philosophy of mind. He is more plausibly taken to support a view that the two are nonhierarchically interdependent, which, in any case, is the view I will defend.

5 Cf. Parfit, "Later Selves and Moral Principles," pp. 139–40.

6 Cf. David Lewis, "Survival and Identity," in *The Identities of Persons*, Amélie Oksenberg Rorty, ed. (Berkeley: Univ. of California Press, 1976), pp. 17–40; and Bernard Williams, "The Self and the Future," *Philosophical Review* 79 (April 1970): 2, reprinted in *Personal Identity*, John Perry, ed. (Berkeley: Univ. of California Press, 1975), pp. 179–98.

7 Parfit, "Later Selves," p. 140.

8 Amélie Rorty and Barbara Herman suggested this point.

9 As Parfit reminds us, cf. "Later Selves," p. 165, esp. n. 65; Parfit's more direct arguments against the Simple View are developed elsewhere, e.g., in his "Personal Identity," *Philosophical Review* 80 (January 1971): 3–27.

10 Bernard Williams has plausibly challenged Parfit on the applicability of the diminished scope claim to the case of promising. Cf. "Persons, Character, and Morality," in *The Identities of Persons*, pp. 197–216. C. A. J. Coady has persuaded me that Parfit's discussion of the Russian nobleman depends for its plausibility on an untenably rigid view of promising. Cf. "Later Selves," pp. 145ff.

11 This claim is not quite true, as Parfit notes, since even on the Simple View we may have *other* ways of attenuating the force of the principles or overriding them.

12 Parfit, "Later Selves," p. 143.

13 Ibid., p. 147.

14 Ibid., p. 148.

15 Miles Morgan first brought this point clearly to my attention.

16 When is a fact a "deep" one? Kripke has suggested that being born of my parents is one of my essential properties. If that status is sufficient to make the fact a "deep" one, it is not enough to make it a morally important one, at least not a generally morally important one. George Smith suggested the example to me.

17 Parfit's formula; "Later Selves," p. 149.
18 Parfit cites David Gauthier, *Practical Reasoning* (Oxford: Clarendon, 1963), p. 126; and John Rawls, *A Theory of Justice* (Cambridge, MA: Harvard, 1971), p. 28.
19 Cf. Parfit, "Later Selves," pp. 149–53.
20 Parfit ("Later Selves," p. 153) cites Rawls, *A Theory of Justice*, pp. 27, 191; also Thomas Nagel, *Possibility of Altruism* (Oxford: Clarendon, 1970), p. 134.
21 Parfit, "Later Selves," p. 153.
22 This point was suggested to me by Barbara Herman.
23 As Amélie Rorty has suggested to me. The point is that there may be only an historical, not conceptual, tie of some deontological views to strong views of personal identity.
24 Rawls seems to attribute such an argument to Parfit (cf. Rawls, "Independence of Moral Theory," p. 19, n. 6), although he does not explicitly do so. In any case, Parfit refrains from advancing his claims about the implications of the Complex View as anything more than a possible defense of utilitarianism. (Cf. "Later Selves," p. 165, n. 65.)
25 Cf. Rawls, "Independence of Moral Theory," pp. 17–19. Rawls points out that even the utilitarian view must keep a strong enough criterion of personal identity to calculate the effect through time of causal influences on persons that alter their capacity for satisfaction.
26 Cf. Rawls, "Independence of Moral Theory," pp. 15–20.
27 Ibid., p. 19.
28 With reference to premises (3) and (5), see my "Reflective Equilibrium and Archimedean Points," *Canadian Journal of Philosophy* 10 (1980): 1:83–103 for a discussion of the role of Rawls' theory of the person in the wide reflective equilibrium that characterizes justice as fairness. Premise (4) amounts to agreement with some parts of Parfit's argument, though not necessarily with Parfit's claim, challenged above, that making personal identity a less deep metaphysical fact is *evidence* or support for the utilitarian view.
29 Rawls, "Independence of Moral Theory," p. 19.
30 Ibid., p. 20.
31 Which is not to say that it is "just" a question of value, and therefore not a fact at all, because it is not a determinate matter of nonmoral fact; see my remarks in the next section.
32 Cf. Hilary Putnam, "Meaning of 'Meaning'" and "Explanation and Reference," in his *Mind, Language and Reality*, vol. 2 (Cambridge: Cambridge University Press, 1975), ch. 11 and 12; see also Saul Kripke, "Naming & Necessity," in G. Harman and D. Davidson, eds., *The Semantics of Natural Language* (Dordrecht: Reidel, 1972), p. 253–355. I intend to leave open the question whether persons are a natural kind or a genus including a number of natural kinds (humans, martians, dolphins, etc). Moreover, I think there may be difficulties treating persons as a natural kind if the critical description of them is purely functional, but I cannot go into these issues here.
33 Bernard Williams' discussion of our attitude toward suffering through exotic changes is an exception (there are others as well) to my generaliza-

tion. Cf. Williams, "The Self and the Future," *Philosophical Review* 79 (April 1970): 161–80, reprinted in Perry, ed., *Personal Identity*, pp. 179–98.

34 By "social" theory, here, I include certain parts of social psychology and sociology which are relevant to exploring how we view personality change through time, given that we have certain *interests* in doing so.

35 Rawls, "Independence of Moral Theory," p. 20.

36 See, for example, Norman Daniels, "IQ, Heritability & Human Nature," *PSA 1974, BU Studies in the Philosophy of Science*, vol. 32, R. S. Cohen, C. A. Hooker, A. C. Michalos, and J. W. Van Evra, eds. (Dordrecht: Reidel, 1976), pp. 143–80.

37 The Plasticity Thesis is, of course, more general than, and not committed to, any historical materialist thesis.

38 I believe the methodology I will sketch is a fair reconstruction (and clarification) of Rawls', whether it departs in detail from his views or not, and is a promising approach to the problems of theory acceptance in ethics. See my "On Some Methods of Ethics and Linguistics," *Philosophical Studies* 37 (1980): 21–36, my "Wide Reflective Eqilibrium and Theory Acceptance in Ethics," *Journal of Philosophy* 76 (May 1979): 256–82, and my "Reflective Equilibrium and Archimedean Points" for more detailed discussion of the method.

39 A partial equilibrium is part of a wide equilibrium; it holds between a component theory or set of principles and some relevant subset of the considered judgments.

40 One way to satisfy it would be for (a') to contain moral judgments different in type from those in (a). For example, if (a) contains moral judgments about rights and entitlements, (a') will not, whatever others it does contain. We might then say that judgments about rights and entitlements can be founded on these other moral notions. I am indebted to George Smith for helpful discussion of the independence constraint. It is discussed in greater detail in my "Reflective Equilibrium and Archimedean Points," where I argue that positing a deep "right-based" theory, involving a right to equal respect, risks violating the independence constraint. Cf. Dworkin, "The Original Position," *University of Chicago Law Review* 40 (Spring 1973): 500–33, reprinted in N. Daniels, ed., *Reading Rawls* (New York: Basic Books, 1975), pp. 16–53.

41 In my "Reflective Equilibrium and Archimedean Points," I argue that many disagreements about the justificational force of the contract argument can be resolved when the problem is viewed in this way and the independence constraint is respected.

42 See Bernard Williams, "Persons, Character, and Morality," in Rorty, *Identities of Persons*, pp. 197–216. Incidentally, Williams overdraws the contrast between his view of character and "projects" and Rawls' notion of a rational plan of life. But the issue requires closer examination.

43 At least one is not forced to infer relativism is true, as some Marxists have thought who have advanced a special version of the Plasticity Thesis.

44 For some remarks on these questions, see my "Wide Reflective Equilibrium and Theory Acceptance in Ethics," pp. 273–82.

Chapter 8

Reflective equilibrium and justice as political

1. POLITICIZING JUSTICE: PLURALISM AND STABILITY

In *A Theory of Justice* (hereafter *Theory*), Rawls argues that justice as fairness provides an Archimedean point from which to assess the justice of social institutions (Rawls 1971, 260–3). If a contractarian agreement on principles of cooperation were tied too closely to the actual interests and desires of persons, for example, if no veil of ignorance were present, then it would not provide such an Archimedean point. People are shaped by the institutions under which they live, and a contract reflecting their known interests would be mired too much in the effects of those institutions to provide critical leverage. Traditional alternative ways of anchoring that Archimedean point, such as a priori or perfectionist assumptions about the nature of persons and the social order, are also unattractive for several reasons. For one, such assumptions usually are too general to yield a useable contract. Alternatively, idealized contractors may seem so unreal to us that we cannot identify with them or their choices. Finally, the assumptions may be too narrowly held to provide a basis for common agreement. How, then, is that Archimedean point to be established?

If Rawls' Original Position had been based only on the weakest assumptions about human rationality – that is, if justice were derivable from rationality alone – then it would be clear how the Archimedean point was secured. The Original Position, however, rested on more robust assumptions: "reasonable" people had to agree it was an appropriate device for selecting principles of justice because the contract procedure was fair to all participants. In the decade after *Theory* was published, partly in response to claims that justice as fairness rested on a "deep theory" (see Dworkin 1973), Rawls fleshed out the set of beliefs or ideals that one must accept in order to consider the Original Position an appropriate device for selecting among alternative conceptions of justice.

By the time the Dewey Lectures (1980) were published, Rawls had clarified the importance of several key background ideas that had been insufficiently emphasized in *Theory*, even though they were modeled in the Original Position and were necessary to motivate the construction in justice as fairness. These included the ideal of a "free and equal" moral agent with two basic moral powers; a capacity to form and revise a conception of the good and a sense of justice. Persons so conceived have a "higher-order interest" in securing the development of those powers. The background ideas also included the ideal of a well-ordered society and a conception of procedural justice. The Archimedean point was rooted in acceptance of these beliefs or ideals, and people who find these ideas unacceptable "will be unmoved by justice as fairness even granting the validity of its arguments" (Rawls 1974, 637; see Daniels 1980, 85).

What would lead people to accept these ideas in the "deep theory"? The answer seemed to be this: philosophical arguments involving the comparison of alternative conceptions of justice and their underlying ideas would persuade "us" to converge on these beliefs in wide reflective equilibrium. Although these beliefs were not a priori (indeed, they were revisable), they would, after due reflection, be considered acceptable to a wide majority of people. Ultimately, justification for a conception of justice consisted of that view being contained within a wide reflective equilibrium of an individual's beliefs. The wide reflective equilibrium was a coherent set of considered moral judgments about justice at all levels of generality, principles of justice, deeper background beliefs or ideals of the person and of the role of morality in society, and even general social theory. To achieve wide reflective equilibrium, an individual worked back and forth among all these elements, testing principles against cases, considering philosophical arguments defending different theoretical perspectives, and revising wherever necessary to produce the most acceptable set of beliefs.

Rawls confirms this picture of the task in *Theory* and its focus on the individual undertaking a philosophical task:

> TJ [*Theory*] does not address persons as citizens but rather as individuals trying to work out their own conception of justice as it applies to the basic political and social institutions of democratic society. For the most part their task is solitary as they reflect on their own considered judgments with their fixed points and the several first principles and intermediate concepts and the ideals they affirm. TJ is presented as a work individuals might study in their attempt – admittedly never fully achieved and always to be striven for – to attain the self-understanding of wide reflective equilibrium. (Rawls 1995b, 6)

As we shall see, this characterization and its contrast with the task in *Political Liberalism* contributes to the feeling some people have that the role of philosophical activity changes between the two books and that the politicization of justice and justification involves "philosophical loss" in a sense to be explained in the next section.

In retrospect, it seems quite striking that little attention was paid at this stage of the development of Rawls' thinking [or mine (see Daniels 1979, Ch. 2; 1980, Ch. 3), following and elaborating on his] to the great diversity in beliefs about philosophical, religious, and even moral matters that would have to be incorporated in such wide reflective equilibria. Perhaps the narrowed focus of attention came from the fact that so much of *Theory* was concerned with defeating utilitarianism, and the arguments needed for doing so drew on a narrow spectrum within a shared philosophical tradition. But whatever the explanation, there was little attention paid to the kinds of diversity present in our own society.

Once we focus on that diversity in background beliefs, it seems less plausible to think that the same philosophical arguments about the acceptability of justice as fairness and its deeper components would be persuasive to all, regardless of their starting points. The very criteria for what would count as a good philosophical argument would be affected by some of those background beliefs. The point was made by a number of critics, of course, that people holding certain fundamentalist religious views, for example, would find themselves unable to commit themselves to the principles of justice (see White 1991, Ch. 10). These cases might have been dismissed as marginal, however. For example, one important adequacy test that a conception of justice must pass, according to *Theory*, is that it be feasible in this sense: it must be possible in general for people who grow up under social institutions governed by it to be motivated to comply with it. But stability does not require the compliance of everyone, regardless of how far out of the mainstream their views might be. Insofar as these exceptions are thought relevant to the stability test, then perhaps they could just be ignored (cf. Barry 1995). This dismissal, however, meant not taking seriously enough the implications of the more general problem of pluralism.

The fact of pluralism is pervasive and deep and cannot be simply ignored. Especially under conditions of freedom of thought and expression, the very conditions protected by the principles characterizing justice as fairness, people are likely to develop quite varied solutions to the complex moral and philosophical issues that humans seek answers to. Suppose we restrict our concerns in worrying about convergence or stability to people who are "reasonable" in this sense: they are concerned to live with others on fair terms, assuming that the others are so willing; they also understand that to be fair the terms of cooperation must be ones that other free and equal persons can accept (Rawls 1993, 48–54; cf. Cohen 1994a, 1537). Reasonable people, we should also suppose, will then recognize that others who share this concern to cooperate on acceptable terms will be led to disagreements on many issues because of what Rawls calls the "burdens of judgment" (1993, 54–58). These burdens include the following conditions: the conflicting and complex evidence that bears on issues, the disagreements about how to weight considerations, the vagueness of some of our concepts, the effects of the totality of a person's experience on how that person weights considerations, and the multiplicity of normative considerations that are relevant and from which a selection must be made in any specific case. We are driven, Rawls concludes, to accept *reasonable pluralism* about many matters of importance. This is a basic fact of political life, and even among reasonable people, we will find disagreements that threaten the original suggestion that philosophical argument could produce convergence on the same wide reflective equilibrium.

The specific feature of his theory that, by the late 1980s, seemed to Rawls most incompatible with the fact of pluralism was his account of stability, one of two conditions of adequacy he imposes on theories of justice in *Theory* (the other is acceptability in wide reflective equilibrium). As I noted earlier, a theory of justice must yield a stable social arrangement, at least compared to alternative conceptions. People raised in a well-ordered society governed by a conception of justice must be able to abide by the commitments of that conception without unacceptable strain. Justice must engage their motivations.

Rawls is not here concerned about the general fact that acting morally will sometimes involve a sacrifice of individual self-interest. He is not worried about the traditional skeptic, who asks "Why should I be just rather than pursue my own rational advantage?" Rather, he has in mind the moral person who will say, "Why should I be just, since justice is not as important as salvation" or "why should I be just, since justice is not as important as establishing a caring community?" Such persons are presumably willing to sacrifice their self-interest on occasion to the demands of morality. The problem is that they also sacrifice justice to other moral concerns, since they do not give the priority to justice over other values that justice as fairness requires. Over time, given the burdens of judgment, people will be raised in and attracted to diverse moral conceptions of this sort, even though they also share a common framework of institutions governed by, say, justice as fairness. Stability is threatened if concerns about justice are overridden in these ways by enough people who are influenced by these comprehensive moral and religious views.

147

In *Theory*, Rawls (1971, S. 86) argued that there was a "congruence" between acting in accordance with justice and the good for people. This argument, however, seems to have invoked particular views about the good of autonomy that are characteristic of certain comprehensive liberal views, such as Mill's or Kant's (see Freeman 1994; Cohen 1994a; Rawls 1995a; but see Barry 1995 for reservations about the scope of this appeal to a comprehensive view). People holding other comprehensive moral views, or views that did not share this particular assessment of the good of autonomy, would have a different view of the strains of commitment. For example, liberal Catholics would not accept the Kantian view of the importance of autonomy. They might, nevertheless, have other reasons for accepting the principles of justice, for example, that the principles manifest God's natural law (see Freeman 1994, 632).

How, then, can the Archimedean point be secured? How can it be maintained as a stable point? If we cannot assume that (even reasonable) people with diverse comprehensive views can be led by reasoned philosophical argument, or rather, by some specific set of such arguments, to stable convergence on justice as fairness, how can convergence, including stability, be achieved? What is the deepest form of stability that can be achieved, given reasonable pluralism? This is the central question raised by *Political Liberalism* (hereafter *Liberalism*).

Rawls' answer to this problem is to recast justice as fairness as a "free standing" *political* conception of justice. The key ideas out of which justice as fairness (or other alternative reasonable political conceptions of justice) are constructed, for example, the idea that citizens are free and equal, are now taken to be shared elements of our political life, that is, of a public, democratic culture. These ideas are already held or accepted by most people who share that culture, whatever other views they diverge on. In effect, it is not philosophy alone – aided by universal reason – that has led people to converge on these ideas but a shared set of institutions and history.

Rawls (1993, 145; 1995a, 149) suggests that we think of the political conception of justice as fairness as a "module" with its own internal principles, reasons, and standards of evidence. For example, justice as fairness includes the two principles of justice ordered in a particular way. Together these ordered principles, illuminated by the shared background ideas and publicly defendable standards of evidence and reasoning, specify the content of "public reason" as it is used to deliberate about matters of justice. This module should be complete: it should give "reasonable" answers to a broad range of questions about "constitutional essentials and basic questions of justice" (1995a, 142). These answers are "reasonable," however, in light of the kinds of reasons to which the political conception is restricted. In effect, the justification for these answers only goes so far: it appeals only to reasons contained in the public view. Rawls calls this "pro tanto justification." To say that a claim about what is just is justified "pro tanto," however, is not yet to say that it is a fully justified belief for a particular person. The criterion for full justification ultimately remains acceptability in wide reflective equilibrium (1995a, 141–43), and pro tanto justification deliberately refrains from seeking such deeper justification. (I later introduce the term "political reflective equilibrium" to characterize the limited results of pro tanto justification as compared to full justification.) By not seeking or alluding to deeper justification, pro tanto justification does not alienate those who have different reasons for accepting the module.

The module is ultimately justified for people in quite different ways, depending on other aspects of the comprehensive views they hold in wide reflective equilibrium. Rawls calls this "full justification" (1995a, 143). No uniform or universal philosophical argument produces a shared rationale for, and convergence on, the module. Instead, it is incorporated for different reasons within the distinct wide reflective equilibria that coexist in a pluralist society. Within the public domain, where we debate matters of justice, we need not – indeed we should not – appeal to those deeper justifications at all. We simply build on people's agreement with the basic ideas and restrict their reasoning about matters of justice to the kinds of considerations internal to the political conception of justice. We restrict them to "public reason."

We obtain the greatest stability we can for a political conception of justice, Rawls argues, answering his central question in *Liberalism*, when there is the right type of "overlapping consensus" on it, that is, when there is overlapping consensus for the right reasons. People with different comprehensive moral views must justify for themselves, by their own lights, that is, in their own wide reflective equilibria, the acceptability of the module. Their rationales will thus differ in ways that reflect their other philosophical, moral, and religious beliefs. Some may insist, for example, that there is "moral truth"; others deny it. Some might see the principles of justice as forms of divinely given natural law; others may see it as a human construction. Ultimately, people are justified in accepting justice as fairness if it is acceptable to them in the different wide reflective equilibria they can achieve.

If there is *general* acceptance in this way of the module within the different "reasonable" comprehensive views in a society, Rawls says that we have "general" reflective equilibrium (1995a, 141, n. 16). It is obvious that general reflective equilibrium is not itself a shared wide reflective equilibrium – except for the overlap on the module. Rawls now explicitly rejects the account of stability he offered in *Theory*, namely, that there is general convergence on a wide reflective equilibrium with comprehensive liberal commitments. On that (rejected) view, justice was a good for each person because each viewed autonomy as a particularly important good and autonomy was adequately respected by justice as fairness. On the revised view, justice is now a good for each on his or her own terms, which may not at all include the Kantian or Millian view of the good of autonomy, and justice is ascribed a priority over other values that reflects what is acceptable in light of those other nonpolitical values. The context and strength of this priority may thus vary from person to person, depending on their views in wide reflective equilibrium. The emphasis that different comprehensive views give to such issues as sexual behavior or family control over moral education means that the boundary between the political and nonpolitical varies across wide reflective equilibria. Whatever the pressures are that lead to convergence on the module, so that an overlapping consensus is formed, they are not sufficient to force convergence on a single wide reflective equilibrium, that is, on a shared, general equilibrium.

Before turning in the next section to the question of philosophical loss alluded to earlier, it will help to distinguish several strands of the argument about stability and to show how these elements fit together. In both *Theory* and *Liberalism*, Rawls retains the same "feasibility" condition on the acceptability of a theory of justice. Specifically, a conception of justice is feasible if it can produce a stable, well-ordered society (as compared to alternative conceptions of justice). What changes between *Theory* and *Liberalism*, as a result of taking reasonable pluralism seriously, is the way in which individuals fit justice as fairness within their overall systems of moral (and other) beliefs. In *Liberalism*, Rawls emphasizes how the key ideas in justice as fairness are present as "free standing" ideas in the public culture formed by the institutions governed by that (political) conception of justice. Institutions play an educative role about the value of those ideas, and this provides opportunity and pressure for individuals with reasonable comprehensive views to elaborate those views in ways that accommodate them to the political conception, providing for overlapping consensus for the right reasons (more on this educative role later).

What is sometimes confusing, however, is that Rawls develops another line of argument in *Liberalism* (1993, 158–67) that is aimed at showing how a broader and deeper consensus – an overlapping consensus for the right reasons – could develop from an initial narrower agreement on some constitutional procedures. Notice that this line of argument attempts to answer the question, How can we get to (stable) convergence on an overlapping consensus if we don't start with one? That is, since we clearly lack such an overlapping consensus, how do we get there from here? But the original question behind the stability test – in both *Theory* and *Liberalism* – is, How do we stay there once we achieve a well-ordered society? How are these two different questions, or their answers, related?

I believe they are related in this way: telling a plausible story about how we might get there from here makes it more plausible that we could stay there once we got there, since getting there is generally harder than staying there. The story about how we might develop a wider and deeper overlapping consensus should make it seem more plausible that, if we were raised in a well-ordered society governed by a political conception of justice as fairness, we could maintain our commitments to giving priority to justice despite the fact of reasonable pluralism.

The reader should not be confused, however, by the shift in questions. The question, How do we get there from here? cannot replace the original question in the stability test, How do we stay committed to a just social order, given reasonable pluralism? In *Liberalism* and in more recent writings, Rawls (see 1995b) also emphasizes that there may be an overlapping consensus on certain key ideas in the democratic culture without there being agreement that, say, justice as fairness is the most reasonable interpretation of those ideas. Rawls suggests (see 1995b) that considerable stability might obtain even in such a situation, although there would also be continuing dispute about some constitutional essentials and matters of basic justice. It is arguable, for example, that the United States is in just such a situation. If there is reasonable stability under these conditions, then we might expect that stability for a well-ordered society governed by a political conception of justice as fairness might also be stable. Once again, the argument about nonideal contexts may be evidentiary for the stability argument about the ideal context.

2. PHILOSOPHICAL LOSS?

Some people have reacted to the politicization of justice with a sense of philosophical loss. This was my own reaction, at least initially. They complain that philosophy is demoted when justice is politicized. Others have thought the approach requires a form of moral schizophrenia or, better, a form of multiple personality disorder. Justification is bifurcated: we keep a tally or ledger of reasons appropriate for justification in the public domain, and then we have a separate ledger of reasons we can use in a broader moral domain. We are divided into double bookkeepers for moral purposes. What kind of moral integrity is there if we keep two sets of moral books? These are serious concerns.

Perhaps the sense of philosophical loss can be explicated by appealing to the metaphor about an Archimedean point with which we began.

If, on the original view, philosophical argument alone could be persuasive to people with diverse views and could lead them to converge on the deep theory underlying justice as fairness, then it seemed reasonable to think that justice as fairness constituted an Archimedean point. It was not mired in the actual interests and desires of people in a specific setting, thereby avoiding the Scylla of infection by existing institutions. It was also not based on a priori or perfectionist premises, thus avoiding the Charybdis of unacceptable generality and abstraction. But if the ideas out of which the political conception of justice are constructed must already be embedded in a shared democratic culture, then why are they not "mired" in existing institutions in ways that challenge their credentials as an Archimedean point? Can we really use them to criticize the justice of existing institutions if they are the products of the very culture that produces those institutions? Can we be sure we have agreement on more than a mere compromise, a modus vivendi, or the results of historical accident or a stage of class struggle? Can we be sure our theory captures what is truly just, what anyone thinking clearly and critically could come to recognize as just, rather than what people with a particular history have been acclimated to think of as just? (In *Theory*, Rawls says little, one way or the other, about the origins of these ideas in a democratic culture; the underlying assumption seems to be that these ideas, wherever they came from, would emerge as justifiable in light of philosophical arguments. Cf. Rawls 1995b, 6, quoted early in Section 1 of this chapter.)

Alternatively, can we really be sure there is stable agreement on the same module, the same conception of justice, if people find "it" acceptable for such different reasons and in light of such different considerations? How complete will the contents of the module be if there is divergence about the priority the view is given on many issues? What is it like to "justify" matters in the political domain solely by reference to the contents of public reason when nonpolitical values clearly have a bearing on those matters, at least as judged by some comprehensive moral views? Can people say to themselves, "Although I have fundamental values and beliefs that bear on this issue of behavior, I will refrain from raising them and consider only the reasons permitted by public reason?" Is this moral double bookkeeping a kind of multiple moral personality disorder? Perhaps Supreme Court justices can put on a public hat and refrain from introducing their nonpolitical values into their reasoning (though historically, this is not obvious), but can each of us as citizens really wear two morally distinct hats in this way?

In the politicization of justice, have we lost our grip on both the notions of justice and justification we thought we had in the earlier view? In the remainder of this essay, I want to explore these issues in greater detail. In the next section, I begin by comparing more carefully the notion of justification in the early and late theories. I return in sections 4 and 5 to consider replies to some of these questions.

3. WIDE REFLECTIVE EQUILIBRIUM: BEFORE AND AFTER POLITICIZATION

A point to emphasize at the outset is that, in both early and late theories, the heart of the account of justification remains an appeal to *wide reflective equilibrium*. Details may vary about what the wide reflective equilibria will look like, but Rawls remains committed to a broadly coherentist view of justification. Specifically, justice as fairness is justified for an individual – both before and after politicization – if it is the conception of justice that is most acceptable to her, given all her other beliefs, in wide reflective equilibrium. (I will say nothing here to clarify the notion of "coherence" except to note that it is intended to be more robust than an appeal to mere logical consistency; for example, inference to the best explanation will be crucial in much development of ethical theory, as it is in science. I also note that Rawls' commitments to constructivism fit within his appeal to a coherentist account of justification in general.)

In appealing to this coherentist view of justification in *Theory*, Rawls felt he was making justification in ethics accord with an account of justification quite broad in its use and appeal. He noted that the idea was originally cited by Goodman as an account of justification for logic, both deductive and inductive (Rawls 1971, 20). In this chapter, I will not consider the important philosophical controversies that surround this coherentist approach in general. Instead, I concentrate on how those modifications of it that result from politicization bear on the issues of philosophical loss and justificatory schizophrenia.

To assess the effects of politicization on the *contents* of wide reflective equilibrium, we should be as clear as possible about just what the justice as fairness "module" contains when we achieve general and wide equilibrium in an overlapping consensus. This module, Rawls insists, is invariant between *Theory* and *Liberalism*. Although some critics have suggested that Rawls has backed away from some of the implications of fair equality of opportunity or the difference principle, Rawls explicitly denies this interpretation. He does so with some exasperation:

> Some think the difference principle is abandoned entirely, others that I no more affirm justice as fairness than any other political conception of justice. And they do so despite the fact that early on I say that justice as fairness is held intact (modulo the account of stability) and affirmed as much as before in TJ . . . If I had dropped something as central as

the difference principle, I like to think I would have said so. (1995b, 2, n. 1)

I believe the confusion in some readers arises from the fact that a political conception of justice using the same democratic ideas that justice as fairness uses might not combine them in the optimal way Rawls believes his conception achieves. Rawls says that justice as fairness is the "most reasonable," not the only reasonable conception based on those ideas.

The module for justice as fairness consists of the following elements: (1) the Original Position, with all of its constraints on knowledge and motivation; (2) the lexically ordered principles of justice that contractors choose in the Original Position, assuring equal basic liberties, fair equality of opportunity, and inequalities that work to the maximum advantage of those who are worst off; (3) several key background ideas: the idea of free and equal moral agents, each having two fundamental moral powers, namely, the capacity to form and revise a conception of the good and to develop a sense of justice; the idea of society as a fair scheme of social cooperation; the idea of a well-ordered society, that is, a society effectively regulated by a public conception of justice; and a conception of procedural justice. The key background ideas are contained in the module because they provide the rationale for the specific design of the Original Position. This rationale for the construction of the Original Position must be a part of justice as fairness itself.

We come to the first important difference between the wide reflective equilibria in *Theory* and *Liberalism* when we note that the key background ideas are themselves in need of justification. We accept them, and they are justified, in light of other things we believe in wide reflective equilibrium. The full rationale for these key background ideas cannot be part of justice as fairness, for then agreement on the module would necessarily involve agreement for the same reasons in wide equilibrium. That wider agreement is exactly what the fact of reasonable pluralism, emphasized in *Liberalism*, makes politically impossible (in the foreseeable future). In *Theory*, philosophical arguments comparing alternative conceptions were presumed to lead "us" to accept the same background ideas for the same reasons. In *Liberalism*, justice as fairness is called a "free standing" view to signal the fact that it is severed from its (full) rationale or justification, which will vary from reasonable comprehensive view to reasonable comprehensive view.

To sharpen our understanding of the change in wide reflective equilibria before and after politicization, it will help to illustrate more concretely what it means to say that a key idea, for example, that persons are free and equal, is now construed as "political" and "free standing." It will also help to illustrate just how different wide reflective equilibria could provide distinct rationales for the same free-standing idea. Cohen's (1994a, 1522–25) discussion of both points is remarkably clear and helpful, and I draw on it in the next two paragraphs.

A central feature of justice as fairness, captured in the use of a veil of ignorance in the Original Position, is the distinction between "relevant" and "irrelevant" features of persons. The veil blocks out such "irrelevant" features as sex, race, class position, talents and skills, and even a person's specific conception of what is good in life. In this way it models a "relevant" feature of persons, that they can form and revise conceptions of the good, and it blocks out an irrelevant one, that they happen to think in some particular way about what is good. In *Theory*, however, the impression is created that the boundary between relevant and irrelevant features is drawn at least partly in terms of a comprehensive liberal view, such as Kant's or Mill's. For example, the suggestion that all will view the exercise of autonomy as an intrinsic good, which appears in the discussion of the nature of the good of autonomy in the argument for congruence and stability, is plausible as a liberal claim about our "nature" and thus about what distinguishes relevant from irrelevant features. In *Liberalism*, the same boundary is drawn, but now "irrelevant" or "contingent" features of persons carry no metaphysical overtones or allusions to comprehensive moral views. They simply refer to features that are not relevant to political argument, and we can tell which these are by "systematizing and extending reasonably familiar ideas about the justification of political arrangements in a democratic society . . . we look to settled ideals and convictions about basic democratic institutions, and to settled understandings about the justification of public norms in a democratic society, and then draw the relevant–irrelevant distinction by reference to the characteristics of persons that play a role in those ideas, convictions, and understandings" (Cohen 1994a, 1523). A feature of persons can then be called "contingent" and mean only that it is not important for political purposes, not that someone can exist without it (as Sandel 1982 seems to suggest).

In *Liberalism*, Rawls asks us to imagine an overlapping consensus of four different reasonable comprehensive views, each of which incorporates justice as fairness, though for different reasons. Cohen (1994a, 1527) suggests how three of these might endorse the idea that citizens are free in the sense that is modeled by the veil of ignorance, namely, that they are free to form and revise their conceptions of a good life and that they have an interest in establishing conditions that permit them to do so. A Kantian morality would support freedom in this sense because it calls for reflective deliberation about ends and requires us to respect people as autonomous choosers. A utilitarian concerned with the conditions that promote long-term happiness would also respect the interest we have in being able to revise our ends in life. A religious conception that endorsed free faith would accept the conception of freedom here because religious obligations cannot be fulfilled unless people genuinely are persuaded of the religious values (Cohen 1994a, 1527, cites Locke's "A Letter Concerning Toleration" as an example of this view). The rationale for the key idea is dramatically different in each wide reflective equilibrium, but the same idea is justified for someone occupying any of these different equilibria. Saying it is justified in this way means that it is truly accepted for its fit with other deeply held values and beliefs, not simply that it is accepted as a matter of compromise or begrudging accommodation.

To summarize our observations so far, consult Table 8.1. In it we note that the justice as fairness module is identical in content in both *Theory* and *Liberalism*. In *Liberalism*, however, the module is called "free standing." The first important difference in the wide reflective equilibria before and after politicization is that the rationale for the module in *Liberalism* is said to be specific to each wide reflective equilibrium. In contrast, in *Theory* the rationale is based on shared philosophical arguments, including the Kantian view of autonomy that played a role in the original argument for convergence.

The second important difference in the contents of wide reflective equilibria in *Theory* and *Liberalism* is that in *Liberalism*, the wide reflective equilibria contained in the overlapping consensus must each contain beliefs about the fact of reasonable pluralism, including an account of the burdens of judgment. Each thus contains an understanding and acceptance of the fact that reasonable people may disagree on fundamental moral matters and yet be reasonable in the sense that they are willing to cooperate with others on terms acceptable to others who share the same concern for cooperation. Each also accepts the idea that it is wrong to coerce people to comply with values they reasonably do not accept (cf. Cohen 1994a, 1528, 1539). In *Liberalism*, Rawls (1993, 217) argues that people should vote (at least regarding constitutional essentials and other basic questions of justice) on the basis of what public reason, not their nonpolitical values, requires. Even voting, he contends, involves a share in the coercive power of the state, and it should not be exercised in ways that involve imposing nonpolitical values that reasonable people may reject.

These beliefs about reasonable pluralism are crucial, as we shall see, to responding to the worries about philosophical loss and justificatory schizophrenia. For now, it is sufficient to note that these beliefs must be explicit within those wide reflective equilibria that form the overlap-

Table 8.1. *The contents of wide reflective equilibrium in* Theory *and* Liberalism

Theory	Liberalism
Original Position; Principles of justice; Free and equal agents; Well-ordered society; Procedural justice	Original Position; Principles of justice; Free and equal agents; Well-ordered society; Procedural justice
(*N.B.* Not free standing)	(*N.B.* Free standing "module")
Philosophical arguments justifying key elements of justice as fairness, including autonomy argument needed for congruence argument	Rationale for key elements of justice as fairness
(*N.B.* Shared rationale)	(*N.B.* Rationale specific to each wide reflective equilibrium)
	Account of reasonableness and burdens of judgment
	Rationale for boundary between public and nonpublic; specifics of boundary
Rest of moral and religious views	Rest of moral and religious views
Considered moral judgments, all levels	Considered moral judgments, all levels

ping consensus on justice as fairness in *Liberalism*. In *Theory*, in contrast, this component of wide reflective equilibrium was not made explicit, even though Rawls was not unaware of the fact of pluralism.

Although acceptance of reasonable pluralism must show up in each wide reflective equilibrium in the overlapping consensus, there need not be, and are probably not, identical accounts of it. Someone who believes in moral truth, for example, might well accept reasonable pluralism as a practical concession, something we might in time overcome or reduce with great moral progress. Someone who believes that God has revealed the truth, but only to some, and that it takes faith to understand that truth, might also accept the idea of reasonable pluralism. Such a believer might accept the fact that faith and the revelation that comes with it cannot be coerced. Someone who rejects the notion of moral truth for philosophical reasons lying elsewhere in his wide reflective equilibrium would see reasonable pluralism as a more fundamental fact of moral life.

The third crucial difference between the wide reflective equilibria in

Liberalism and *Theory* is the drawing, as a result of politicization, of a boundary between political and nonpolitical moral beliefs and the provision of a rationale for that boundary. From within each wide reflective equilibrium containing justice as fairness, there must be an acceptance of a boundary between "public reason" and nonpolitical moral views and values. It is important to see, however, that this boundary will probably be drawn in different ways by people holding different comprehensive views because of the influence of other beliefs in these wide equilibria. Differences in the conception of the burdens of judgment and reasonable pluralism, which we noted were possible, could contribute to this variation. But there are other sources of variation as well.

There are two kinds of variation possible in the way the public/ nonpublic boundary is drawn. First, there may be variation in the degree and scope of priority given to political over nonpolitical values among different comprehensive views. Second, there may be variation in the response to cases where the public reason does not give determinate or clear answers. Both sorts of variation may lead people to intrude their nonpolitical values into public debate about matters of justice. Some people will see these intrusions as justifiable; others, as not. This suggests that the scope and content of public reason is something about which there will be reasonable disagreement and protracted controversy.

An example may help to make these points more concrete. People in different wide reflective equilibria, each accepting justice as fairness and the political values it contains, might give different degrees of priority to some of those political values depending on nonpolitical values in the rest of their wide reflective equilibrium. In *Wisconsin v. Yoder*, the Supreme Court ruled that the Old Order Amish were not bound by a state law requiring that children be sent to school through age fifteen. The Amish argued that their agrarian communities did not require that level of schooling and that the emphasis placed on education by the state law threatened to disrupt their community life. Suppose, for the sake of argument (and contrary to fact), that Wisconsin institutions were themselves governed by the political conception of justice as fairness and that the Amish as well generally accept that conception, endorsing it from within their own more comprehensive moral and religious views. They might then say that *normally* they think they should comply with state laws passed in accord with that conception. This law was presumably such a law: we can even imagine that the law had been passed with an eye to securing an educational level for everyone that promoted fair equality of opportunity. In this case, the Amish are complaining that the interference with their other values of community is too great. They cannot ascribe the priority others might give to equality of opportunity over their religious scruples about a simple, agrarian life.

Now this example involving the Amish might not be as clear a case of nonpolitical values overriding political ones as I have described it. Freedom to practice religion is itself a political value of great importance within justice as fairness. The Amish might be construed as protesting that the state law pits two important political values against each other, and they believe that freedom to practice religion should be given more importance than it is assigned in the state law, which gives more importance to promoting equal opportunity (we may suppose). Indeed, this is how the Supreme Court decided the case: it said the harms imposed by loss of the extra education, including harms to equal opportunity, were not sufficiently immediate and beyond dispute as the kinds of harms that ordinarily are appealed to when freedom of religious practice is curtailed, for instance, in compulsory vaccinations of those who have religious scruples against them.

Even if in this example there is room within justice as fairness to decide in favor of the Amish because of a particular view about how to weigh one basic liberty against the value of equality of opportunity (and because there is no evidence the Amish children are denied knowledge of their basic rights), there is also good reason to think that the Amish would have stuck by their beliefs had the Court ruled against them. Their argument need not have been the abstract one about the relative importance of the practice of religion, which falls within the scope of public reason and is what moved the Supreme Court. Their argument could have affirmed the weight they give to the specific nonpolitical value of living the agrarian life they want to lead. This weighing of a nonpolitical value against the political value of equal opportunity would lead them to reject an argument cast solely in terms of conflicting interpretations of the weight of political values alone.

To summarize our discussion so far, we have noted three key differences in the contents of the wide reflective equilibria that are present in *Theory* and *Liberalism*. First, in contrast to the single rationale for the key background ideas in *Theory*, we have distinct rationales provided by the different wide reflective equilibria that form the overlapping consensus. Second, each wide reflective equilibrium in overlapping consensus must contain an account of, and acceptance of, the fact of reasonable pluralism; different comprehensive views may vary in their accounts of and in their basis for acceptance of reasonable pluralism. Third, each wide reflective equilibrium in the overlapping consensus must contain an account of the *boundary* between political and nonpolitical moral values. This account must specify how much priority to give the political over the nonpolitical values and in what contexts.

These accounts too may vary in significant ways. That is why the metaphor of a boundary is invoked: it is not simply a question of priority being given to the political over the nonpolitical but the fact that different comprehensive views will emphasize some nonpolitical values rather than others and differ from each other in where and why the priority of the political is overridden. For the sake of completeness, Table 8.1 notes that wide reflective equilibria in both *Theory* and *Liberalism* also include various beliefs about other moral, religious, and philosophical matters and considered moral judgments at all levels of generality.

4. PHILOSOPHICAL LOSS: CAN WE LOSE WHAT WE NEVER HAD?

I noted in Section 1 that the politicization of justice produced a sense of philosophical loss in some (including me). Philosophy seems to do less and to be thought capable of doing less, that is, less than some of us might have thought or hoped it was supposed to do. Philosophical argument no longer has (if it ever did) the task, or at least the expectation, of moving everyone who can think clearly and rationally about matters, regardless of their starting beliefs, to convergence on justice as fairness. Of course, philosophy still has important tasks. It may persuade those of us who accept key democratic ideas that justice as fairness is the most reasonable political conception combining them. It also plays a role within each of our comprehensive views in helping us to provide a rationale for justice as fairness (or another reasonable political conception). Indeed, Rawls (1993, 159) emphasizes, the gaps or "looseness" in our systems of beliefs leave room for philosophical imagination to flesh out the needed rationale. What is distinctive about Rawls' account after politicization, however, is the major role assigned not to philosophy but to an institutional mechanism that, over time, helps groups with different comprehensive views to accommodate themselves to justice as fairness.

We should distinguish any sense of loss from whether there is a real loss, that is, from whether there is a real change in the task assigned philosophy before and after politicization. I think there are elements of *Theory* that suggest, or at least leave the door open, to a more robust set of expectations from philosophy and philosophical argument than is present in *Liberalism*. But I think these elements operate less at the level of insistence or commitment and more at the level of suggestion, or even less, by leaving certain hopes or expectations in place by not showing they are unrealistic. *Theory* may have encouraged a philosopher's dream, at least by leaving room for it, and the loss produced by politicization may be the reluctance to be wakened from that dream-world.

One point where the suggestion of a shift in philosophical roles is strongest comes in the *role* assigned to wide reflective equilibrium before and after politicization. (In the previous section I considered the changes in the *content* of the equilibria, not their roles.) It will help to explore this in some detail. In *Theory*, contractors in the Original Position, operating under constraints on motivation and knowledge, select the first and second principles of justice in preference to alternative conceptions of justice, such as utilitarianism or various combinations of utilitarianism and other principles. These principles must cohere in (wide) reflective equilibrium with "our" considered moral judgments about the justice of cases and institutions.

This appeal to wide reflective equilibrium is a crucial adequacy test Rawls imposes on the theory of justice. If the chosen principles do not match our considered moral judgments, we must think about revising the Original Position and the principles it yields until we arrive at a conception of justice that coheres in wide reflective equilibrium with our considered moral judgments. This adequacy test led Hare and others (mistakenly, I believe) to complain that the Original Position was "rigged" and added nothing to the process of justification (see Hare 1973; Daniels 1980). The appeal to wide reflective equilibrium as an adequacy test was iterative. Through repetition, we flesh out and refine the chosen conception of justice, making it more determinate as we go, and we show that it and its refinements are acceptable to "us" in wide reflective equilibrium, that is, that we are justified in believing them. (It remained, then, to apply the feasibility test by showing that the otherwise acceptable theory was stable and did not produce relatively unacceptable strains of commitment for people who grew up in a society governed by it.)

The specific content of justice as fairness is thus made determinate through this process in which all of us are invited to participate. All of us are, in effect, put in the driver's seat for purposes of theory construction and justification. This is the philosopher's dream I alluded to earlier (and which I earlier quoted Rawls as encouraging; cf. Rawls 1995b, 2). All of us are in this position because it is, after all, "our" considered moral judgments in wide reflective equilibrium that constitute the adequacy test. Indeed, in our dream, we may imagine that the philosopher's wide reflective equilibrium can stand in as proxy for everyone's – we are just being reflectively analytic whereas others are less disciplined. In applying the test, we may make revisions, not only in the construction of justice as fairness, but elsewhere in our system of beliefs. We make these revisions in light of philosophical reflection on alternative views and their merits compared to the ones we begin with. This is the process through which philosophical argument will persuade us, if it can, to converge on justice as fairness in a shared wide reflective equilibrium.

Rawls nowhere says that this process will produce convergence on justice as fairness. He nowhere says that if we do not start with the basic ideas of free and equal persons or of a well-ordered society that we can be made to accept them through philosophical deliberation. Indeed, as I noted above, he says that if we do not share those ideas, we will not find justice as fairness attractive or justified. He hoped these ideas were widely shared, but he also knew they had a moral content some might find controversial; they were clearly more robust than simple assumptions about human rationality. But the appeal to acceptability in wide reflective equilibrium by all people willing to engage themselves in the process of theory construction and justification involved the suggestion that philosophical activity was capable of producing the needed acceptance and thus justification among all reflective persons.

There is no direct analogue to this use of wide reflective equilibrium as an adequacy test in the politicized version of Rawls' theory. The original appeal to wide reflective equilibrium in *Theory* had two functions: Through iteration, it made the conception determinate, and it assured "us" that the determinate conception counted as just by "our" lights, that it was justified for each of us. After politicization, there is no "we" capable of playing both roles at once. Instead, we face the diversity in comprehensive views implied by reasonable pluralism. Of necessity, the different tasks assigned the original adequacy test are divided after politicization, specifically into pro tanto justification, which we use to flesh out and make the political conception determinate and complete, and full justification, through which each of us establishes that the determinate conception is justifiable in light of our other beliefs. This shift has much to do with the sense of philosophical loss, for it takes "us" out of the philosophical driver's seat the original adequacy test suggested "we" occupied. To support my view, we must examine more carefully what Rawls says about the different forms of justification after politicization.

The original adequacy test involved finding out whether a conception of justice, such as justice as fairness, gives determinate and complete answers to questions about justice – as judged by us in wide reflective equilibrium. Pro tanto justification avoids the problem of the dissolving "us" by restricting the process of fleshing out the conception to the types of reasons and reasoning permitted in the public conception itself. It is justification that goes only so far – up to the boundaries of the political conception of justice in question. It avoids any kinds of reasons or appeals to values that come from other beliefs we hold in wide reflective equilibrium.

Pro tanto justification allows us to see whether the conception is complete, that is whether it gives "reasonable answers" to a broad range of questions about justice (1995a, 142–43). But "reasonable answer" here does not mean, "acceptable to each of us in wide reflective equilibrium," which was its meaning in the original adequacy test. This is true even though Rawls says that the "overall criterion of the reasonable is general and wide reflective equilibrium" (1995a, 141). Instead, a reasonable answer is one that involves a *reasonable balance* of the political values involved in this conception, as judged by the kinds of reasons and reasoning endorsed by that conception itself. From the fact that an answer is "reasonable" in light of these political considerations alone, it does not follow that an individual will find it reasonable in light of everything else she believes in wide reflective equilibrium.

Rawls offers us little help in the way of examples to clarify what is involved in showing that an answer is a "reasonable" or "balanced" one. His one illustration, the brief discussion of abortion, is presented in a footnote (1993, 243, n. 43). (It is really offered as an illustration of what is meant by balancing values, not a real argument about abortion.) Suppose, Rawls says, that three important political values (among others) are present in a well-ordered society: "the due respect for human life, the ordered reproduction of political society over time, including the family in some form, and finally the equality of women as equal citizens." Rawls then says that "any reasonable balance" of these ideas would involve granting a woman a right to terminate pregnancy in the first trimester. Presumably, denying that right would mean giving excessive weight to one of the three values, the due respect we owe to human life, and no weight at all to the equality of women. Bringing in other nonpublic values or beliefs to justify the special weight assigned to respect for human life, for example, beliefs about the fetus having a nonoverridable right to life from the moment of conception, would clearly be departing from answers given by public reason and pro tanto justification. It is exactly these views about the beginnings of personhood that reasonable people disagree about, and so insisting on one interpretation of that view to the exclusion of other public values is to act unreasonably. In this case, the failure to give a "balanced" answer that incorporates all the relevant public values stems directly from ignoring the fact that other reasonable people cannot accept the weighting involved.

Whether or not this specific example about abortion in the first trimester seems plausible, other aspects of the abortion view would quickly become problematic. Does permitting late second trimester abortion for reasons other than a threat to maternal health or life, for example, to avoid serious defects in a fetus, constitute a "reasonable balance" of these values? Does public funding of early abortion, through Medicaid or in military hospitals, constitute a necessary recognition of the equality of women, or does it involve undervaluing respect for human life by forcing those who give much greater weight to such respect to fund abortions they do not approve of? It becomes less obvious that the internal structure of the political conception Rawls described actually tells us what constitutes a reasonable balance of values in these cases. That uncertainty raises a question whether we do smuggle in our wider sense of reasonableness, deriving from our considered judgments in our various wide reflective equilibria, in all of these judgments about reasonable balance, including the one Rawls takes to be settled. The answer to this question may depend on how robust and detailed the settled convictions are that arise through clear cases of the exercise of public reason.

We might think of the exercise of public reason involved in pro tanto justification as establishing a *political reflective equilibrium*. There is an equilibrium among the kinds of considerations relevant to giving reasons in, say, justice as fairness, and judgments about the "reasonableness" of specific implications of the view for questions of basic justice. Any reasonable political conception of justice might yield such a political reflective equilibrium. Judgments about justice made within that political equilibrium are justified for people only pro tanto; they may be overridden in full justification, once all values, and not just political ones, are taken into consideration. Justification pro tanto, that is, the justification that results from being in political reflective equilibrium alone, thus falls short of full justification and it lacks the justificatory force involved in Rawls' original appeal to wide reflective equilibrium in *Theory* as an adequacy test. Lloyd (1994) points out, however, that even the "shallow" justification that refrains from appealing to any justifications from comprehensive views has considerable force, so that pro tanto justification will be compelling on many issues.

Consider now the second function of the original adequacy test, namely, showing that a conception of justice gives answers to questions about justice that we find acceptable in light of everything else we believe. This function is now assigned to full justification (and full justification in turn is crucial to establishing an overlapping consensus for the right reasons). In Section 2, we took care to sort out just what kinds of beliefs would be contained in any wide reflective equilibrium that contained justice as fairness as a module. These wide equilibria will differ from each other in important details, even where there is overlap on important components, because of the ineliminable diversity in comprehensive views that results from the burdens of judgment. Still, as in the original adequacy test, a conception of justice is justified for individuals if it coheres in wide reflective equilibrium with all the rest of their beliefs. It is in full justification, then, that we really test the "reasonableness" of claims about justice – that is, their reasonableness in light of all the kinds of reasons we think are relevant, not just the political ones.

Rawls intends the notion of full justification to be perfectly general: we can imagine an individual in any time or place assessing whether a particular conception of justice fits with his or her other beliefs in wide reflective equilibrium. In this regard, it resembles the adequacy test involving wide reflective equilibrium in *Theory*. Nevertheless, the central question of *Liberalism*, as we noted, concerns how deep a form of stability is possible. Rawls' answer, pointing to an overlapping consensus of reasonable wide reflective equilibria, thus places the discussion of full justification by appeal to reflective equilibrium in a particular context, one primarily concerned with how people raised in a society governed by a particular conception can stably adhere to it given the burdens of judgment. The stability argument presupposes that people are raised in a society governed by, say, justice as fairness: it is there as a given for them to embrace or reject. In contrast, in *Theory*, the appeal to wide reflective equilibrium as an adequacy test is made in the context of asking, quite generally and apart from the stability test, How can we come to converge on a theory with a determinate content and accept it?

Rawls' answer in *Liberalism* to the stability question emphasizes the role of *institutions* operating over time on *groups* that share certain comprehensive views. Institutions play an "educative role," as Cohen (1994a, 1530) emphasizes: "the formation of moral-political ideas and sensibilities also proceeds less by reasoning or explicit instruction – which may be important in the formation of comprehensive moral views – than by mastering ideas and principles that are expressed in and serve to interpret these institutions" (Cohen 1994a, 1531). For example, the idea of political equality is manifest in many features of democratic institutions, explicitly in claims about equality before the law and equal civil rights, but also implicitly, in the way in which citizens are forced to win others to their projects in a political and market context. These practices put pressure on people holding various comprehensive views to accommodate the idea of others as equal persons and even as reasonable ones (Cohen 1994a, 1532). People become attached to ideas they become familiar with and understand through these experiences. But this attachment need not be thought of as mere indoctrination; it is reasonably viewed as the result of learning and education.

The institutional mechanism Rawls describes at once explains why some convergence is possible and why there is not full convergence on all elements of the comprehensive views (see Cohen 1994a, 1533). The institutional pressures go only so far. They put pressure on us to accommodate to the political values in the conception governing our institutions, but these pressures do not reach far enough to compel accommodation in beliefs that govern our other beliefs and the institutions that dominate the nonpublic parts of our lives. We get, then, an explanation – however anthropological it sounds – to the question why we do not have adequate forces at work to produce overall convergence, even if we get partial convergence in overlapping consensus. (Remember, this whole discussion is part of ideal theory and is intended to help us answer the original question about stability, namely, Can we maintain a motivation to comply with this conception of justice, given that we are raised under institutions governed by it? Rawls is not here explaining how we could initially produce convergence on an overlapping consensus for the right reasons.)

Since Rawls is at such pains to explain how, over time and through institutional mechanisms, the basis for accommodation of comprehensive views is achieved, it is easy to see why the *iterative* nature of the original appeal to reflective equilibrium as an adequacy test drops out of the account. No doubt, at the same time that comprehensive views accommodate themselves to a political conception, there is some struggle against some of its features, and the public conception also evolves over time in response to some of that struggle. But this historical process is a far cry from the iterative role that was ascribed to the original adequacy test in *Theory*, and it is particularly far from the role ascribed to the individual seeking wide reflective equilibrium, as opposed to groups seeking to make their political surroundings accommodate to them.

I believe the sense of philosophical loss is explained, at least in part, by this shift from a philosopher's dream, an iterative process of construction and justification involving all of us, to a social and political process in which, over time, people holding diverse views maintain an overlapping consensus on a public conception of justice. The shift may, however, be partly an illusion created by the different problems Rawls focuses on in his earlier and later work. Further confusion may be added by the discussion of nonideal contexts ("How might we get to overlapping consensus for the right reasons if we do not yet have it but only share some democratic ideas?"), to which I alluded in discussing stability at the end of Section 1.

In *Theory*, much of the discussion necessarily focuses on the construction of a new theory and what the process of justifying it must look like. In *Liberalism*, the focus is on the stability argument. The stability argument supposes we already have a determinate theory and are simply assessing how reasonable people with diverse views can accommodate to the conception of justice that is already determinate within their culture. If that is the basic problem *Liberalism* addresses, then it is not surprising that Rawls does not engage us in the process of theory construction in the same way he did when his project had a different central problem. Still, it is hard to see how "full justification" can play the iterative role in theory construction and justification that Rawls assigned to the original adequacy test involving wide reflective equilibrium, except over time and in the context of evolving modifications of social institutions through political disagreement, struggle, and reform. Though philosophy is not absent from that process – it plays a crucial role within and between comprehensive views in securing accommodation – it is not so clearly central as in the philosopher's dream. If philosophy can really only have that reduced role, then the sense of loss is the sorrow of waking from a pleasant dream.

We can sharpen the effect of that awakening by posing this question: Can someone be justified in rejecting "reasonableness" in wide reflective equilibrium? The answer seems to be "yes." That is because "reasonableness" is given a fairly specific content in terms of beliefs and commitments (see Section 1, this chapter). (We are not simply asking, without equivocation, "Is it reasonable to be unreasonable?") Reasonable comprehensive views in wide reflective equilibrium will contain an account of the burdens of judgment and a willingness to submit matters of justice to consideration in terms of reasons that are acceptable to other reasonable people. Unreasonable people, for example, those holding views that leave no room for seeking terms of cooperation with others on grounds that others can reasonably accept, will not share these specific elements. Some members of certain fundamentalist religious sects, for example, might ascribe overriding weight to the belief that God's will should dominate human political relations. For them justice – on terms reasonable to others who are reasonable – holds no appeal at all.

How troubling is this result? We may suppose that the fundamentalist listens to reasons that fit well within his system of beliefs. We may suppose he commits no logical fallacies and we may even suppose that he is not epistemologically irresponsible in adhering to beliefs for which there is counterevidence he can be held responsible for taking into account, given other things he believes. Then such a person would not be justified in accepting justice as fairness (or some other reasonable political conception). But this outcome should be no more troubling to us than the fact that someone might – given a certain history, set of beliefs, experiences, and culture – be justified in believing the earth is flat or the sun orbited the earth. Neither skepticism nor relativism is an inevitable consequence of this coherence account of justification, and the fact that sound philosophical argument will not necessarily persuade all who are sufficiently reflective, regardless of their initial beliefs, is not to abandon philosophy.

There is a further analogy between the political view of justice and a position taken by some in the philosophy of science. Important features of scientific method, it is sometimes claimed (see Boyd 1988), do not really facilitate progress in science unless a certain threshold is reached. Some "approximately true" theory must be adopted. Then, given appropriate methodological scruples, significant further progress can be made.

Certain democratic ideas constitute a similar threshold, in Rawls' view. We may not be led to them whatever our starting point by reflection and philosophical argument alone, but if we acquire them in a democratic culture where they are embodied in our institutions, then political philosophy can help us refine them into a more reasonable, perhaps an optimally reasonable, conception of justice. And if that conception governs our well-ordered society, philosophical analysis and discussion helps us to accommodate our other views, given their "looseness," to the conception. Philosophy may not be capable of leading us from the desert to a full-blown convergence on justice as fairness, as it might have appeared it was supposed to do in *Theory*, any more than scientific method can lead Robinson Crusoe to quantum mechanics, but it has not been replaced by moral anthropology either.

5. MORAL DOUBLE-BOOKKEEPING AND INTEGRITY

The politicization of justice means that we must bifurcate our justificatory practice. We must draw a line between the domain of public reason, that is, matters involving constitutional essentials and other issues of basic justice, and the rest of our moral, religious, and philosophical beliefs. Can we keep two moral ledgers in this way without threatening moral integrity? Points that have emerged in our analysis of reflective equilibrium after politicization help us to answer this question positively: there need be no threat to moral integrity. Before turning to those points, however, it will help to comment on the fact that there are other contexts in which we engage – fruitfully and without a loss of integrity – in analogous double-bookkeeping.

In many churches and synagogues (but by no means all) there is an unspoken rule governing sermons: they may address the moral dimensions of social and political issues, but they must do so without becoming enmeshed in "politics," specifically party politics. I once asked a rabbi why he refrained from drawing the connection between his moral discussions and their implications for a particular election and the positions of the candidates. His reply was that he felt competent to explain how his religious and moral tradition contained implications for some of our social practices and policies, but "so many other factors" go into party allegiances and preferences that "intelligent, reflective people" who shared the same moral views could disagree about them. He specifically mentioned the intricacies of economics and political science, the difficulty of interpreting historical events, and complexity of making judgments about the character of individual politicians.

It is worth paraphrasing his explanation in more detail. He said, "I have my carefully thought out views on those subjects, and I am sure I am right, but I would not presume to impose them on my congregation, even though I have the pulpit. Many of its most thoughtful members disagree about them, and if I tie my moral conclusions to my political ones, people whom I might influence morally will be lost to me. Some disagree with me about my interpretation of the moral tradition, but we have more common ground to carry out our discussion about such issues. These moral issues are ones we have struggled with in our families and communities for many generations, and they are debated extensively in the rabbinic literature. We may disagree, but at least we can hope for basic agreement because of our shared commitments and experiences. But politics – that's too complicated!"

Perhaps some clergy might keep politics out of their sermons solely to protect their position within their congregation. That might, at least in some instances, be a compromise that threatened moral integrity. The rationale offered by this rabbi, however, does not threaten integrity, at least generally.

The boundary the rabbi draws between the moral and the political, however, has some ironic contrasts with Rawls'. From within a shared tradition, supported by its own institutions over long periods of time, some moral issues will seem clear and resolvable by reference to shared assumptions, whereas political ones may not. In his discussion of overlapping consensus and stability, Rawls makes the opposite point: shared democratic institutions produce a framework for political agreement about constitutional essentials and basic matters of justice, but complexity will show up beyond the public domain. The rabbi is not, however, restricting the political domain in the same way Rawls does, and some of the contrast in their positions derives from that fact. (For the rabbi, the political concerns all aspects of party politics and not just fundamental issues of justice.) A second ironic contrast is that Rawls is interested in protecting agreement in the domain of public reason by excluding sources of disagreement that fall outside of it, whereas the rabbi is excluding "politics" in order to protect agreement in the nonpublic domain.

The main point, however, is not the differences between the boundaries that Rawls and the rabbi draw. It is the fact that in various private associations, including ones that claim significant moral authority, people draw justificatory boundaries of the sort that Rawls does and for somewhat similar reasons. The point should be familiar to all of us, since we all assume roles, professional or otherwise, in which we must distinguish our own values from the values it is appropriate to invoke given the role we must play. For example, each of us in our capacities as parents, teachers, or advisors must sometimes separate our own values from those appropriately appealed to in the context of giving advice to our children, students, advisees, or clients.

Rawls points us toward another example of boundary drawing common in our tradition: the special place we give to rules of evidence in the law (1993, 221). We are interested in protecting a right to a fair trial, and to do so we devise a complex set of procedures for introducing and evaluating evidence in trials. The effect of these rules is that sometimes not all relevant information will be available to a jury. We are less interested in the "whole truth," however it is obtained, than we are in assuring a mechanism for fair trials. More generally, we adjust our standards of what we count as relevant authorities and procedures of reasoning to the task we have at hand in various private associations. We only allow certain authorities powers to deliberate in certain institutions, for instance, in educational institutions deliberating curriculum design or in religious institutions debating a matter of doctrine. As Rawls notes, "The criteria and methods of these nonpublic reasons depend in part on how the nature (the aim and point) of each association is understood and the conditions under which it pursues its ends" (1993, 221).

Politicization should not, then, be criticized merely for drawing a boundary that bifurcates justificatory practices. We do that commonly and for good reason at many points in our lives, both in private and public contexts. The challenge to integrity must be more specific if it is to be serious, and that leads us back to some of the points that emerged in our discussion of wide reflective equilibrium.

To consider whether the boundary between public reason and nonpublic values threatens moral integrity, we must consider two cases. One case involves the situation in an overlapping consensus for the right reasons. For example, suppose that justice as fairness is a module within various wide reflective equilibria established by people with differing comprehensive views. The second case is one in which there are alternative conceptions of justice held by people who at least share some common democratic ideas, but there is not yet an overlapping consensus on a shared conception. (Notice that this second case does not arise in ideal theory, where we are thinking about the original stability question. It is relevant to stability in nonideal contexts, as I noted at the end of Section 1.) Our analysis so far has concentrated on the first case, and we begin with it here.

A wide reflective equilibrium that contains justice as fairness (for example) as a module, must also contain three other elements that bear on the concern about a threat to integrity. The equilibrium contains a rationale for the key background ideas involved in justice as fairness. We saw how people sharing different equilibria might provide their own different justifications for thinking of people as free moral agents with an interest in conditions protecting that freedom. This means that the basic ideas involved in public reason, as defined by the shared conception of justice as fairness, are not themselves "moral compromises" begrudgingly made. The values contained in the shared conception are values for the person in wide reflective equilibrium, and this means the person is fully justified in acting in accord with those values. Specifically, the person can say that, normally speaking, decisions made by institutions duly constituted according to justice as fairness are decisions the individual is fully justified in accepting.

The second element of the wide equilibrium is the acceptance of an account of the burdens of judgment and the reasonableness of others who may differ in their nonpublic values. This acceptance of reasonable pluralism is itself justified for each person in wide reflective equilibrium, albeit in somewhat different ways. The effect of each person accepting reasonable pluralism is that each has respect for the kinds of reasons others can be expected to accept and reasons others would not accept. An element of this acceptance of reasonable pluralism is the moral belief that it is wrong to use the coercive power of the state to impose constraints on others for reasons that they can reasonably reject. If constraints – including those that result from the effects of voting – are to be imposed, they must be defensible on grounds all can reasonably accept. Because each person thus has a rationale or justification for accepting reasonable pluralism, each has a general reason for bifurcating justification in the way the public–nonpublic boundary requires. There is no threat to integrity if the rationale for drawing the boundary itself is ultimately justified within the agent's total system of beliefs and values.

Finally, the third element each must have in wide reflective equilibrium is a specification of the priority each will give to public values over nonpublic ones. This boundary must reflect differences in the nonpublic values and in the specifics of the priority permitted, given the differences in the rationales for this boundary that must exist in wide reflective equilibrium. Each might be able to say that "normally" priority will be given to the decisions made by just institutions, although how each characterizes exceptions will vary depending on features of the different comprehensive views.

Because there is variation in the rationales and in the exceptions to what is "normally" taken to be justifiable priority for public values, even in a stable overlapping consensus there will be ongoing disagreement on some issues. Rawls (1995a, 148–49) notes, for example, that Quakers may conscientiously object to democratic decisions to wage war, viewing that outcome of an otherwise acceptable set of institutions as warranting conscientious objection, without being forced to conclude that those democratic institutions are themselves unacceptable. The institutions may, on the whole, represent the best way to realize other Quaker values, which include a concern for basic rights and fundamental interests of other people (1995a, 149). To take another example: someone who thinks abortion is morally wrong might accept the "balance of public reasons" that recognizes a woman's right to a first trimester abortion (see Section 4) but conscientiously resist being asked to contribute resources (through public funding) to facilitate such abortions (for those on Medicaid or at military bases, for example).

Another troubling example is this one: is permitting voluntary religious expression in the schools consistent with avoiding the "establishment" of religion? If the great majority in a school is of the same religion, does this put undue pressure on those who are of different religions or have no religious beliefs at all? One reason this type of example is troubling is that it is not clear that public reason will give an unequivocal answer. The account may not be complete with respect to all these questions. In such a case, the overlapping consensus does not preclude the intrusion of nonpublic values into the debate, and different comprehensive views will find it important for different reasons and in different degrees to intrude their own nonpublic solutions on these matters.

The permeability of the public–nonpublic boundary goes beyond these cases of incompleteness, because reasonable people ultimately must justify how much priority to give public reason and public values in their own terms. How much friction results, and how much instability is threatened, is largely an empirical matter: it depends on the composition of the overlapping consensus. Since ultimate authority for how to weigh public against nonpublic values must rest with the individual and must be justifiable to her in light of all of her values, there is no general threat to integrity from the drawing of the boundary or its unevenness.

Finally, we must consider the case (in nonideal theory) in which we do not have an overlapping consensus on the same political conception of justice, although we have some overlap on key democratic ideas and thus on some of the elements of public reason. I take it this is the situation in the United States today: there is agreement on many constitutional essentials, much less agreement on many basic questions of justice, and diverse conceptions of justice, each of which draws in its own way on important democratic ideas. For example, Rawls would argue that justice as fairness is the *most reasonable* way to combine fundamental ideas in our democratic tradition (Rawls 1995b, 2). He claims that this conception makes sense of some of our settled convictions about justice, for example, about the importance of certain basic liberties and that it allows us to leverage those points of agreement so that we resolve remaining points of disagreement, for instance, about acceptable forms of social and economic inequality (see Cohen 1989). Justice Scalia no doubt has a different conception of justice that he invokes; Justice O'Connor has yet another.

In this context, where there is less agreement on the content and limits of public reason, dispute about appropriate and inappropriate appeals to nonpublic values will be more intense and harder to resolve. Nevertheless, Rawls argues that considerable stability may result even in this situation, since each political conception that is affirmed is reasonable and all reasonable comprehensive views affirm one such conception or another (see Rawls 1995b, 2ff.). He further suggests that over time the most reasonable conception among the family of reasonable political conceptions will form a core around which other members of the family will tend to gather "at a decreasing (or not increasing) distance" (1995b, 3). This claim about stability in a nonideal context, if it is plausible, adds weight to the claim that the most reasonable view (justice as fairness) will be stable in a well-ordered society. More effective institutional forces would be at work in the well-ordered society to educate people about the value of justice and its key ideas than in the nonideal context.

The question before us, however, is this: What threat is there to moral integrity where there is no overlapping consensus on the same political conception and each of us attempts to respect a boundary between public and nonpublic values in justifying claims about constitutional essentials and basic questions of justice? Let us suppose, as we did in the case of overlapping consensus for the right reasons, that reasonable people will include in their respective wide reflective equilibria some account of the burdens of judgment and reasonable pluralism. Suppose that they will also include some boundary that they draw and justify in their own terms between public and nonpublic uses of reason. Compared to the case in which there is overlapping consensus on the same political conception of justice, there will be less agreement about where appeals to nonpublic values violate the boundary and where there are justifiable exceptions. Still, there is no additional threat to moral integrity in this case. The acceptance of a particular boundary between public and nonpublic values is made by each person in wide reflective equilibrium. The public–nonpublic boundary is fully justified for each person, and each has adequate reasons for respecting it. The fact that there is no consensus on the same political conception does not affect the fact that the boundary each draws in light of his own acceptance of a reasonable political conception is itself fully justified for him.

Whether or not there is overlapping consensus, then, there is no threat to moral integrity, provided people justify the drawing of a public–nonpublic boundary in ways that derive from their own views in wide equilibrium. The politicization of justice and of justification is not a threat to moral integrity. Nor does it impose unacceptable philosophical loss, even if it forces us to revise some of our expectations. Wide reflective equilibrium, and thus justification, remains alive and well after politicization.

ACKNOWLEDGEMENT

I wish to thank Joshua Cohen, Erin Kelly, and John Rawls for extremely helpful discussion of earlier drafts of this essay.

REFERENCES

Barry, Brian. 1995. "John Rawls and the Search for Stability," *Ethics* 105(July):874–915.

Boyd, Richard N. 1988. "How to Be a Moral Realist," In Sayre-McCord, Geoffrey. *Essays on Moral Realism*. Ithaca: Cornell University Press, pp. 181–228.

Cohen, Joshua. 1989. "Democratic Equality," *Ethics* 99(July):727–51.

Cohen, Joshua. 1994a. "A More Democratic Liberalism," *Michigan Law Review* 92:6:1506–43.

Cohen, Joshua. 1994b. "Pluralism and Proceduralism," *Chicago-Kent Law Review* 69:3:589–618.

Daniels, Norman. 1975. *Reading Rawls*. New York: Basic Books.

Daniels, Norman. 1979. "Wide Reflective Equilibrium and Theory Acceptance in Ethics," *Journal of Philosophy* 76:5:256–82.

Daniels, Norman. 1980. "Reflective Equilibrium and Archimedean Points," *Canadian Journal of Philosophy* 10:1:83–103.

Dworkin, Ronald. 1973. "The Original Position," *University of Chicago Law Review* 40:3(Spring):500–33. Reprinted in Daniels 1975, pp. 16–52.

Freeman, Samuel. 1994. "Political Liberalism and the Possibility of Just Democratic Constitution," *Chicago-Kent Law Review* 69:3:619–68.

Greenawalt, Kent. 1994. "On Public Reason," *Chicago-Kent Law Review* 69:3:669–90.

Hare, R. M. 1973. "Rawls' Theory of Justice," *Philosophical Quarterly* 23(April):144–55 and 23(July):241–51. Reprinted in Daniels 1975, pp. 81–107.

Lloyd, S. A. 1994. "Relativizing Rawls," *Chicago-Kent Law Review* 69:3:709–36.

Rawls, John. 1971. *A Theory of Justice*. Cambridge, MA: Harvard University Press.

Rawls, John. 1974. "Independence & Moral Theory," *Proceedings and Addresses of the American Philosophy Association* 48:5–22.

Rawls, John. 1980. "Kantian Constructivism in Moral Theory," *Jounal of Philosophy* 77:515–72.

Rawls, John. 1993. *Political Liberalism*. New York: Columbia University Press.

Rawls, John. 1995a. "Reply to Habermas," *Journal of Philosophy* 92:3:132–80.

Rawls, John. 1995b. "A *Theory of Justice* and *Political Liberalism* and Other Pieces: How Related?" Draft (5/6/95) of comments to be presented at October 1995 Santa Clara Conference on Rawls' work.

Sandel, Michael J. 1982. *Liberalism and the Limits of Justice*. Cambridge: Cambridge University Press.

White, Stephen L. 1991. *The Unity of the Self*. Cambridge, MA: MIT Press.

PART II

Chapter 9

Health-care needs and distributive justice

1. WHY A THEORY OF HEALTH-CARE NEEDS?

A theory of health-care needs should serve two central purposes. First, it should illuminate the sense in which we – at least many of us – think health care is "special," that it should be treated differently from other social goods. Specifically, even in societies in which people tolerate (and glorify) significant and pervasive inequalities in the distribution of most social goods, many feel there are special reasons of justice for distributing health care more equally. Some societies even have institutions for doing so. To be sure, others argue it is perverse to single out health care in this way, or that if we have reasons for doing so, they are rooted in charity, not justice. But in any case, a theory of health-care needs should show their connection to other central notions in an acceptable theory of justice. It should help us see what kind of social good health-care is by properly relating it to social goods whose importance is similar and for which we may have a clearer grasp of appropriate distributive principles.

Second, such a theory should provide a basis for distinguishing the more from the less important among the many kinds of things health care does for us. It should tell us which health-care services are "more special" than others. Thus, a broad category of health-services functions to improve quality of life, not to extend or save it. Some of these services restore or compensate for diminished capacities and functions; others improve life quality in other ways. We do draw distinctions about the urgency and importance of such services. Our theory of health-care needs should provide a basis for a reasonable set of such distinctions. If we can assume some scarcity of health-care resources,[1] and if we cannot (or should not) rely just on market mechanisms to allocate these resources, then we need such a theory to guide macro-allocation decisions about priorities among health-care needs.

In short, a theory of health-care needs must come to grips with two widely held judgments: that there is something especially important about health care, and that some kinds of health care are more important than others. The philosophical task is to assess, explain, and justify or modify these distinctions we make about the importance of different wants, interests, or needs. After considering a preliminary objection to the claim that we need a theory of health-care needs (Section 2), I shall offer an account of basic needs in general (Section 3) and health-care needs in particular (Section 4). These needs are important to maintaining normal species functioning, and in turn, such normal functioning is an important determinant of the range of opportunity open to an individual. This connection to opportunity helps clarify the kind of social good health care is and provides the basis for subsuming health-care institutions under principles of distributive justice (Sections 5 and 6).

2. A PRELIMINARY OBJECTION

Before turning to the theory, I would like to address one objection to the project as a whole, for there is reason to think that talk about health-care needs and their priorities both is avoidable and undesirable. The objection, which challenges the assumption that we cannot rely on medical markets even where there is adequate income redistribution, can be put as follows: Suppose we could agree on a theory of distributive justice that gives us a notion of a *fair income share*. Then individuals could protect themselves against the risk of needing health care by voluntary insurance schemes. Each person would be responsible for buying insurance at a level of protection he or she desires. No one (except children and the congenitally handicapped) has a *claim* on social resources to meet health-care needs unless he is prudent enough to buy the relevant insurance (which does not preclude charity). Resource allocation to meet demand, expressed through varying insurance packages, can be accommodated by the medical market, provided appropriate competitive conditions obtain. In this way there is protection against expensive but rare needs for health care, for which relatively inexpensive insurance can be bought; so too, common but inexpensive services can either be risk shared through insurance or paid out of pocket without great sacrifice, if preferred. But expensive and potentially common "needs" – for example, to be provided with artificial hearts or to be cryogenically preserved – would not become a drain on social resources since individuals who want protection against the risks of facing them would have to buy expensive insurance out of their own fair shares. This way of meeting health needs does not create a bottomless pit into which we are forced to drain all available social resources.[2]

Sometimes needs-based theories are criticized because they give us too small a claim on social resources, providing only a floor on deprivation.[3] In contrast, the objection we face here warns against granting precedence to the satisfaction of needs because we then allow too great a claim on social resources. I postpone until Section 6 considering how a need-based theory can avoid this problem. Similarly, I shall not here defend the assumption that medical markets fail to be acceptable allocative mechanisms.[4] Instead, I would like to suggest that the insurance scheme fails to obviate the need for a theory of health-care needs.

The key assumption underlying this scheme is that the prudent citizen will be able to buy a *reasonable* health-care insurance package from his fair share. Such a package can meet the health-care needs it is *reasonable for people to want to be protected against*. However, if some fair shares turn out to be inadequate to pay the premium for such a package, then there is something unacceptable about them. Intuitively, they are not fair to those people. But we can describe such a benefit package, and thus determine minimum constraints on a fair share, only if we already use a notion of basic or reasonable health-care needs, the ones it is rational for a prudent person to insure against. So the "fair share plus insurance" approach only *appears* to avoid talk about health-care needs. Either it must smuggle such a theory in when it arrives at constraints on fair shares, or else it is open to the objection the shares are not fair.

There is another way in which a theory of health-care needs is implicit in the insurance-scheme market approach: the approach puts health-care needs on a par with other wants and preferences and allows them to compete for resources with no constraints other than market mechanisms operating.[5] But such a stance, far from avoiding the need to develop a theory of needs, already *is* a view of health-care needs. It sees them as one kind of preference among many, with no special claim on social resources except that which derives from strength of preference. To be sure, where strength of preference is high, needs may be met, but strength may vary in ways that fail to reflect the importance we ought (and usually do) ascribe to health care. Such a market view needs justification, and it is not a justification simply to point to the *existence* of such a market.

3. NEEDS AND PREFERENCES

Not all preferences are created equal

Before turning to health-care needs in particular, it is worth noting that the concept of needs has been in philosophical disrepute, and with some good reason. The concept seems both too weak and too strong to get us very far toward a theory of distributive justice. Too many things become needs, and too few. And finding a middle ground seems to involve many of the issues of distributive justice one might hope to resolve by appeal to a clear notion of needs.

It is easy to see why too many things appear to be needs. Without abuse of language, we refer to the means necessary to reach any of our goals as needs. To reawaken memories of Miller's, the neighborhood delicatessen of my childhood, I need only the smell of sour pickles in a barrel. To paint my son's swing set, I need a clean brush.[6] The problem of the importance of needs seems to reduce to the problem of the importance or urgency of preferences or wants in general (leaving aside the fact that not all the things we need are expressed as preferences).

But just as not all preferences are on a par – some are more important than others – so too not all the things we say we need are. It is possible to pick out various things we say we need, including needs for health care, which play a special role in a variety of moral contexts. Taking a cue from T. M. Scanlon's discussion in "Preference and Urgency," we should distinguish *subjective* and *objective* criteria of well-being.[7] We need *some* such criterion to assess the importance of competing claims on resources in a variety of moral contexts. A *subjective* criterion uses the relevant individual's own assessment of how well-off he is with and without the claimed benefit to determine the importance of his preference or claim. An *objective* criterion invokes a measure of importance independent of the individual's own assessment, for example, independent of the *strength* of his preference.

In contexts of distributive justice and other moral contexts, we do *in fact* appeal to some *objective* criteria of well-being. We refuse to rely solely on subjective ones. If I appeal to my friend's duty of beneficence in requesting $100, I will most likely get a quite different reaction if I tell him I need the money to get a root canal than if I tell him I need the money to go to the Brooklyn neighborhood of my childhood to smell pickles in a barrel. Indeed, it is not likely to matter in his assessment of *obligations* that I strongly *prefer* to go to Brooklyn. Nor is it likely to matter if I insist I feel a great *need* to reawaken memories of my childhood – I am overcome by nostalgia. (He might give me the money for either purpose, but if he gives it so I can smell pickles, we would probably say he is not doing it out of any duty at all, that he feels no obligation.) Similarly, if my appeal was directed to some (even utopian) social welfare agency rather than my friend, it would adopt objective criteria in assessing the importance of the request independent of my own strength of preference.

The issue as Scanlon has drawn it, between subjective and objective standards of well-being, is not just a claim about the *epistemic* status of our criteria of well-being. He is surely right that we do not rely on subjective standards of well-being: we do not just accept an individual's assessment of his well-being as the *relevant* measure of his well-being in important moral contexts. But the issue here is not just that such a measure is *subjective* and we use an *objective* measure. Nor is the issue that we may be skeptical about the feasibility of developing an objective interpersonal measure of satisfaction, and so we use another measure. Suppose we had an intersubjectively acceptable way of determining individual levels of well-being, where well-being is viewed as the level of satisfaction of the individual's *full range of preferences*. That is, suppose we had some deep social-utility function that enabled us to compare different persons' levels of satisfaction, given the full range of their preferences and the social goods they have available. Such a scale would be the wrong scale to use in a broad range of moral contexts involving justice and the design of social institutions – at least it is not just an improvement on the scale we do in fact use. We would continue to use a far narrower scale of well-being, one that *does not include the full range of kinds of preferences* people have. So the real issue behind Scanlon's insightful discussion is the choice between objective *truncated* or selective scales of well-being and either objective or subjective *full-range* or "satisfaction" scales of well-being.[8] I shall return shortly to consider why the truncated scale *ought to be* (and not just *is*) the measure used in issues of social justice.

One indication that we appeal to an objective, truncated standard is that I might say the root canal, but not the smell of pickles in a barrel, is something I *really* need (assuming the dentist is right). It is a *need* and not just a desire. The implication is that some of the things we claim to need fall into special categories which give them a weightier moral claim in contexts involving the distribution of resources (depending, of course, on how well-off we already are within those categories of need).[9] Our task is to characterize the relevant categories of needs in a way that *explains* two central properties these special needs have. First, these needs are *objectively ascribable*: we can ascribe them to a person even if he does not realize he has them and even if he denies he has them because his preferences run contrary to the ascribed needs. Second, and of greater interest to us, these needs are *objectively important*: we attach a special weight to claims based on them in a variety of moral contexts, and we do so independently of the weight attached to these and competing claims by the relevant individuals. So our philosophical task is to characterize the class of things we need which has these properties and to do so in such a way that we explain why such importance is attached to them.

Needs and species-typical functioning

One plausible suggestion for distinguishing the relevant needs from all the things we can come to need is David Braybrooke's distinction between "course-of-life needs" and "adventitious needs." *Course-of-life needs* are those needs which people "have all through their lives or at certain stages of life through which all must pass." *Adventitious needs* are the things we need because of the particular contingent projects (which may be long-term ones) on which we embark. Human course-of-life needs would include food, shelter, clothing, exercise, rest, companionship, a mate (in one's prime), and so on. Such needs are not themselves deficiencies, for example, when they are anticipated. But a deficiency with respect to them "endangers the normal functioning of the subject of need *considered as a member of a natural species.*"[10] A related suggestion can be found in McCloskey's discussion of the human and personal needs we appeal to in political argument. He argues that needs "relate to what it would be detrimental to us to lack, *where the detrimental is explained by reference to our natures as men and specific persons.*"[11]

The suggestion here is that the needs which interest us are those things we need in order to achieve or maintain species-typical normal functioning. Do such needs have the two properties noted earlier? Clearly they are objectively ascribable, assuming we can come up with the appropriate notion of species-typical functioning. (So, incidentally, are adventitious needs, assuming we can determine the relevant goals by reference to which the adventitious needs become determinate.) Are these needs objectively important in the appropriate way? In a broad range of contexts we do treat them as such – a claim I shall not trouble to argue. What is of interest is to see *why* being in such a need category gives them their special importance.

A tempting first answer might be this: whatever our specific chosen goals or tasks, our ability to achieve them (and consequently our happiness) will be diminished if we fall short of normal species functioning. So, whatever our specific goals, we need these course-of-life needs, and therein lies their objective importance. We need them whatever else we need. For example, it is sometimes said that whatever our chosen goals or tasks, we need our health, and so appropriate health care. But this claim is not strictly speaking true. For many of us, some of our goals, perhaps even those we feel most important to us, are not necessarily undermined by failing health or disability. Moreover, we can often adjust our goals – and presumably our levels of satisfaction – to fit better with our dysfunction or disability. Coping in this way does not necessarily diminish happiness or satisfaction in life.

Still, there is a clue here to a more plausible account: impairments of normal species functioning reduce the range of opportunity we have within which to construct life plans and conceptions of the good we have a reasonable expectation of finding satisfying or happiness producing. Moreover, if persons have a high-order interest in preserving the opportunity to revise their conceptions of the good through time, then they will have a pressing interest in maintaining normal species functioning by establishing institutions – such as health-care systems – which do just that. So the kinds of needs Braybrooke and McCloskey pick out by reference to normal species functioning are objectively important because they meet this high-order interest persons have in maintaining a normal range of opportunities. I shall try to refine this admittedly vague answer, but first I want to characterize health-care needs more specifically and show that they fit within this more general framework.

4. HEALTH-CARE NEEDS

Disease and health

To specify a notion of health-care needs, we need clear notions of health and disease. I shall begin with a narrow, if not uncontroversial, "biomedical" model of disease and health. The basic idea is that health is the absence of disease, and diseases (I here include deformities and disabilities that result from trauma) are *deviations from the natural functional organization of a typical member of a species.*[12] The task of characterizing this natural functional organization falls to the biomedical sciences, which must include evolutionary theory since claims about the design of the species and its fitness to meeting biological goals underlie at least some of the relevant functional ascriptions. The task is the same for man and beast with two complications. For humans we require an account of the species-typical functions that permit us to pursue biological goals as social animals. So there must be a way of characterizing the species-typical apparatus underlying such functions as the acquisition of knowledge; linguistic communication and social cooperation. Moreover, adding mental disease and health into the picture complicates the issue further, most particularly because we have a less well-developed theory of species-typical mental functions and functional organization. The "biomedical" model clearly presupposes we can, in theory, supply the missing account and that a reasonable part of what we now take to be psychopathology would show up as diseases.[13]

The biomedical model has two controversial features. First, the deviations that play a role in the definition of disease are from species-typical functional organization. In contrast, some treat health as an idealized level of fully developed functioning, as in the WHO defini-tion.[14] Others insist that the notion of disease is strictly normative and that diseases are deviations from socially preferred functional norms.[15] Still, the WHO definition seems to conflate notions of health with those of general well-being, satisfaction, or happiness, overmedicalizing the domain of social philosophy. And, historical arguments which show that "deviant" functioning – for example, "Drapetomania" (the running-away disease of slaves) or masturbation – have been medicalized and viewed as diseases do not establish the strongly nor-mative thesis that deviance from social norms of functioning consti-tutes disease. So I shall accept the first feature of the model, noting, of course, that the model does not exclude normative judgments *about* diseases, for example, about which are undesirable or which excuse us from normally criticizable behavior and justify our entering a "sick role." These judgments circumscribe the normative notion of illness or sickness, not the theoretically more basic notion of disease (which thus admittedly departs from looser ordinary usage).[16]

Second, pure forms of the biomedical model also involve a deeper claim, namely that species-normal functional organization can itself be characterized without invoking normative or value judgments. Here the debate turns on hard issues in the philosophy of biology.[17] Fortu-nately, these need not detain us since my discussion does not turn on so strong a claim. It is enough for my purposes if the line between disease and the absence of disease is, for the general run of cases, *uncontroversial* and ascertainable through publicly acceptable methods, for example, primarily those of the biomedical sciences. It will not matter if there is some relativization of what counts as a disease category to some features of social roles in a given society, and thus to some normative judgments, provided the core of the notion of species-normal functioning is left intact. The model would still, I presume, count infertility as a disease, even though some or many individuals might prefer to be infertile and seek medical treatment to render them-selves so. Similarly, unwanted pregnancy is not a disease. Again, dys-functional noses are diseases, since noses have normal species functions and anatomy. If the dysfunction or deformity is serious, it might war-rant treatment as an illness. But deviation of nasal anatomy from indi-vidual or social conceptions of beauty does not constitute disease.[18]

Thus the modified biomedical model still allows me to draw a fairly sharp line between uses of health-care services to prevent and treat diseases and uses to meet other social goals. The importance of such other goals may be different and may rest on other bases, for example, in the induced infertility or unwanted pregnancy cases. My intention is to show which principles of justice are relevant to distributing health-care services where we can take as fixed, primarily by nature, a gener-

ally uncontroversial baseline of species-normal functional organization. If important moral considerations enter at yet another level, to
determine what counts as health and what disease, then the principles
I discuss and these others must be reconciled, a task the biomedical
model makes unnecessary at this stage and which I want to avoid here
in any case. Of course, a complete theory, which I do not pursue, would
presumably have to establish priorities among principles governing the
meeting of health-care needs and principles for using health-care services to meet other social or individual goals, for example the termina-
tion of unwanted pregnancy or the upgrading of the beauty of the
population.[19]

Though I have deliberately selected a rather narrow model of disease and health, at least by comparison to some fashionable construals,
health-care needs emerge as a broad and diverse set. Health-care needs
will be those things we need in order to maintain, restore, or provide
functional equivalents (where possible) to normal species functioning.
They can be divided into:

(1) adequate nutrition, shelter
(2) sanitary, safe, unpolluted living and working conditions
(3) exercise, rest, and other features of healthy life-styles
(4) preventive, curative, and rehabilitative personal medical services
(5) nonmedical personal (and social) support services

Of course, we do not tend to think of all these things as included
among health-care needs, partly because we tend to think narrowly
about personal medical services when we think about health care.
But the list is not constructed to conform to our ordinary notion of
health care but to point out a functional relation between quite
diverse goods and services and the various institutions responsible for
delivering them.

Disease and opportunity

The *normal opportunity range* for a given society will be the array of "life
plans" reasonable persons in it are likely to construct for themselves.
The range is thus relative to key features of the society – its stage of
historical development, its level of material wealth and technological
development, and even important cultural facts about it. Facts about
social organization, including the conception of justice regulating its
basic institutions, will of course determine how that total normal range
is distributed in the population. Nevertheless, that issue of distribution
aside, normal species-typical functioning provides us with one clear
parameter relevant to defining the normal opportunity range. Consequently, impairment of normal functioning through disease constitutes

a fundamental restriction on individual opportunity relative to the normal opportunity range.

There are two important points to note about the normal opportunity range. Obviously some diseases constitute more serious curtailments of opportunity than others relative to a given range. But because normal ranges are society relative, the same disease in two societies may impair opportunity differently and so have its importance assessed differently. Thus the social importance of particular diseases is a notion we plausibly ought to relativize between societies, assuming for the moment that impairment of opportunity is a relevant consideration. Within a society, however, the normal opportunity range abstracts from important individual differences in what might be called *effective opportunity*. From the perspective of an individual with a particular conception of the good (life plan or utility function), one who has developed certain skills and capacities needed to carry out chosen projects, *effective* opportunity range will be a subspace of the normal range. A college teacher whose career and recreational skills rely little on certain kinds of manual dexterity might find his effective opportunity diminished little compared to what a skilled laborer might find if disease impaired that dexterity. By appealing to the normal range I abstract from these differences in effective range, just as I avoid appeals directly to a person's conception of the good when I seek a measure for the social importance (for claims of justice) of health-care needs.[20]

What emerges here is the suggestion that we use impairment of the normal opportunity range as a fairly crude measure of the relative importance of health-care needs at the macro level. In general, it will be more important to prevent, cure, or compensate for those disease conditions which involve a greater curtailment of normal opportunity range. Of course, impairment of normal species functioning has another distinct effect. It can diminish satisfaction or happiness for an individual, as judged by that individual's conception of the good. Such effects are important at the micro level – for example, to individual decision making about health-care utilization. But I am here seeking the appropriate framework within which to apply principles of justice to health care at the macro level. So we shall have to look further at considerations that weigh against appeals to satisfaction at the macro level.

5. TOWARD A DISTRIBUTIVE THEORY

Satisfaction and narrower measures of well-being

So far my discussion has been primarily descriptive, not normative. As Scanlon suggests, we do not in fact use a full-range satisfaction criterion of well-being when we assess the importance or urgency of individual claims on our resources. Rather, we treat as important only a narrow range of kinds of preferences. More specifically, preferences that bear on the fulfillment of certain kinds of needs are important components of this truncated scale of well-being. In a broad range of moral contexts, we give precedence to claims based on such needs, including health-care needs, over claims based on other kinds of preferences. The Braybrooke and McCloskey suggestion gives us a general characterization of this class of needs: deficiency with regard to them threatens normal species functioning. More specifically, we can characterize health-care needs as things we need to maintain, restore, or compensate for the loss of normal species functioning. Since serious impairments of normal functioning diminish our capacities and abilities, they impair individual opportunity range relative to the range normal for our society. If we suppose people have an interest in maintaining a fair and roughly equal opportunity range, we can give at least a plausible *explanation* why they think health-care needs are special and important (which is not to say we actually do distribute them accordingly).

In what follows, I shall urge a normative claim: we ought to subsume health care under a principle of justice guaranteeing fair equality of opportunity. Actually, since I cannot here defend such a general principle without going too deeply into the general theory of distributive justice, I shall urge a weaker claim: *if* an acceptable theory of justice includes a principle providing for fair equality of opportunity, then health-care institutions should be among those governed by it. Indeed, I shall sketch briefly how one general theory, Rawls' theory of justice as fairness, might be extended in this way to provide a distributive theory for health care. *But my account does not presuppose the acceptability of Rawls' theory.* If a rule or ideal code utilitarianism, or some other theory, establishes a fair equality of opportunity principle, my account will probably be compatible with it (though some of the argument that follows may not be).

In order to introduce some issues relevant to extending Rawls' theory, I want to consider an issue we have thus far left hanging. *Should* we, for purposes of justice, use the objective, truncated scale of well-being we happen to use rather than a full-range satisfaction scale? Clearly, this too is a general question that takes us beyond the scope of this essay. Moreover, it is unlikely that we could establish conclusively a case against the satisfaction scale by considering the health care context alone. For example, a utilitarian proponent of a satisfaction or enjoyment scale might claim that the general tendencies of different diseases to diminish satisfaction provides, at worst, a rough equivalent to the "impairment of opportunity" criterion I am proposing.[21] Still, it is worth suggesting some of the considerations that weigh against the use of a satisfaction scale.

We can begin by pointing to a special case where our moral judgment would incline us against using a satisfaction scale, namely the case of "social hijacking" by persons with expensive tastes.[22] Suppose we judge how well-off someone is by reference to the full range of individual preferences in a satisfaction scale. Suppose further that moderate people adjust their tastes and preferences so that they have a reasonable chance of being satisfied with their share of social goods. Other more extravagant people form exotic and expensive tastes, even though they have comparable shares to the moderates, and, because their preferences are very strong, they are desperately unhappy when these tastes are not satisfied. Assume we can agree intersubjectively that the extravagants are less satisfied. Then if we are interested in maximizing – or even equalizing – satisfaction, extravagants seem to have a greater claim on further distributions of social resources than moderates. But something seems clearly unjust if we deny the moderates equal claims on further distributions just because they have been modest in forming their tastes. With regard to tastes and preferences that *could have been otherwise* had the extravagants chosen differently, it seems reasonable to hold them *responsible* for their own low level of satisfaction.[23]

A more general division of responsibility is suggested by this hijacking case. Rawls urges that we hold *society* responsible for guaranteeing the individual a fair share of basic liberties, opportunity, and all-purpose means, like income and wealth, needed for pursuing individual conceptions of the good. But the *individual* is responsible for choosing his ends in such a way that he has a reasonable chance of satisfying them under such just arrangements.[24] Consequently, the special features of an individual's conception of the good – here his extravagant tastes and resulting dissatisfaction – do not give rise to any special claims of justice on social resources. This suggestion about a division of responsibility is really a claim about the *scope* of theories of justice: just arrangements are supposed to guarantee individuals a reasonable share of certain basic social goods which constitute the relevant – truncated – scale of well-being for purposes of justice. The immediate object of justice is not, then, happiness or the satisfaction of desires, though just institutions provide individuals with an acceptable framework within which they can seek happiness and pursue their interests. But individuals remain responsible for the choice of their ends, so there is no injustice in not having sufficient means to reach extravagant ends.

Obviously, a full defense of this claim about the scope of justice and the social division of responsibility, and thus about the reasons for using a truncated scale of well-being, cannot rest on isolated intuitions about cases like the hijacking one. In Rawls' case, a full argument involves the claim that adopting a satisfaction scale commits us to an unacceptable view of persons as mere "containers" for satisfaction, one that departs significantly from our moral practice.[25] Because I cannot pursue these issues here, beyond suggesting there are problems with a satisfaction scale, I am content to show there is a systematic, plausible alternative to using a satisfaction scale (and ultimately to utilitarianism) whose acceptability depends on more general issues. Consequently I stick with my weaker, conditional claim above.

Rawls' argument for a truncated scale is, of course, for a specific scale, one composed of his primary social goods. But my talk about a truncated scale has focused on talk about certain basic needs, in particular, things we need to maintain species-typical normal functioning. Health-care needs are paradigmatic among these. The task that remains is to fit the two scales together. My analysis of the relation between disease and normal opportunity range provides the key to doing that.

Extending Rawls' theory to health care

Rawls' *index of primary social goods* – his truncated scale of well-being used in the contract – includes five types of social goods: (a) a set of basic liberties; (b) freedom of movement and choice of occupations against a background of diverse opportunities; (c) powers and prerogatives of office; (d) income and wealth; (e) the social bases of self-respect. Actually, Rawls uses two simplifying assumptions when using the index to assess how well-off (representative) individuals are. First, income and wealth are used as approximations to the whole index. Thus the two principles of justice[26] require basic structures to maximize the long-term expectations of the least advantaged, estimated by their income and wealth, given fixed background institutions that guarantee equal basic liberties and fair equality of opportunity. More importantly for our purposes, the theory is *idealized* to apply to individuals who are "normal, active and fully cooperating members of society over the course of a complete life."[27] There is no distributive theory for health care because no one is sick.

This simplification seems to put Rawls' index at odds with the thrust of my earlier discussion, for the truncated scale of well-being we in fact use includes needs for health care. The primary goods seem to be *too truncated* a scale, once we drop the idealizing assumption. People with equal indices will not be equally well-off once we allow them to differ in health-care needs. Moreover, we cannot simply dismiss these needs as irrelevant to questions of justice, as we did certain tastes and preferences. But if we simply build another entry into the index, we raise special issues about how to arrive at an approximate weighting of the index items.[28] Similarly, if we treat health-care services as a specially important primary social good, we abandon the useful generality of the notion of a primary social good. Moreover, we risk generating a long list of such goods, one to meet each important need.[29] Finally, as I argued earlier in answer to Fried's proposal about insurance schemes, we cannot just finesse the question whether there are special issues of justice in the distribution of health care by assuming fair shares of primary goods will be used in part to buy decent health-care insurance. A constraint on the adequacy of those shares is that they permit one to buy reasonable protection – so we must already know what justice requires by way of reasonable health care.

The most promising strategy for extending Rawls' theory without tampering with useful assumptions about the index of primary goods simply includes health-care institutions among the background institutions involved in providing for fair equality of opportunity.[30] Once we note the special connection of normal species functioning to the opportunity range open to an individual, this strategy seems the natural way to extend Rawls' view that *the subject* of theories of social justice are the *basic institutions* which provide a framework of liberties and opportunities within which individuals can use fair income shares to pursue their own conceptions of the good. Insofar as meeting health-care needs has an important effect on the distribution of health, and more to the point, on the distribution of opportunity, the health-care institutions are plausibly included on the list of basic institutions a fair equality of opportunity principle should regulate.[31]

Including health-care institutions among those which are to protect fair equality of opportunity is compatible with the central intuitions behind wanting to guarantee such opportunity in the first place. Rawls is primarily concerned with *the opportunity to pursue careers* – jobs and offices – that have various benefits attached to them. So equality of opportunity is *strategically* important: a person's well-being will be measured for the most part by the primary goods that accompany placement in such jobs and offices.[32] Rawls argues it is not enough simply to eliminate formal or legal barriers to persons seeking such jobs – for example, race, class, ethnic, or sex barriers. Rather, positive steps should be taken to enhance the opportunity of those disadvantaged by such social factors as family background.[33] The point is that none of us *deserves* the advantages conferred by accidents of birth – either the genetic or social advantages. These advantages from the "natural lottery" are morally arbitrary, and to let them determine individual opportunity – and reward and success in life – is to confer arbitrariness on the outcomes. So positive steps, for example, through the educational system, are to be taken to provide fair equality of opportunity.[34]

But if it is important to use resources to counter the advantages in opportunity some get in the natural lottery, it is equally important to use resources to counter the natural disadvantages induced by disease (and since class-differentiated social conditions contribute significantly to the etiology of disease, we are reminded disease is not just a product of the natural component of the lottery). But this does not mean we are committed to the futile goal of eliminating all natural differences between persons. Health care has as its goal normal functioning and so concentrates on a specific class of obvious disadvantages and tries to eliminate them. That is its *limited* contribution to guaranteeing fair equality of opportunity.

The approach taken here allows us to draw some interesting parallels between education and health care, for both are strategically important contributors to fair equality of opportunity. Both address needs which are not equally distributed between individuals. Various social factors, such as race, class, and family background, may produce special learning needs; so too may natural factors, such as the broad class of learning disabilities. To the extent that education is aimed at providing fair equality of opportunity, special provision must be made to meet these special needs. Here educational needs, like health-care needs, differ from other basic needs, such as the need for food and clothing, which are more equally distributed between persons. The combination of unequal distribution and the great strategic importance of the opportunity to have health care and education puts these needs in a separate category from those basic needs we can expect people to purchase from their fair income shares.

It is worth noting another point of fit between my analysis and Rawls' theory. In Rawls' contract situation, a "thick" veil of ignorance is imposed on contractors choosing basic principles of justice: they do not know their abilities, talents, place in society, or historical period. In selecting principles to govern health-care resource-allocation decisions, we need a thinner veil, for we must know about some features of the society, for example, its resource limitations. Still, using the normal opportunity range and not just the effective range as the baseline has the effect of imposing a plausibly thinned veil. It reflects basic facts about the society but keeps facts about individuals' particular ends from unduly influencing social decisions. Ultimately, defense of a veil depends on the theory of the person underlying the account. The intuition here is that persons are not defined by a particular set of interests but are free to revise their life plans. Consequently, they have an interest in maintaining conditions under which they can revise such plans, which makes the normal range a plausible reference point.

Subsuming health-care institutions under the opportunity principle can be viewed as a way of keeping the system as close as possible to the original idealization under which Rawls' theory was constructed, namely, that we are concerned with normal, fully functioning persons with a complete life-span. An important set of institutions can thus be viewed as a first defense of the idealization: they act to minimize the likelihood of departures from the normality assumption. Included here are institutions which provide for public health, environmental cleanliness, preventive personal medical services, occupational health and safety, food and drug protection, nutritional education, and educational and incentive measures to promote individual responsibility for healthy life-styles. A second layer of institutions corrects departures from the idealization. It includes those which deliver personal medical and rehabilitative services that restore normal functioning. A third layer attempts, where feasible, to maintain persons in a way that is as close as possible to the idealization. Institutions involved with more extended medical and social support services for the (moderately) chronically ill and disabled and the frail elderly would fit here. Finally, a fourth layer involves health care and related social services for those who can in no way be brought closer to the idealization. Terminal care and care for the seriously mentally and physically disabled fit here, but they raise serious issues which may not just be issues of justice. Indeed, by the time we get to the fourth layer moral virtues other than justice become prominent.

6. WORRIES AND QUALIFICATIONS

I would like to address two kinds of worries that arise in response to the approach to equality of opportunity that I have been sketching, though no doubt there are others.[35] One is that the account cannot be *exhaustive* of distributive issues in health care – the connection to opportunity is but one consideration among many. A second worry is that the appeal to opportunity is not a *useable* one – it commits us to too much or fails to tell us what we are committed to. Both worries emphasize the degree to which my account is programmatic.

One way to put the first worry is that my account makes the "specialness" of health care rest on quite abstract considerations. After all, when we reflect on the importance of health-care needs, many other factors than their effects on opportunity come to mind. Some might say health care in a direct and simple way reduces pain and suffering – and no fancy analysis of opportunity is needed to show why people value reducing them. Still, much health care affects quality of life in other ways, so the benefit of reducing pain and suffering is not general enough for our purposes. Moreover, some suffering, for example, some emotional suffering, though a cause for concern, does not obviously become a concern of justice. Others may point to psychological or cultural bases for our viewing health care as special, for example, disease reminds us of the fragility of life and the limits of human existence. But even if this point is relevant to sociological or psychological explanations of the importance some of us attribute to some kinds of health care, I have been attempting a different kind of analysis, one that can be used to justify and not just explain the importance attached to health care. So I have abstracted a central *function* of health care, the maintenance of species-typical function, and noted its central *effect* on opportunity. As a result, we are in a better position to frame distributive principles that account for the special way we treat health care because we can now say what kind of a social good health care is, namely one that maintains normal opportunity range. My analysis, while not exhaustive, focuses on that general benefit which is most relevant from the point of view of distributive justice.

Still, this qualification does not settle the first worry, which can be raised in another way. Within the confines of Rawls' theory, fair equality of opportunity – and Rawls' principle guaranteeing it – is concerned solely with access to jobs and offices. In contrast, my notion of normal opportunity range is far broader. To be sure, the narrower notion, whatever its problems, is far clearer than the broader one. But if we stick with the narrower one, we immediately import a strong age bias into our distributive theory. The opportunity of the elderly to enter jobs or offices is not impaired by disease since they are beyond, as the crass phrase goes, their "productive" years. Thus fair equality of opportunity narrowly construed seems open to one of the standard objections raised against "productivity" measures of the value of life.[36]

There are two ways to respond to this problem while still adhering to the narrower construal of opportunity. One is to admit that equality of opportunity is only one among several considerations that bear on the justice of health-care distribution. Still, even on this view, it is an important consideration with broad implications for health-care delivery. Fleshing out this response would require showing how the opportunity principle fits with these other considerations. A stronger response is to claim that the domain of basic considerations of *justice* regarding health care is exhausted by the equal opportunity principle. Other moral considerations may bear on distribution, but claims of justice will be based on the narrowly construed opportunity principle. This response bites the bullet about the age effect.

If we turn to the broader construal of equality of opportunity, using the notion of normal opportunity range, the problem reemerges, as do the weaker and stronger responses, but there may be more flexibility. The problem reemerges because it might seem that the young will always suffer greater impairment of opportunity than the elderly if health-care needs are not met. But a further alternative suggests itself: it may be possible to make the normal opportunity range relative to age. On this view, for each age (stage of life) there is a normal opportunity range, but it reflects basic facts about the life cycle and a society's responses to it. Consequently, diseases may have different effects on the young and elderly and their importance will be assessed differently.[37] This approach may avoid the most serious objections about age bias. It still leaves open the weak claim that the opportunity principle is only one consideration among many or the stronger claim that it circumscribes the scope of basic claims of justice. The stronger claim may seem more plausible since the opportunity principle has broader scope on this construal. But employing the broader construal brings with it other serious problems: do arguments which establish the priority of fair equality of opportunity on the narrow construal with its competitive aspect extend to the broader notion? These issues and alternatives require more careful discussion than they can be given here.

The second worry, about what commitments the appeal to equal opportunity generates, also has several sources. Certain "hard" cases raise the issue sharply. What does asking for the restoration of normal opportunity range mean for the terminally ill, on whom we lavish exotic life-prolonging technology, or for the severely mentally retarded? We are not required to pour all our resources into the worst cases, for that would undermine our ability to protect the opportunity of many others. But I am not sure what the approach requires here, if it delivers an answer at all. Similarly, the approach provides little help with another sort of hard case, the resource-allocation decisions in which we must choose between services which remove serious impairments of opportunity for a few people and those which remove significant but less serious impairments from many. But these shortcomings are not special to the approach I sketch: distributive theories generally founder on such cases. It seems reasonable to test my approach first in the cases where we have a better understanding of what kind of health care is owed. In any case, I do not rule out here the strong response sketched earlier to the worry about exhaustiveness, namely that our problem with at least the first kind of hard case derives from the fact that it takes us beyond the domain of justice into other considerations of right.

The second worry also has more fundamental sources. Suppose supplying a car to everyone who cannot afford one would do more to remove individual impairments of normal opportunity range than supplying certain health-care services to those who need them. Does the opportunity approach commit us now to supply cars instead of treatments?[38] The example is an instance of a far more general problem, namely, that socioeconomic (and other) inequalities affect opportunity (broadly or narrowly construed), not just the health-care and educational needs we have picked out as strategically important. But my approach does not require me to deny that certain inequalities in wealth and income may conflict with fair equality of opportunity and that guaranteeing fair equality of opportunity may thus constrain acceptable inequalities in these goods. Rather, my approach rests on the calculation that certain institutions meet needs which quite generally have a central impact on opportunity range and which should therefore be governed directly by the opportunity principle.

Finally, the second worry can be traced to the fear that health-care needs are so *expansive* (and expensive), given the advance of technology, that they create a bottomless pit. Fried, for example, argues that recognizing individual right claims to the satisfaction of health-care needs would force society to forgo realizing other social goals. He cautions we would end up worshipping the opportunity to pursue our goals but having to forgo the pursuit. Here we have the other form of the social hijacking argument, hijacking by needs rather than preferences.[39]

Two points can be offered in response to Fried's version of the second worry. First, the narrow model I have given of health-care needs excludes some of the kinds of cases Fried uses to demonstrate the threat of the bottomless pit. Thus Fried's example of retarding the effects of normal aging does not emerge as a *need* on my analysis, since normal aging does not involve a departure from normal species functioning. Such uses of health-care technology may be thought important in a particular society. Then, arguments about the relative merits of this use of scarce resources may be advanced. But such arguments would not rest on claims about basic health-care needs and thus may have different justificatory force. Still, technology does expand the ways (and costs) we have of meeting genuine health-care needs. So my account of needs at best reduces but does not eliminate Fried's worry.

Second, there is a difference between Fried's account of individual rights and entitlements and the one I am assuming here (which is quite Rawlsian). Fried is worried that if we posit a fundamental individual right to have needs satisfied, no other social goals will be able to override the right claims to all health care needs.[40] But no such fundamental right is *directly* posited on the view I have sketched. Rather, the particular rights and entitlements of individuals to have certain needs met are specified only *indirectly*, as a result of the basic health-care institutions acting in accord with the general principle governing opportunity. Deciding which needs are to be met and what resources are to be devoted to doing so requires careful moral judgment. The various institutions which affect opportunity must be weighed against each other. Similarly, the resources required to provide for fair equality of opportunity must be weighed against what is needed to provide for other important social institutions. Clearly, health-care institutions capable of protecting opportunity can be maintained only in societies whose productive capacities they do not undermine. The bugaboo of the bottomless pit is less threatening in the context of such a theory. The price paid is that we are less clear – in general and abstracting from the application of the theory to a given society – just what the individual claim comes to. The price is worth paying.

These worries emphasize the sense in which my account is sketchy and programmatic. It is worth a reminder that my account is incomplete in other ways. I have not argued that opportunity-based considerations are the only ones that should bear on the design of health-care systems. Other important social goals – some protected by right claims or other claims of need – may require the use of health-care technology. I have not considered when, if ever, these needs or rights take precedence over other wants and preferences or over some health-care needs.[41] Similarly, there is the question whether the demand for equality in health care extends beyond some decent adequate minimum – which we may suppose is defined by reference to fair equality of opportunity. Should those health-care services not considered basic be allowed to operate on a market basis? Should we insist on equality even here? These issues are not addressed by my analysis.[42]

Finally, my account is incomplete because I have concentrated on social obligations to maintain and restore health and have ignored individual responsibility to do so. But there is substantial evidence that individuals can do much to avoid incurring risks to their health – by avoiding smoking, excess alcohol, and certain foods, and by getting adequate exercise and rest. Now, nothing in my approach is incompatible with encouraging people to adopt healthy life-styles. The harder issue, however, is deciding how to distribute the burdens that result when people "voluntarily" incur extra risks and swell the costs of health care by doing so (by over 10 percent, on some estimates). After all, the consequences of such behavior cannot be easily dismissed as the arbitrary outcome of the natural lottery. Should smokers be forced to pay higher insurance premiums of special health-care taxes? I do not believe my account forces us to ignore the source of health-care risks in assigning such burdens. But at this point little more can be said because much here depends on very specific details of social history. In the United States, government subsidies of the tobacco industry, the legality of cigarette advertising, the legality of smoking in public places, and special subculture pressures on key groups (for example, teenagers) all undermine the view that we have clear-cut cases of informed, individual decision making for which individuals must be held fully accountable.

7. APPLICATIONS

The account of health-care needs sketched here has a number of implications of interest to health planners. Here I can only note some of them and set aside the many difficulties that face drawing implications from ideal theory for nonideal settings.[43]

Access

My account is compatible with (but does not imply) a multitiered health-care system. The basic tier would include health-care services that meet important health-care needs, defined by reference to their effects on opportunity. Other tiers would include services that meet less important health-care needs or other preferences. However the upper tiers are to be financed – through cost sharing, at full price, at "zero" price[44] – there should be no obstacles, financial, racial, sexual, or geographical to *initial access* to the system as a whole.

The equality of initial access derives from basic facts about the sociology and epistemology of the determination of health-care needs.[45] The "felt needs" of patients are (unreliable) initial indicators of real health-care needs. Financial and geographical barriers to initial access – say to primary care – compel people to make their own determinations of the importance of their symptoms. Of course, every system requires some patient self-assessment, but financial and geographical barriers impose different burdens in such assessment on particular groups. Indeed, where sociological barriers exist to people utilizing services, positive steps are needed (in the schools, at work, in neighborhoods) to make sure unmet needs are detected.

It is sometimes argued that the difficult access problems are ones deriving from geographical barriers and the maldistribution of physicians within specialties. In the United States, it is often argued that achieving more equitable distribution of health-care providers would unduly constrain physician liberties. It is important to see that no fundamental liberties need be violated. Suppose that the basic tier of a health-care system is redistributively financed through a national health insurance scheme that eliminates financial barriers, that no alternative insurance for the basic tier is allowed, and that there is central planning of resource allocation to guarantee needs are met. To achieve a more equitable distribution of physicians, planners *license those eligible for reimbursement* in a given health-planning region according to some reasonable formula involving physician–patient ratios.[46] Additional providers might practice in an area, but they would be without benefit of third-party payments for all services in the basic tier (or for other tiers if the national insurance scheme is more comprehensive). Most providers would follow the reimbursement dollar and practice where they are most needed.

Far from violating basic liberties, the scheme merely puts physicians in the same relation to market constraints on job availability that face most other workers and professionals. A college professor cannot simply decide there are people to be taught in Scarsdale or Chevy Chase or Shaker Heights; he must accept what jobs are available within universities, wherever they are. Of course, he is "free" to ignore the market, but then he may not be able to teach. Similarly, managers and many types of workers face the need to locate themselves where there is need for their skills. So the physician's sacrifice of liberty under the scheme (or variants on it, including a National Health Service) is merely the imposition of a burden already faced by much of the working population. Indeed, the scheme does not change in principle the forces that already motivate physicians; it merely shifts where it is profitable for some physicians to practice. The appearance that there is an enshrined liberty under attack is the legacy of an historical accident, one more visible in the United States than elsewhere, namely, that physicians have been more independent of institutional settings for the delivery of their skills than many other workers, and even than physicians in other countries. But this too shall pass.

Resource allocation

My account of health-care needs and their connection to fair equality of opportunity has a number of implications for resource-allocation issues. I have already noted that we get an important distinction between the use of health-care services to meet health-care needs and their use to meet other wants and preferences. The tie of health-care needs to opportunity makes the former use special and important in a way not true of the latter. Moreover, we get a crude criterion – impact on normal opportunity range – for distinguishing the importance of different health-care needs, though I have also noted how far short this falls of being a solution to many hard allocation questions. Three further implications are worth noting here.

There has been much debate about whether the United States' health-care system overemphasizes acute therapeutic services as opposed to preventive and public health measures. Sometimes the argument focuses on the relative-efficacy and cost of preventive, as opposed to acute, services. My account suggests there is also an important issue of distributive justice here. Suppose a system is heavily weighted toward acute interventions, yet it provides equal access to its services. Thus anyone with severe respiratory ailments – black lung, brown lung, asbestosis, emphysema, and so on – is given adequate and comprehensive services as needed. Does the system meet the demands of equity? Not if they are determined by the approach of fair equality of opportunity. The point is that people are differentially at risk of contracting such diseases because of work and living conditions. Efficacy aside, preventive measures have distinct distributive implications from acute measures. The opportunity approach requires we attend to both.

My account points to another allocational inequity. One important function of health-care services, here personal medical services, is to restore handicapping dysfunctions, for example, of vision, mobility, and so on. The medical goal is to cure the diseased organ or limb where possible. Where cure is impossible, we try to make function as normal as possible, through corrective lenses or prosthesis and rehabilitative therapy. But where restoration of function is beyond the ability of medicine per se, we begin to enter another area of services, nonmedical social support (we move from (4) to (5) on the list of health-care needs in Section 4). Such support services provide the blind person with the closest he can get to the functional equivalent of vision – for example, he is taught how to navigate, provided with a seeing-eye dog, taught braille, and so on. From the point of view of their impact on opportunity, medical services and social support services that meet health-care needs have the same rationale and are equally important. Yet, for various reasons, probably having to do with the profitability and glamor of personal medical service and careers in them as compared to services for the handicapped, our society has taken only slow and halting steps to meet the health-care needs of those with permanent disabilities. These are matters of justice, not charity; we are not facing conditions of scarcity so severe that these steps to provide equality of opportunity must be forgone in favor of more pressing needs. The point also has implications for the problem of long-term care for the frail elderly, but I cannot develop them here.

A final implication of the account raises a different set of issues, namely, how to reconcile the demands of justice with certain traditional views of a physician's obligation to his patients. The traditional view is that the physician's direct responsibility is to the well-being of his patients, that (with their consent) he is to do everything in his power to preserve their lives and well-being. One effect of leaving all resource-allocation decisions in this way to the micro-level decisions of physicians and patients, especially where third-party payment schemes mean little or no rationing by price, is that cost-ineffective utilization results. In the current cost-conscious climate, there is pressure to make physicians see themselves as responsible for introducing economic considerations into their utilization decisions. But the issue raised here goes beyond cost-effectiveness. My account suggests that there are important resource-allocation priorities that derive from considerations of justice. In a context of moderate scarcity, this suggests it is not possible for physicians to see as their ideal the maximization of the quality of care they deliver regardless of cost: pursuing that ideal upsets resource-allocation priorities determined by the opportunity principle. Considerations of justice challenge the traditional (perhaps mythical) view that physicians can act as the unrestrained agents of their patients. The remaining task, which I pursue elsewhere, is to show at what level the constraints should be imposed so as to disturb as little as possible of what is valuable about the traditional view of physician responsibility.[47]

These remarks on applications are frustratingly brief, and fuller development of them is required if we are to assess the practical import of the account I offer. Nevertheless, I think the account offers enough that is attractive at the theoretical level to warrant further development of its practical implications.

NOTES

Research for this paper was supported by Grant Number HS03097 from the National Center for Health Services Research, OASH, and by a Tufts Sabbatical Leave. I am also indebted to the Commonwealth Fund, which sponsored a seminar on this material at Brown University. Earlier drafts benefited from presentations to the Hastings Center Institute project on Ethics and Health Policy (funded by the Kaiser Foundation), a NCHSR staff seminar, and colloquia at Tufts, NYU Medical Center, University of Michigan, and University of Georgia. Helpful comments were provided by Ronald Bayer, Hugo Bedau, Richard Brandt, Dan Brock, Arthur Caplan, Josh Cohen, Allen Gibbard, Ruth Macklin, Carola Mone, John Rawls, Daniel Wikler, and the Editors of *Philosophy & Public Affairs*. This essay is excerpted from my *Just Health Care* (Cambridge: Cambridge University Press, 1985).

1 The objection that health-care resources are scarce only because we waste money on frivolous things presupposes distinctions which a theory of needs should illuminate.

2 I paraphrase Charles Fried, *Right and Wrong* (Cambridge: Harvard University Press, 1978), pp. 126ff. See my comments on Fried's proposal in "Rights to Health Care: Programmatic Worries," *Journal of Medicine and Philosophy* 4, no. 2 (June 1979): 174–91. I ignore here an issue of paternalism which Fried may have wanted to pursue but which is better raised when fair shares are clearly large enough to purchase a reasonable insurance package: Should the premium purchase be compulsory?

3 Needs-based theories cut two ways. Egalitarians use them to criticize the failure of inegalitarian systems to meet basic human needs. Inegalitarians

use them to justify providing only minimally for basic needs while allowing significant inequalities above the floor. Here I resist the temptation to respond to the inegalitarian by expanding the category of needs to consume such inequalities.

4 Arrow's classic paper traces the anomalies of the medical market to the uncertainties in it. My analysis has a bearing on the further moral issue, whether health care ought to be marketed even in an ideal market. Cf. Kenneth Arrow, "Uncertainty and the Welfare Economics of Medical Care," *American Economic Review* 53 (1963): 941–73.

5 The presence of people with preferences for more-than-reasonable coverage may result in inflationary pressures on the premium for "reasonable" insurance packages. So interference in the market is likely to be necessary to protect the adequacy of fair shares.

6 For emphasis, we often refer to things we simply desire or want as things we need. Sometimes we invoke a distinction between noun and verb uses of "need," so that not everything we say we need counts as a *need*. Any distinction we might draw between noun and verb uses depends on our purposes and the context and would still have to be explained by the kind of analysis I undertake above.

7 T. M. Scanlon, "Preference and Urgency," *Journal of Philosophy* 77, no. 19 (November 1975): 655–69.

8 The difference might not be in the *extent* but in the *content* of the scale. An objective full-range satisfaction scale might be constructed so that some categories of (key) preferences are lexically primary to others; preferences not included on a truncated scale never enter the full-range scale except to break ties among those equally well-off on key preferences. Such a scale may avoid my worries, but it needs a rationale for its ranking. The objection raised here to full-range satisfaction measures applies, I believe, with equal force to happiness or enjoyment measures of the sort Richard Brandt defends in *A Theory of the Good and the Right* (Oxford: Oxford University Press, 1979), ch. 14.

9 See Scanlon, "Preference and Urgency," p. 660.

10 David Braybrooke, "Let Needs Diminish that Preferences May Prosper," in *Studies in Moral Philosophy*, American Philosophical Quarterly Monograph Series, No. 1 (Blackwells: Oxford, 1968), p. 90 (my emphasis). Personal medical services do not count as course-of-life needs on the criterion that we need them all through our lives or at certain (developmental) stages, but they do count as course-of-life needs in that deficiency with respect to them may endanger normal functioning.

11 McCloskey, unlike Braybrooke, is committed to distinguishing a narrower noun use of "need" from the verb use. See J. H. McCloskey, "Human Needs, Rights, and Political Values," *American Philosophical Quarterly* 13, no. 1 (January 1976): 2f (my emphasis). McCloskey's proposal is less clear to me than Braybrooke's: presumably our natures include species-typical functioning but something more as well. Moreover, McCloskey is more insistent than Braybrooke in leaving room for *individual natures*, though Braybrooke at least leaves room for something like this when he refers to the needs that we may have by virtue of individual temperament. The

hard problem that faces McCloskey is distinguishing between things we need *to develop our individual natures* and things we come to need in the process of what he calls "self-making," the carrying out of projects one chooses, perhaps in accordance with one's nature but not just by way of developing it.

12   The account here draws on a fine series of articles by Christopher Boorse; see "On the Distinction between Disease and Illness," *Philosophy & Public Affairs* 5, no. 1 (Fall 1975): 49–68; "What a Theory of Mental Health Should Be," *Journal of the Theory of Social Behavior* 6, no. 1: 61–84; "Health as a Theoretical Concept," *Philosophy of Science* 44 (1977): 542–73. See also Ruth Macklin, "Mental Health and Mental Illness: Some Problems of Definition and Concept Formation," *Philosophy of Science* 39, no. 3 (September 1972): 341–65.

13   Boorse, "What a Theory of Mental Health Should Be," p. 77.

14   "Health is a state of complete physical, mental, and social well-being, and not merely the absence of disease or infirmity." From the Preamble to the Constitution of the World Health Organization. Adopted by the International Health Conference held in New York, 19 June–22 July 1946, and signed on 22 July 1946. *Off. Rec. Wld. Health Org.* 2, no. 100. See Daniel Callahan, "The WHO Definition of 'Health,'" *The Hastings Center Studies* 1, no. 3 (1973): 77–88.

15   See H. Tristram Engelhardt, Jr., "The Disease of Masturbation: Values and the Concept of Disease," *Bulletin of the History of Medicine* 48, no. 2 (Summer 1974): 234–48.

16   Boorse's critique of strongly normative views of disease is persuasive independently of some problematic features of his own account.

17   For example, we need an account of functional ascriptions in biology [see Boorse, "Wright on Functions," *Philosophical Review* 85, no. 1 (January 1976): 70–86]. More specifically, we need to be able to distinguish genetic variations from disease, and we must specify the range of environments taken as "natural" for the purpose of revealing dysfunction. The latter is critical to the second feature of the biomedical model: for example, what range of social roles and environments is included in the natural range? If we allow too much of the social environment, then racially discriminatory environments might make being of the wrong race a disease; if we disallow all socially created environments, then we seem not to be able to call dyslexia a disease (disability).

18   Anyone who doubts the appropriateness of treating some physiognomic deformities as serious diseases with strong claims on surgical resources should look at Frances C. MacGreggor's *After Plastic Surgery: Adaptation and Adjustment* (New York: Praeger, 1979). Even where there is no disease or deformity, there is nothing in the analysis I offer that precludes individuals or society from deciding to use health-care technology to make physiognomy conform to some standard of beauty. But such uses of health technology will not be justifiable as the fulfillment of health-care *needs*.

19   My account has the following bearing on the debate about Medicaid-funded abortions. Nontherapeutic abortions do not count as health-care needs, so if Medicaid has as its only function the meeting of the health-care

needs of the poor, then we cannot argue for funding the abortions just like any other procedure. Their justifications will be different. But if Medicaid should serve other important goals, like ensuring that poor and well-off women can equally well control their bodies, then there is justification for funding abortions. There is also the worry that not funding them will contribute to other health problems induced by illegal abortions.

20 One issue here is to avoid "hijacking" by past preferences which themselves define the effective range. Of course, effective range may be important in microallocation decisions.

21 Presumably, he must also claim that we improve satisfaction more by treating and preventing disease than by finding ways to encourage people to adjust to their conditions by reordering their preference curves.

22 I draw on Rawls' unpublished lecture, "Responsibility for Ends," in the following three paragraphs.

23 Here again the utilitarian proponent of the satisfaction scale may issue a typical promissory note, assuring us that maximizing satisfaction overall requires institutional arrangements that act to minimize social hijacking.

24 The division presupposes, as Rawls points out in response to Scanlon, that people have the ability and know they have the responsibility to adjust their desires in view of their fair shares of (primary) social goods. See Scanlon, "Preference and Urgency," pp. 665–66.

25 Satisfaction scales leave us no basis for not wanting to *be* whatever person, construed as a set of preferences, has higher satisfaction. To borrow Bernard Williams' term, they leave us with no basis for insisting on the *integrity* of persons. See Rawls, "Responsibility for Ends." The view that issues here turn in a fundamental way on the nature of persons is pursued in Derek Parfit, "Later Selves and Moral Principles," *Philosophy and Personal Relations*, ed. Alan Montefiore (London: Routledge & Kegan Paul, 1973): 137–69; Rawls, "Independence of Moral Theory," *Proceedings and Addresses of the American Philosophical Association* 48 (1974–1975): 5–22; and Daniels, "Moral Theory and the Plasticity of Persons," *Monist* 62, no. 3 (July 1979): 265–87.

26 See *A Theory of Justice* (Cambridge: Harvard University Press, 1971), p. 302.

27 Rawls, "Responsibility for Ends."

28 Some weighting problems will have to be faced anyway; see my "Rights to Health Care" for further discussion. Also see Kenneth Arrow, "Some Ordinalist Utilitarian Notes on Rawls's Theory of Justice," *Journal of Philosophy* 70, no. 9 (1973); 245–63. Also see Joshua Cohen, "Studies in Political Philosophy," Ph.D. diss. (Harvard University, 1978), Part III and Appendices.

29 See Ronald Greene, "Health Care and Justice in Contract Theory Perspective," in *Ethics & Health Policy*, ed. Robert Veatch and Roy Branson (Cambridge, MA: Ballinger, 1976), pp. 111–26.

30 The primary social goods themselves remain general and abstract properties of social arrangements – basic liberties, opportunities, and certain all-purpose exchangeable means (income and wealth). We can still simplify matters in using the index by looking solely at income and wealth – assuming a background of equal basic liberties and fair equality of oppor-

tunity. Health care is not a primary social good – neither are food, clothing, shelter, or other basic needs. The presumption is that the latter will be adequately provided for from fair shares of income and wealth. The special importance and unequal distribution of health-care needs, like educational needs, are acknowledged by their connection to other institutions that provide for fair equality of opportunity. But opportunity, not health care or education, is the primary social good.

31 Here I shift emphasis from Rawls when he remarks that health is a *natural* as opposed to *social* primary good because its possession is less influenced by basic institutions. See *A Theory of Justice*, p. 62. Moreover, it seems to follow that where health care is generally inefficacious – say, in earlier centuries – it loses its status as a special concern of justice and the "caring" it offers may more properly be viewed as a concern of charity.

32 The ways in which disease affects normal opportunity range are more extensive than the ways in which it affects opportunity to pursue careers, a point I return to later.

33 Of course, the effects of family background cannot all be eliminated. See *A Theory of Justice*, p. 74.

34 Rawls allows individual differences in talents and abilities to remain relevant to issues of job placement, for example, through their effects on productivity. So fair equality of opportunity does not mean that individual differences no longer confer advantages. Advantages are constrained by the difference principle. See my "Merit and Meritocracy," *Philosophy & Public Affairs* 7, no. 3 (Spring 1978): 206–23.

35 For example, appeals to equality of opportunity have historically played a conservative, deceptive role, blinding people to the injustice of class and race inequalities in rewards. Historically, appeals to the ideal of equal opportunity have implicitly justified strong competitive individual relations. More concretely, we often find institutions, like the United States educational system, praised as embodying (at least approximately) that ideal, whereas there is strong evidence the system functions primarily to replicate class inequalities. See my "IQ, Heritability and Human Nature" in *Proceedings of the Philosophy of Science Association*, 1974, ed. R. S. Cohen (Dordrecht: Reidel, 1976), pp. 143–80; and, with J. Cronin, A. Krock, and R. Webber, "Race, Class and Intelligence: A Critical Look at the IQ Controversy," *International Journal of Mental Health* 3, no. 4: 46–123; and S. Bowles and H. Gintis, *Schooling in Capitalist America* (New York: Basic Books, 1976).

36 See E. J. Mishan, "Evaluation of Life and Limb: A Theoretical Approach," *Journal of Political Economy*, 79, no. 4 (1971): 687–705; Jan Paul Acton, "Measuring the Monetary Value of Life Saving Programs," *Law and Contemporary Problems* 40, no. 4 (Autumn 1976): 46–72; Michael Bayles, "The Price of Life," *Ethics* 89, no. 1 (October 1978): 20–34.

37 It would be interesting to know if this age-relativized opportunity range yields results similar to that achieved by the Rawlsian device of a veil. If people who do not know their age are asked to design a system of health-care delivery for the society they will be in, they would presumably budget their resources in a fashion that takes the special features of each

stage of the life cycle into account and gives each stage a reasonable claim on resources.

38 Using medical technology to enhance normal capacities or functions – say strength or vision – makes the problem easier: the burden of proof is on proposals that give priority to altering the normal opportunity range rather than protecting individuals whose normal range is compromised.

39 See Fried, *Right and Wrong*, ch. 5. The problem also worries Braybrooke, "Let Needs Diminish."

40 It is not clear to me how much Fried's side-constraints resemble Nozick's.

41 See n. 19 above.

42 Except where conditions of extensive scarcity leave basic health-care needs unmet and so no room for less important uses of health-care services, or except where the existence of a market-based health-care system threatens the ability of the basic system to deliver its important product.

43 I discuss these difficulties in "Conflicting Objectives and the Priorities Problem," In Peter Brown, Conrad Johnson, and Paul Vernier, eds., *Income Support: Conceptual and Policy Issues* (Totowa, NJ: Rowman & Littlefield, 1981). My *Just Health Care* (Cambridge: Cambridge University Press, 1985) develops some applications in detail.

44 The strongest objections to such mixed systems is that the upper tier competes for resources with the lower tiers. See Claudine McCreadie, "Rawlsian Justice and the Financing of the National Health Service," *Journal of Social Policy* 5, no. 2 (1976): 113–31.

45 See Avedis Donabedian, *Aspects of Medical Care Administration* (Cambridge: Harvard University Press, 1973).

46 I ignore the crudeness of such measures. For fuller discussion of these manpower distribution issues see my "What Is the Obligation of the Medical Profession in the Distribution of Health Care?" *Social Science and Medicine* 15F (1981): 129–35.

47 See Avedis Donabedian "The Quality of Medical Care: A Concept in Search of a Definition," *Journal of Family Practice* 9, no. 2 (1979): 277–84; and Daniels, "Cost-Effectiveness and Patient Welfare," in Marc Basson, ed., *Ethics, Humanism and Medicine*, vol. 2 (New York: Aldon Liss, 1981), pp. 159–70.

Chapter 10

Equality of what: Welfare, resources, or capabilities?[1]

1. THE TARGET OF EGALITARIAN CONCERNS

Many of us have egalitarian concerns. To some extent, that is, at some cost, we prefer a world in which goods – powers, liberties, opportunities, wealth, health – are more equally distributed to one in which they are not. At least to some extent, we are willing to forego delivering a greater benefit to someone who is already better off in order to deliver a lesser benefit to someone who is worse off. Whether we are strictly concerned with equality or merely with giving priority to the claims of those who are worse off, we face the question, What is the ultimate target of our egalitarian concerns?[2]

Three apparently distinct targets have been proposed as answers to this question. First, when we urge specific egalitarian reforms, we are really trying to make people equally happy or *satisfied*, or at least to guarantee them *equal opportunity for such welfare*. This is the claim made by Richard Arneson and (with qualifications) by G. A. Cohen.[3] Rejecting welfare-based targets, others say the target of our egalitarian concerns is assuring people greater equality in the *resources* needed to pursue their ends. Ronald Dworkin argues in this vein,[4] and John Rawls' Difference Principle gives priority to those who are worse off according to an index of primary social goods.[5] A third view is that the target of our egalitarian concerns is the positive freedom or *capability* of people to do or be what they choose. Amartya Sen rejects both welfare- and resource-based accounts in favor of this target.[6]

In what follows, I will not attempt to resolve this dispute about the ultimate target of our egalitarian concerns. For one thing, I am not sure that the task of a theory of justice involves answering this question about the ultimate target of our egalitarian concerns in the way in which it is posed here. Our egalitarian concerns might, for example, have different targets in different contexts. Though Arneson, Cohen, Dworkin, and Sen seem committed to some version of the encompass-

208

ing question about targets, it is not clear to me that Rawls is, even though his arguments for primary goods and against welfare-based claims about well-being began the dispute. Rawls may not believe there is a unified target of egalitarian concerns because our interests in equality or equal treatment may differ for purposes of political philosophy and in other moral contexts, e.g., in a family or other private association (see Section 4 below). Nevertheless, I want to explore some issues raised by the dispute, and I want to do so by examining some recent criticisms of a central feature of Rawls' theory of justice as fairness, namely, his claim that an index of primary social goods is the appropriate measure of relative well-being for purposes of political philosophy. This approach fits well with the history of the debate about targets, for it was Rawls' criticisms of welfare-based measures of well-being and introduction of the primary social goods that began the dispute.

I am interested in criticisms of the primary goods (and Rawls' use of them) that come from two different directions, in the sense that they are defenses of distinct targets. Each says that the primary goods are inflexible or insensitive to some kind of variability in people. This variability keeps people from converting primary goods with equal efficiency into what is of ultimate moral concern. As a result, the primary goods inadequately capture the force of our egalitarian concerns, leading us to treat people similarly when a relevant inequality still exists among them.

One line of criticism of the primary social goods is that they fail to capture a fundamental moral intuition that underlies our concerns about equality (that is, about permissible inequalities). The intuition is that whenever we are made worse off through no fault of our own, or as the result of nothing that we could control, then we have a legitimate initial claim on others for assistance or compensation for our misfortune. Rawls' use of primary goods keeps us from responding to certain ways in which individuals with the same primary goods may be made worse off with regard to their opportunity for welfare through no fault of their own, and so his principles of justice will not be responsive to this central egalitarian intuition. Arneson and Cohen, in developing this line of criticism, further argue that the underlying intuition is one that Rawls himself appeals to elsewhere in his theory.[7]

The other line of criticism is that individuals vary in their ability to convert primary goods into what is really important to them, namely, the freedom or capability to do or to be (to function as) what they choose. This variability in the ability of people to convert primary goods into capabilities suggests that the primary goods are "inflexible" and ultimately miss what is of fundamental moral concern, namely, greater equality of capabilities. Sen, who develops this line of criticism, suggests there is an element of "fetishism" in Rawls' use of primary goods.[8] What is of ultimate concern here is not the primary goods, but capabilities, which are the result of a *"relationship* between persons and goods."[9] Though welfare-based accounts are mistaken about what is of ultimate concern (Sen agrees with Rawls in rejecting them), at least they, like Sen's capabilities, avoid fetishism.

I shall argue that neither of these lines of criticism shows us that a theory of justice using primary social goods misses the target of our egalitarian concerns, at least for purposes of the just design of basic social institutions. To be sure, judging the well-being of representative individuals by reference to an index of primary goods is a very *abstract* measure of well-being. Rawls intends it only to capture the well-being of people insofar as they are thought of as citizens who share an interest in cooperation for mutual advantage in a well-ordered, pluralist society, who function normally over a complete life, and who are "free" and "equal." They are free and equal in the specific sense that they have two basic moral powers, the power to form and revise a conception of the good and the capacity for a sense of justice.[10] The primary goods thus meet the needs and interests of citizens, conceived in this abstract and idealized way. Nevertheless, this does not make them "fetishist" and "inflexible," as Sen argues, and I suggest in the next section how we can appropriately flesh out the primary goods so that the principles of justice avoid these criticisms. In the third section, I argue that accounts that focus on "equal opportunity for welfare (or advantage)" run afoul of Rawls' insistence that individual conceptions of the good are incommensurable, that is, with the fact of pluralism. I also respond to Arneson's and Cohen's arguments that the primary goods are inflexible because they force us to ignore the legitimate complaints of people who are worse off than others because some of their preferences or values, which they have through no fault of their own, put them at a disadvantage.

Though I believe I can defend the primary goods against these criticisms about inflexibility, a deeper issue about justification remains. These criticisms arise from a basic disagreement between Rawls and his critics about the domain of justice and the relevance of comprehensive moral views to the construction of a *political* conception of justice, one that is not a compromise with what justice ideally requires. I comment briefly on this issue in the last section.

2. CAPABILITIES AND THE INFLEXIBILITY OF PRIMARY GOODS

Sen's central objection to the primary goods builds on a criticism originally made by Arrow, who noted that people who were ill or disabled might be worse off than others despite enjoying the same index of primary social goods.[11] More generally, people vary in their ability to convert primary goods into well-being. As a result, if we take the primary goods as the appropriate measure of well-being for purposes of justice, we may treat people unfairly. There are really two related claims here.[12] First, the variability among persons implies that the primary goods are an *inflexible* measure of well-being, ignoring variations that matter. Second, this inflexibility should count as strong evidence that the primary goods are the wrong quality space in which to work: we are not ultimately concerned with goods – primary or not – but with what people, given their variability, can do and be with those goods (thus Sen's charge of fetishism). I will first respond to the charge about variability and inflexibility; then it may be possible to address the claim that justice is concerned with capabilities.

One source of variability in the conversion of primary goods into well-being is that introduced by the different conceptions of the good, including different preferences and values, held by individuals. How satisfied people are with their lot in life – how much *welfare* they have, as judged by utilitarian and other welfarist theories – will depend not only on the primary goods available to them, but on their preferences.[13] Some people will be inefficient converters of primary goods into welfare because their conceptions of the good make them hard to satisfy. For example, if someone has expensive tastes, e.g., for expensive wines, and is unhappy because she cannot be satisfied on her share of primary goods, then our egalitarian concerns do not seem to pull us in the direction of thinking she has a legitimate claim on us because we have not adequately provided for her welfare. Indeed, we resist what seems like "hijacking" by expensive tastes. Sen agrees with Rawls that it is an advantage of the primary goods that they ignore *this* source of variability, because, like Rawls, he rejects welfare as an appropriate measure of well-being or relative advantage for purposes of justice. (I return to these matters in the next section where I discuss the retreat from "equality of welfare" to "equal opportunity for welfare" in the face of these antihijacking sentiments.)

What does trouble Sen is the other kind of variability that also bothered Arrow: some individuals are inefficient converters of primary goods into relative advantage or well-being because they are ill or handicapped. Similarly, there may be variability in the nutritional needs of individuals – e.g., between those with low or high metabolic rates, or between pregnant women and others. In contexts of serious poverty, these nutritional differences would lead to significant differences in relative advantage. A theory that judges the well-being of individuals by an index of primary social goods ignores this variability. Sen remarks that the "Charybdis of overrigidity threatens us as much as the Scylla of subjectivist variability, and we must not lose sight of the important personal parameters in developing an approach to well-being."[14] To some extent, Rawls invites Sen's criticism, since he explicitly sets aside and ignores the variability among individuals that is introduced by disease and disability.[15] Rawls' view is that, if we can solve the problem of justice for the idealized case that ignores this variability, then maybe we can extend the solution to more complex cases. I shall suggest shortly that Rawls' best response to Sen lies in such an extension of the basic theory; but I am getting ahead of myself.

Sen's own account of relative advantage or well-being concentrates on the concept of "functioning." How well-off we are depends on what we can do and be, that is, on how we function. For example, "doings" and "beings" include "activities (like eating or reading or seeing), or states of existence or being, e.g., being well nourished, being free from malaria, not being ashamed by the poverty of one's clothing or shoes."[16] Sen suggests that we represent "the focal features of a person's living" by an n-tuple of different types of functionings; each component of the n-tuple reflects the extent of the achievement of a particular functioning. The n-tuple is thus not just an array of kinds of functionings, but it includes a measure of the level of achievement of each functioning in the array. Sen suggests that a person's *capability* can be represented by the set of n-tuples of functionings from which the person can choose any one n-tuple. In this way, the "capability set" stands "for the actual freedom of choice a person has over alternative lives that he or she can lead."[17]

Given the same index of primary goods, a handicapped or ill individual may not enjoy the same capability set or freedom of choice as someone who is normal. I believe the attraction of Sen's criticism comes from this central set of examples. The example of nutritional differences seems problematic only if we assume that an assignment of primary goods will not allow individuals to accommodate, without undue sacrifice, their differences in metabolic needs. In many parts of the world this assumption does fail, because people lose entitlements to food and not simply because of natural shortages of resources, as Sen persuasively argues.[18] Still, I think that an acceptable extension of Rawls' theory to handle the cases of disease and disability can be further extended to accommodate the problem of nutritional differences, though I will say nothing further about nutrition here.

Before turning to the examples of disease and disability, it is worth noting that Sen says little, at least in the context of this line of criticism of Rawls, about another important kind of individual variability, namely, variability in the natural bases for talents and skills. Someone who is naturally manually dextrous can convert a given level of pri-

mary goods into a larger or better capability set than someone who
is not (and is in all other ways the same). It is not clear what Sen wants
to do about this source of inequality in capability sets or freedoms.
It is not obvious that any simple adjustment to resources can eliminate
this source of inequality in capabilities. My guess is that Sen would
probably try to mitigate the effects of this inequality in some way,
acknowledging that he cannot eliminate it. But that is just what Rawls
does.

Rawls is, of course, explicitly concerned with this source of variability. The Difference Principle acts to *mitigate* but not to eliminate
(which may be impossible) the effects on those with the worst talents
and skills by ensuring that inequalities tend to work maximally to their
advantage. Rawls' approach is to let the variability that results from the
distribution of talents and skills work to everyone's advantage – that is
what the "democratic equality" interpretation of the Second Principle
involves. The pursuit of fair equality of opportunity does not require
leveling all differences in talents or skills, though we are required to
mitigate the effects of this inequality. In judging a theory of justice,
then, this form of inflexibility of the primary goods does not seem a
fatal obstacle. Flexibility can be found elsewhere.[19]

Let us return to the central examples of inflexibility, namely, the
problems raised by disease and disability. Sen is suggesting that the
primary goods leave us incapable of responding to the health-care
needs of those with disease and disability, especially since Rawls has
assumed these conditions away in order to arrive at a core theory for
"fully functioning" citizens. I want to show that a plausible extension of
Rawls' theory can accommodate, with appropriate flexibility, concerns
about disease and disability; I draw on my earlier work on justice and
health-care needs.[20]

I begin with a narrow, if not uncontroversial, "biomedical" model:
the basic idea is that health is the absence of disease, and diseases (I
include deformities and disabilities that result from trauma) are *deviations from the normal functional organization of a typical member of a
species.*[21] The task of characterizing this natural functional organization
falls to the biomedical sciences. The concept of disease that results is
not merely a statistical notion; rather, it draws on a theoretical account
of the design of the organism. In the case of people, we require an
account of the species-typical functional organization that permits us to
pursue biological goals as *social* animals: our various cognitive and
emotional functions must be included. Similarly, we must include mental disease and health into the picture, even though we have a less well-
developed theory of species-typical mental functions. This biomedical
model has controversial features that I ignore here.[22] By appealing to it,
however, I can draw a fairly sharp line between uses of health-care

services to prevent and treat diseases – that is, uses that keep people functioning normally – and uses that meet other individual or social goals. Though I use a rather narrow model of disease and health, at least by comparison to some fashionable views, health-care needs emerge as a broad and diverse set. Health-care needs will be those things we need in order to maintain, restore, or provide functional equivalents (where possible) to normal species function. They include (1) adequate nutrition and shelter; (2) sanitary, safe, unpolluted living and working conditions; (3) exercise, rest, and some other features of life-style; (4) preventive, curative, and rehabilitative personal medical services; and (5) nonmedical personal and social support services. The task of extending Rawls' theory seems difficult in part because it is hard to see how to fit provision of these diverse and extensive needs within the "inflexible" framework of the principles and the primary goods.

I want to emphasize a relationship between normal functioning and opportunity, one of the primary social goods. Impairments of normal species functioning reduce the range of opportunity open to the individual in which he may construct his "plan of life" or conception of the good. Life plans for which we are otherwise suited are rendered unreasonable by impairments of normal functioning. Consequently, if persons have a fundamental interest in preserving the opportunity to revise their conceptions of the good through time, then they will have a pressing interest in maintaining normal species functioning by establishing institutions, such as health-care systems, which do just that.

This point can be made more precise. The *normal opportunity range* for a given society is the array of life plans reasonable persons in it are likely to construct for themselves. The normal range is thus dependent on key features of the society – its stage of historical development, its level of material wealth and technological development, and even important cultural facts about it. This is one way in which the notion of normal opportunity range is socially relative. Facts about social organization, including the conception of justice regulating its basic institutions, will also determine how that total normal range is distributed in the population. Nevertheless, normal species functioning provides us with one clear parameter affecting the share of the normal range open to a given individual. It is this parameter which the distribution of health care affects.

The share of the normal range open to an individual is also *determined in a fundamental way by his talents and skills*. Fair equality of opportunity does not require that opportunity be equal for all persons. It requires only that it be equal for persons with similar skills and talents. Thus individual shares of the normal range will not in general be equal, even when they are fair to individuals. As I noted earlier, within justice as fairness, unequal chances of success which derive from unequal talents may be compensated for in other ways, by the constraints on inequality imposed by the Difference Principle. What is important here, however, is that impairment of normal functioning through disease and disability restricts an individual's opportunity relative to that portion of the normal range his skills and talents would have made available to him were he healthy.[23] If an individual's fair share of the normal range is the array of life plans he may reasonably choose, given his talents and skills, then disease and disability shrinks his share from what is fair. Thus restoring normal functioning through health care has a particular and limited effect on an individual's share of the normal range. It lets him enjoy that portion of the range to which his full array of talents and skills would give him access, assuming that these too are not impaired by special social disadvantages (e.g., racism or sexism).

Two points about the normal opportunity range should be emphasized. First, some diseases constitute more serious curtailments of opportunity than others relative to a given range, and the normal range is defined in a socially relative way. Thus the social importance of a particular disease is a notion that is itself socially relative. Second, the normal range abstracts from important individual differences in which I will call *effective opportunity*. From the perspective of an individual who has a particular plan of life and who has developed certain skills accordingly, the effective opportunity range will only be a part of her fair share of the normal range. For purposes of justice, we ignore the individual assessments of the importance of a given function that derive from particular conceptions of the good.[24]

The suggestion that derives from this analysis of the effect of disease and disability on an individual's fair share of the normal opportunity range is that health-care systems should be governed by the principle protecting fair equality of opportunity. In fact, as I have argued elsewhere,[25] fair equality of opportunity must be protected over the lifespan of each individual. Since the impact of disease or disability on opportunity range may vary at each stage of life, our system must prudently allocate health-care resources by protecting an individual's fair share of the normal opportunity range at each stage of life. In this way we arrive at a fair distribution of health-care resources between age groups.

It is important to notice that my notion of normal opportunity range is broader than the primary good of opportunity, as Rawls describes it in his discussion of the original position. There opportunity is primarily concerned with access to jobs and careers, which are taken to be the central matters of concern for citizens, construed as free and equal moral agents possessing certain fundamental moral powers. Does this extension of Rawls' theory do violence to the more restrictive notion of primary goods involved in the discussion of the Original Position?

I think not. As we move from the original position to the constitutional and legislative stages of Rawls' theory, we have available more information about the specific conditions in a particular society, and the primary goods will be fleshed out and extended in various ways. Rawls suggests that this is true for basic rights and liberties.[26] Similarly, the primary goods of income and wealth should not be confused simply with personal income and private wealth. Providing certain public goods (clean air and water, which are important health-care needs) could be counted as part of each person's income or wealth. The same can be done *ex ante* for the contingent claims each individual can make on necessary medical services, even if *ex post*, the services each person actually gets will depend on the contingencies of disease and disability. But we should not interpret these contingent claims on access to medical services as mere supplements to the income of the least advantaged. Rather, this form of income or wealth (if that is how we, or economists, count it) – the health-care system with this design – is necessary if fair equality of opportunity is to be assured and citizens are to be kept normal, fully functioning members of society.[27]

There are some important similarities and contrasts between the approach sketched here and Sen's. Sen's capability sets, for example, resemble my notion of an individual's share of the normal opportunity range. Sen was silent on the issue of whether capability sets should be equal despite the distribution of talents and skills, whereas my account explicitly says shares can be fair even if talents and skills make them unequal. (The effect of this inequality is mitigated by the Difference Principle.) My account also focuses attention on departures from *normal functioning* that shrink shares below what is fair.

This is a crucial restriction, and nothing in the structure of Sen's account matches this restriction. The effect is to make us concerned only with certain sources of the inequality of capabilities open to individuals. What is of urgent moral concern to us is not assuring equality of capability in some global way, in all of its dimensions, but the more modest goal of protecting individuals from certain impairments of their capabilities. The reference to a normal range of functioning is crucial and captures what I believe underlies our sense of the urgency of meeting health-care needs for disease and disability. We are not, for example, concerned with shortfalls from some notion of optimal or enhanced capabilities: if I cannot run a 3:50 mile, I do not view myself as handicapped in ways that give rise to claims on society for assistance or compensation for my lack of optimal capabilities. Under justice as fairness, the distribution of talents and skills works to everyone's advantage through the mitigating effects of the Difference Principle. We have special claims on others only when our functioning falls short of the normal range (remember, *normal* is not a statistical notion). We respond to inequalities in capability sets in different ways, depending on the source of the inequality. Properly extended, Rawls' theory captures just the structure of our responses in a plausible way. It is quite unclear, in contrast, just how Sen wants to work with his notion of capability sets or freedoms.[28]

Sen wants to use the claim about the inflexibility of the primary goods to show that these goods placed us in the wrong space for purposes of justice. He argues that we should really be concerned with a certain relationship between goods and persons, namely, capabilities, not primary goods alone. It is now possible to respond to this second claim.

In his recent work, Rawls argues that the primary goods are justified because they are what citizens need to exercise their fundamental moral powers as free and equal citizens. These powers include a sense of justice and the capacity to form and revise a conception of the good. This model of moral agents, Rawls argues, is a *political* conception, one central to the liberal democratic tradition. Viewed in this way, the primary goods *are* connected to a space in which we are concerned about *capabilities:* the capabilities of citizens functioning normally over the course of their whole lives.[29] Understood in this way, the target of egalitarian concerns is more similar for Sen and Rawls than it appeared from Sen's criticism of Rawls' fetishism.

As we relax the assumption that we are concerned only with normally functioning citizens – as we introduce the variability that troubled Sen – then we must flesh out the details of the primary goods and the application of the principles. Flexibility can be appropriately introduced. Nevertheless, priority is given to keeping the society as close as possible to the goal of having normally functioning citizens: that is where the underlying political conception drives us. Addressing the problem of health-care needs through the primary good of opportunity, that is, through the fair equality of opportunity clause of the Second Principle, keeps us focused on the normal range of capabilities.

What is not driving Rawls' view, however, is some underlying, comprehensive moral view: that positive freedom or capability, in all its dimensions, is of concern for purposes of justice. This point is analogous to Rawls' insistence that his concern for basic liberties is not the result of allegiance to some comprehensive moral view about the importance of autonomy or liberty. Basic liberties as well as fair equality of opportunity derive their moral importance from their relationship to the political ideal of citizens as free and equal moral agents with certain basic powers. The primary goods are not defended on the grounds that they approximate a dimension of basic moral value (like positive freedom or capability). Rather, they are defended because of their connection to the limited political ideal of a free and equal citizen.[30] It is especially important for justification here that the *same* underlying political notions, such as that citizens are "free" and "equal," unify our account of how to distribute both liberties and economic goods.[31]

3. EQUAL OPPORTUNITY FOR WELFARE

I want to turn my attention to the other line of criticism of primary goods. Here too the primary goods are being accused of being insensitive to a type of variability among people, in particular variability among the preferences people have. For example, some people may have more expensive tastes than others and so be less efficient converters of primary goods into satisfaction or welfare. For the same assignment of primary goods, such people will be less well-off than people with more modest tastes (or values).

In response to this line of objection to the primary goods, Rawls has suggested that individuals "be held responsible" for their ends, whereas society is responsible for providing the just framework of all-purpose means within which individuals can pursue their conceptions of the good.[32] Dworkin argues for a similar point in his discussion of the case of Louis, who has been given resources sufficient to yield him equal enjoyment to others.[33] Louis now imagines cultivating a more expensive set of tastes. Louis should know that if he cultivates these tastes, and then is compensated because his enjoyment drops, his compensation will come at the cost of lower enjoyment for others. Choosing this outcome, Dworkin urges, would be unfair of Louis, and he would not deserve compensation under these conditions. Now Rawls never offers an argument similar to this one; he makes no such appeal to an intuitive notion of fairness or desert. Nor is it clear that when Rawls says we should "hold people responsible" for their tastes, he is assuming that people actually chose to have the preferences they have and that they can always, at least over time and with some cost or effort, revise them.

The line of objection to the primary goods we are now considering, however, does make the issue of choice of preferences or control over preferences central to egalitarian concerns. Arneson and Cohen, as I noted earlier, have both argued for accounts that make choice central and explicit (the "foreground" choice, as Cohen puts it).[34] The suggestion that emerges is this: our egalitarian concerns do not require that we be compensated for being worse off than others when it is our chosen preferences (tastes or values) that make us worse off. We are considered to have chosen a value with which we were raised if we would not be willing to renounce it. For example, if I did not choose to be raised in a religion that makes me feel guilty about sex, but I nevertheless would not choose to have been raised in some other way, then I am in effect affirming the values that lead me to feel guilty, and I should not be compensated as a result of egalitarian concerns for my well-being.

Choice here is central. If I am made worse off because gambles I have made have turned out badly, that is, I have had poor *option luck*, then egalitarian concerns are not triggered. If I fare worse than others because of matters outside my control, then I am a victim of poor *brute luck*, and egalitarian concerns are appropriately brought to bear.[35] If this claim is right – and I will return to challenge it shortly – then Rawls' suggestion that we should "hold people responsible for their ends" seems in need of qualification, for now people did not choose, and so should not really be responsible, for all their preferences.[36]

If we think that the moral principle underlying our egalitarian concerns is simply that we have legitimate claims on others whenever we are worse off than they through no fault of our own, then it might be possible to capture that intuition with a version of a welfare-based theory. Arneson argues that this principle is accommodated if we make the target of egalitarian concerns *equal opportunity for welfare*, where *welfare* means only *preference satisfaction*. Equal opportunity for welfare obtains when each person faces "an array of options that is equivalent to every other person's in terms of the prospects for preference satisfaction it offers."[37] We should picture this in the following way. Imagine that we represent a person's life as a decision tree in which all possible life histories are represented. Equal opportunity for welfare obtains if the best path on each person's life tree *ex ante* has the same expected payoff in preference satisfaction. Branches in the tree represent all possible choices, including choices about which preferences to act on or to develop.[38]

The fact that equal opportunity for welfare (or Cohen's "equal access to advantage") allows us to make explicit the choice of preferences does not mean it is responsive to Rawls' objections to using satisfaction as a measure of well-being for purposes of justice. (This defense of a welfare-based account seems more responsive to Dworkin's arguments, which I am not primarily concerned with here.) Rawls' objections to such overall measures of satisfaction weigh against its use in equality of opportunity for welfare as well. To decide, for example, that expected preference satisfaction is equal on at least one path on each life tree, we must make at least ordinal or co-ordinal comparisons. That would commit us to there being some social utility function that would let us compare the level of satisfaction each person enjoys on the relevant path. Such a utility function would commit each of us, Rawls argues, to accepting its rankings of our overall satisfaction relative to every other person. But such a function *constitutes* a "shared highest-order preference function."[39] On the basis of such a function, it would be "rational for them to adjust and revise their final ends and desires, and to modify their traits of character and to reshape their realized abilities, so as to achieve a total personal situation ranked higher in the ordering" defined by the function. Rawls' main argument is that this shared highest-order preference function is "plainly incompatible with the conception of a well-ordered society in justice as fairness," in which citizens' conceptions of the good are "not only said to be opposed but to be incommensurable." We start, in other words, with the fact of pluralism. Conceptions of the good "are incommensurable because their final ends and aspirations are so diverse, their specific content so different, that no common basis for judgment can be found."[40] Indeed, Rawls remarks about "holding people responsible for their ends" is raised in the context of defending the primary goods against the charge of inflexibility in the face of varied preferences; it is not itself offered as an argument against a welfare-based account.

I want to pursue a different kind of objection from Rawls' to the equal opportunity for welfare (or equal access to advantage) account. I do not believe that the account captures our egalitarian concerns; indeed, an account based on primary goods, extended to include appropriate health care, seems perfectly adequate. I will argue that unchosen preferences that make us worse off than others do not (generally) arouse egalitarian concerns unless they can be assimilated to the cases of psychological disability, that is, to a departure from normal functioning. In that case, they will merit some form of treatment, but not necessarily other forms of compensation. This does not seem to be what would be implied by an equal opportunity for welfare account.

Suppose John's mother raised him on Mrs. Morgan's Fish Sticks and that as a result he cannot stand the taste of fish.[41] He becomes interested in the quality of his diet and otherwise quite adventuresome in his eating. Nevertheless, he feels deprived that he is denied access to the broad range of food pleasures that would come from eating and enjoying seafood. He feels ill, however, at the very thought of eating fish. We might even suppose this aversion makes him feel he should not pursue a career as a restaurant critic. If his opportunity for welfare falls below that of others because of this aversion, does he have a legitimate egalitarian claim for compensation?

Suppose Jane's mother raised her to believe that a mother's duty is to stay home with her children and that no woman should pursue a career during her childrearing years. Jane no longer believes that, has had a good career, and now faces the choice about what to do about childrearing. But she feels so guilty at the thought of pursuing her career that she ends up staying home with her children. Not only does this mean she is deeply disappointed about her sacrifice of career, but she resents the burden placed on her by her children (and her mother). Since this is fantasy, let us also suppose her husband would rather she bring home the bacon than cook it, but he cannot change her mind. Should she be compensated because her opportunity for welfare (or advantage) is less than others?

I think we should do something to help John or Jane only if their situations really reflect some underlying departure from normal functioning. Ordinarily, we expect that someone who does not like fish copes with his unwanted preference by pursuing his other tastes. There's enough else that he likes that we expect him to adapt to his preferences, whatever their etiology. If John was a compulsive or phobic personality, and the aversion to fish were symptomatic of a more generalized inability to accommodate to his preferences, or to reform and revise them over time, then I would be inclined to offer him some form of therapy for the underlying disorder. If, however, he then said that he really did not want the therapy, but preferred to "cash it in" for a week skiing in Vail, then I would refuse him the alternative. I am not interested in moving him to the point where his opportunity for welfare is equal to others; I am only interested in making sure that he has the mental capability to form and revise his conception of the good in a normal fashion. Beyond that, I hold him responsible for his preferences.

My response to Jane is similar. If she suffers from a more generalized incapacity to form and revise her ends over time, perhaps as the result of some unresolved problems in her relationship with her mother, then I would want her to have access to the appropriate form of therapy or group support. I would not, however, be willing to substitute other forms of compensation aimed at moving her back to equal opportunity for welfare. What does the work here is the belief that there is some underlying handicapping condition.

In considering similar sorts of cases, Dworkin also suggests that compensation is due only if we have a case of a "handicapping taste," because handicaps count as resource deficiencies on Dworkin's view.[42] Cohen suggests that the heart of Dworkin's claim is the idea that the individual is "alienated" from the taste, that it is no longer something the individual identifies with.[43] By itself, Cohen urges, this is an inadequate account. Some people may deserve compensation even if they are not reflective enough to formulate the idea that they are alienated. In other cases, life-hampering tastes are not ones the individual really wants to renounce. Rather, the individual really just feels unlucky in having such a taste, say because it turns out to be an expensive one.

Ultimately, Cohen suggests that identification and disidentification with a taste matter "only if and insofar as they indicate presence and absence of choice."[44]

I think Cohen misses the mark. It is not actual choice that matters, but the underlying capacity for forming and revising one's ends that is at issue. If we have independent reasons to believe that a preference, whether chosen or not, whether identified with or not, cannot be eliminated and is handicapping because of a broader, underlying handicapping condition, then we have reasons to make certain resources available as compensation. It is not the unchosen taste, or the fact that the taste is unchosen, that gives rise to the claim on us. Rather, it is the underlying mental or emotional disability, and the taste, chosen or not, is but a symptom.

My unwillingness to consider converting treatment into other forms of compensation confirms this analysis of the basis for the reaction. It also confirms the view that we are not being motivated by an egalitarian ideal of equal opportunity for welfare or advantage. The structure of our egalitarian concerns does not seem to correspond to a concern for equal opportunity for overall satisfaction. Lack of well-being in some categories counts for a lot; it matters what the source of the shortfall from opportunity for welfare is, not just that there is a shortfall.[45] [A methodological aside: In saying that I (or we) do not respond to cases in ways that the equal opportunity for welfare or advantage views would endorse, I have not thereby shown those views morally unjustifiable; I have only shown that they do not cohere with at least some of my (our) considered judgments about what is morally required. I return in the next section to comment briefly on what kind of evidence we get for or against Rawls' view from such correspondence (or lack of it) with this broad range of egalitarian concerns, given that Rawls' is a theory of justice for basic institutions.]

In his discussion of Dworkin's distinction between preferences and resources, Cohen argues that Dworkin fails to place choice in as central position as it belongs. The cut between considerations that give rise to issues of redistribution is not the cut between preferences and resources, as Dworkin would have it, but between choice and mere luck.[46] Where we have lost chances to gain welfare or advantage as a result of brute luck, and not through any choices of our own, then we have a claim of justice on others. For example, if someone's opportunity for welfare is less than others as a result of unchosen and unreaffirmed religious preferences inculcated in childhood, both Arneson and Cohen believe compensation may be owed. John's aversion to fish and Jane's guilt about the conflict of career and children are other examples in which compensation would be owed, according to the equal opportunity for welfare account. This position is clearly different from Rawls' insistence that we "hold people responsible for their ends," whether or not actual choice underlies a particular preference or not. Earlier I defended Rawls' position by offering a different account of how our intuitions work in these cases. Now I want to offer a reason for thinking that Rawls' suggestion has moral justification, beyond merely appealing to this evidence from judgments about examples.

The interest we have in pursuing our conceptions of the good often requires that we be given considerable liberty to raise our children as we see fit. There are clear costs to this fact; many children will be able to establish command over their own plans of life with considerable difficulty and at some cost. But if we think it is a concern of justice to intervene in each person's life to rectify unequal opportunities for welfare or advantage wherever preferences were not actually chosen, then we must think it is really a task of justice to restrict in many quite intrusive and coercive ways the autonomy we grant people to pursue their plans of life, including their autonomy in childrearing. To be sure, we all believe that parents should not abuse their children or deny them certain fundamental kinds of opportunity. But if we think parents have a responsibility to teach their children to be virtuous and to convey to them what they think is valuable, or at least to model those values for their children, then we can expect children to grow up with some unchosen preferences. Holding people responsible for their ends means that we are acting as if they can exercise their underlying moral power to form and revise their conceptions of the good. We want to back away from "holding people responsible" only if we have reason to think the underlying capacity is compromised, not if we think certain actual choices have not been made. To be committed to rectifying all failures to make actual choices would mean we are committed to compromising one of the central contexts in which the underlying moral power or capacity is exercised, namely, in the autonomy we grant people to raise their children as they see fit.[47]

From this perspective, it is reasonable not to make actual choice central in the manner proposed by Cohen and Arneson, although we are interested in protecting the underlying capacity for choice, at least against certain departures from normal functioning.[48] These considerations show that the moral practice I suggested we exhibit in our attitudes toward John and Jane and in some of the other examples in the literature have more to be said for them than that they merely happen to be what we do. "Holding people responsible for their ends" will be what we do if we are to respect the liberties it is appropriate to grant individuals in the pursuit of the plans of life, including childrearing.

Justice and justification

4. A CONCLUDING REMARK ON JUSTIFICATION

I have defended Rawls' use of primary goods against two lines of criticism, both of which claim the primary goods are inflexible and ignore relevant differences in well-being. Although the initial statement of justice as fairness involves the idealization that people function normally over the whole course of their lives, the theory can be extended (in the legislative stage) to accommodate the reality of disease and disability. My account of health-care needs shows their connection to the primary good of opportunity. This extension of the theory captures much of what motivates Sen's criticism that justice is concerned with the distribution of capabilities and not merely goods.

In response to the other line of criticism, that our egalitarian concerns require that people be aided whenever their unchosen preferences make them worse off in opportunity for satisfaction than others, I claimed that our egalitarian concerns have a different structure. We are concerned about cases like these only when there is an underlying disability or dysfunction that makes us unable to form and revise our plans of life in a normal fashion. Further, we may "hold people responsible" for their ends without being committed to examining which ones were actually chosen; we need only be assured people can function normally for them to be held responsible. In effect, I have argued that an account of justice that appeals to primary goods matches our considered judgments about how to respond to certain sources of variability in well-being, at least for purposes of justice. Neither line of criticism thus gives us adequate reason for abandoning a theory of justice that uses primary social goods as its measure of well-being.

I want to conclude with a brief comment on an important epistemological issue related to this defense of primary goods. Consider the question that began this paper, What is the ultimate target of our egalitarian concerns? I said I would not answer it directly, and I have not, despite my defense of primary goods. I have not answered it directly because it presupposes that all of our egalitarian concerns have one target, and I am skeptical that they are all of a kind. I am not sure they are *uniform* in the sense implied by the question. When I am concerned about responding to the needs and preferences of my children, or of my friends, or of my colleagues in the department I chair, it is not clear to me that my egalitarian concerns are all cut from one uniform moral fabric, and the suspicion that it is not grows stronger when I compare my egalitarian concerns in these contexts with my concerns in wider, public arenas. This skepticism about the uniformity of egalitarian concerns, which I believe I share with Rawls, stands in contrast with the perspective that underlies the positions taken by Sen, Arneson, and Cohen (despite their defenses of different targets). They argue as if one target – capabilities, or equal opportunity for welfare or advantage – comprehensively captures our egalitarian concerns.

Whether or not there is such uniformity affects how we should react to the egalitarian concerns evidenced in certain cases. Suppose that we sometimes do take deficits in opportunity for welfare into account when we think about examples of individuals who suffer from unchosen and unwanted preferences. (My argument in Section 3 responded only to certain examples and could not rule out this possibility.) Perhaps we do this with people we know very well, such as friends or family. Maybe we do this when we understand – or perhaps share – in some detail their conception of the good and when we have fairly reliable knowledge of what is responsible for their dissatisfaction in life, and perhaps where we feel some special responsibility to help them because of our special relationship to them. Would such responses show that a theory of justice governing basic social institutions must respond to the same egalitarian concerns and have the same target? Is my concern for the relative well-being of others in these instances of a piece with the concerns I might express about how society as a whole should react to inequalities in relative well-being for citizens?

Such examples by themselves do not show that there is an unified target underlying our concerns for the relative well-being of others. Nor would they show that our concerns in the public domain were just "approximations" to what interested us in private settings, for example, that it was "only" for administrative reasons that we "compromised" our concerns in the public domain. What should be of moral relevance in the public domain may not be what is of relevance in private domains. What we count as just for basic social institutions may not merely be a necessary departure from what egalitarian concerns "in theory" or "ideally" require. It is an unargued for assumption underlying the question, Equality of what? that there is but one target in all contexts, a target revealed by a uniformity in our firm, considered moral judgments about all contexts in which we are concerned about relative well-being.

This point has epistemological or justificatory implications: it is not clear what kinds of counterexamples to count as evidence in the debate about the target of equality. My showing that *for purposes of justice* we are not and should not be concerned about making choice as central as Cohen would have it does not show that it is an inappropriate focus for egalitarian concerns in other contexts. By the same token, positive evidence that in some individualized contexts we are concerned with actual choices and their impact on opportunity for welfare would not show that this is the target for theories of justice for basic social institutions. Only if we already believed in the uniformity of our egalitarian concerns would examples in one context count as counterexamples to claims about the target in another kind of context. Without the belief in uniformity, we may only have evidence about how to divide our egalitarian concerns into different domains with different targets.

Rawls' claim that principles of justice apply to basic institutions and not to private exchanges opens the door to rejecting the uniformity of egalitarian concerns.[49] His more recent elaboration of the claim that justice as fairness is a *political conception of justice* brings a different set of arguments to bear on the question of uniformity. It will be helpful to paraphrase Rawls' view, since it is an explicit attempt to argue against the uniformity thesis.[50]

Any political conception of justice must accept certain "general facts" of political sociology. These include the following: there is a diversity of comprehensive religious, philosophical, and moral doctrines (the fact of pluralism); only oppressive use of state power could maintain common affirmation of a comprehensive doctrine; a stable democratic regime requires widespread, free support by a substantial majority; and the political culture of stable democracies normally contains fundamental intuitive ideas that can serve as the basis for a political conception of justice. A political conception of justice has three main features. First, although it is a moral conception, it is developed and applied only to a specific subject, the basic institutions of a democratic regime. Second, people accept the political conception on the basis of accepting certain fundamental, intuitive ideas present in the political culture. One such fundamental idea is that society is a fair system of social cooperation over time, across generations; another is that citizens are free and equal persons capable of cooperating over a full life. Third, accepting the political conception does not presuppose accepting a comprehensive moral doctrine; nor is the political conception a "compromise" tailored to fit the range of comprehensive doctrines present in the society. Nevertheless, supporters of divergent comprehensive doctrines can achieve an "overlapping consensus" on an appropriate political conception.[51]

Rawls defends a particular type of political conception of justice: justice as fairness is an example of a *political constructivist* theory. It does not presuppose that there is any prior moral order that a theory of justice purports to correspond to or represent. Rather, principles of justice as the product of a procedure that represents reasonable constraints on how rational agents should reason practically about the terms of social cooperation. The outcome of such a procedure might clearly lead to discontinuity between the target of egalitarian concerns in the sphere of justice and the egalitarian concerns that may be present elsewhere in our (diverse) moral doctrines.

A political conception of justice need not be constructivist, however. We might imagine an alternative political conception that involved an attempt to construct a political conception by "balancing" the political "values" implied by the fundamental intuitive ideas present in the democratic culture. When the appropriate balancing is accomplished, it might be thought we had captured the moral truth appropriate to this domain. Nor should we think that the balance is but a compromise with what is "ideally" egalitarian: the balancing picks out what is just in the political sphere. Still, the target of egalitarian concerns expressed in this balance of political values may not be continuous with the target of egalitarian concerns outside the political sphere. Uniformity fails here too. This means that the points I have been making about the assumption of uniformity are independent of the debate between intuitionists and moral or political constructivists.

My intention here is not to defend Rawls' view that we must seek political conceptions of justice.[52] Rather, I have tried to make explicit how such a view bears on the uniformity thesis that seems to underlie the question, What is the target of our egalitarian concerns? Since uniformity is not established, we are unsure how to construe the evidence from certain kinds of examples that explore our moral intuitions.

One way to understand either Sen's view or the Arneson–Cohen view is as part of a "comprehensive" moral view. If that is true, then the fact that elements of that view do not fit with Rawls' account will not necessarily count against Rawls' view. Rawls' view is not tested by matching it to some such comprehensive moral view. The test is whether those who hold these other moral doctrines can support the project of using the fundamental ideas Rawls' singles out to construct a theory of fair cooperation, despite their disagreements about other issues. They do not even have to accept the fundamental ideas for exactly the same reasons. I will not venture a guess whether or not there is such an "overlapping consensus" among these theorists. I suspect from the style of argument underlying each line of criticism that there is little sympathy with Rawls' notion of a political conception of justice or, in particular, with his political constructivism. I suspect that proponents of each line would think there is not enough of a basis for objectivity in justification if we politicize it in this way. That is not an issue I can address here.

NOTES

1 I have benefited greatly from discussions with Joshua Cohen and John Rawls in preparing this paper.

2 Derek Parfit has argued persuasively (unpublished ms.) that a concern for equality and a concern for giving priority to the worst off are not the same. For my purposes here I count them both as egalitarian concerns, since the distinction is not important to the debate about their target.

3 Cohen is interested in "advantage," a broader notion than mere welfare, but advantage includes welfare. Cf. G. A. Cohen, "On the Currency of Egalitarian Justice," *Ethics* 99 (July 1989): 906–44; Richard J. Arneson, "Equality and Equal Opportunity for Welfare," *Philosophical Studies* 54 (1988): 79–95.

4 Ronald Dworkin, "What is Equality? Part I: Equality of Welfare," *Philosophy and Public Affairs* 10 (Summer 1981): 185–246; "What is Equality? Part 2: Equality of Resources," *Philosophy and Public Affairs* 10 (Fall 1981): 283–345.

5 John Rawls, *A Theory of Justice* (Cambridge: Harvard University Press, 1971); "Social Unity and the Primary Goods," in Amartya Sen and Bernard Williams, eds., *Utilitarianism and Beyond* (Cambridge: Cambridge University Press, 1982), pp. 159–86; "The Priority of Right and Ideas of the Good," *Philosophy and Public Affairs* 17 (Fall 1988): 251–76.

6 Amartya Sen, "Equality of What?" in S. McMurrin, ed., *Tanner Lectures on Human Values*, Vol. 1 (Cambridge: Cambridge University Press, 1980), reprinted in Sen, *Choice, Welfare, and Measurement* (Cambridge: MIT Press, 1982), pp. 353–69; "Well-being, Agency and Freedom: The Dewey Lectures 1984," *Journal of Philosophy* 82 (April 1985): 169–220; *Commodities and Capabilities* (Amsterdam: North-Holland, 1985); "Justice: Means Versus Freedoms," *Philosophy and Public Affairs* 19 (Spring 1990): 111–21.

7 Cf. Arneson, "Primary Goods Reconsidered" *Nous* 24 (June 1990): 429–54.

8 Sen, "Equality of What?" p. 363.

9 Sen, "Equality of What?" p. 366.

10 The derivation of a workable list of the primary goods from these basic *political* notions lying at the heart of liberalism represents a shift from their derivation in *A Theory of Justice*. Cf. Rawls, "Social Unity," p. 165 n. 5 and "The Priority of Right," p. 259 n. 10.

11 Kenneth Arrow, "Some Ordinalist-Utilitarian Notes on Rawls's Theory of Justice," *Journal of Philosophy* 70 (1973): 253ff.

12 Rawls divides the argument in a similar way, and there is considerable agreement between his response to it and mine; cf. "Justice as Fairness: A Briefer Restatement" (unpublished ms., 1989), pp. 118ff.

13 Cf. Arrow, "Ordinalist-utilitarian Notes," pp. 253ff; see Dworkin's excellent discussion of these issues in "Equality of Welfare," pp. 228ff.

14 Sen, "Well-being, Agency and Freedom," p. 196.

15 Rawls says, "It is best to make an initial concession in the case of special health and medical needs. I put this difficult problem aside in this paper and assume that all citizens have physical and psychological capacities within a certain normal range. I do this because the first problem of justice concerns the relations between citizens who are normally active and fully cooperating members of society over a complete life," "Social Unity," p. 168. He appears to endorse my approach to extending his theory to health care needs in "Justice as Fairness: A Briefer Restatement," pp. 122ff.

16 Sen, "Well-being, Agency and Freedom," p. 197.
17 Sen, "Justice: Means versus Freedoms," pp. 113–14.
18 Sen, *Poverty and Famines: An Essay on Entitlement and Deprivation* (Oxford: Clarendon Press, 1981).
19 Sen may believe that producing flexibility in these ways means the theory is responding in an ad hoc manner to what it should have recognized as fundamental from the beginning, namely, variations in capability. It is far from clear, however, that we do or should respond to all variations in capability in the same way or with the same moral justification. I return to this issue briefly in the last section.
20 Daniels, "Health Care Needs and Distributive Justice," *Philosophy and Public Affairs* 10 (1981): 146–79; *Just Health Care* (Cambridge: Cambridge University Press, 1985); and *Am I My Parents' Keeper? An Essay on Justice between the Young and the Old* (New York: Oxford University Press, 1988).
21 My account draws on work by Christopher Boorse; cf. Christopher Boorse, "On the Distinction between Disease and Illness," *Philosophy and Public Affairs* 5 (1976): 49–68; and "Health as a Theoretical Concept," *Philosophy of Science* 44 (December 1977): 542–73.
22 See Daniels, *Just Health Care*, pp. 29ff for further discussion.
23 This is a hefty counterfactual, but I think of it by analogy to what fair equality of opportunity requires in the case of compensatory efforts for those whose talents and skills are misdeveloped, putting them at competitive disadvantage, because of racism or sexism.
24 We thus avoid "hijacking" by past preferences which themselves define the effective range. Of course, impact on the effective range may be important in microallocation decisions, including decisions by individuals whether they want to receive certain services.
25 Daniels, "Am I My Parents' Keeper?" *Midwest Studies in Philosophy* 7 (1982): 517–40; *Am I My Parents' Keeper?* Chs. 3–4.
26 Rawls, "Justice as Fairness: A Briefer Restatement," p. 122.
27 Cf. Rawls, "Justice as Fairness: A Briefer Restatement," pp. 122–23; Daniels, *Just Health Care*, Ch. 3.
28 Sen does offer a detailed discussion to show that we may arrive at a partial ordering of objective evaluations of levels of functioning or well-being or advantage (cf. *Capability and Commodities*, Chs. 5–7). What he says little about, however, is what steps justice obliges us to take in response to differences in capabilities or advantage. My modest claim above is that a plausible development of Rawls' primary goods, combined with his principles of justice, allows us to respond to capability differences in reasonable and recognizable ways.
29 See Rawls, "Social Unity," pp. 168–69.
30 Cf. Rawls, "Priority of Right," p. 259. I believe Sen misunderstands Rawls' point here. Sen argues that no appeal to a comprehensive moral ideal is involved in his use of capabilities because individuals who differ in their conceptions of the good might still think one set of capabilities preferable to another (cf. "Means versus Freedoms," pp. 117–21). But that might be true and Rawls still be correct, Rawls' point is that there is no general or comprehensive moral interest in positive freedom or capability, from the

perspective of this construction in political philosophy; there is only an interest in the capabilities of citizens and what it takes to keep them functioning normally as citizens.

31 Cf. Joshua Cohen, "Democratic Equality," *Ethics* 99 (July 1989): 727–51.
32 Rawls, "Social Unity," pp. 170ff.
33 Dworkin, "Equality of Welfare," pp. 229ff.
34 Cohen, "Currency of Egalitarian Justice," pp. 922, 933.
35 The distinction between these kinds of luck is made in Dworkin, "Equality of Resources," p. 293; cf. Cohen, "Currency of Egalitarian Justice," p. 908.
36 Arneson suggests we restate Rawls' claim so: "To whatever extent it is reasonable to hold individuals personally responsible for their preferences, to that extent adjusting an individual's distributive shares according to how expensive his preferences are to satisfy is unfair" ("Primary Goods Reconsidered," p. 10). He then argues that this modified proposal actually conflicts with the operation of the Difference Principle, since some people (e.g., a Bohemian artist who had the talents and education to be a prosperous business man) might end up among the worst off in lifetime expectations as a result of their own choices. If actual choice is "foregrounded" or made central in the way proposed here, then it may not be fair that the Difference Principle makes the undeserving poor as well-off as possible; it should only help those who are poor through no fault of their own. I will later suggest why Rawls should not make actual choice central in this way, which implies that Rawls should not accept Arneson's modification.
37 Arneson, "Equal Opportunity for Welfare," p. 87.
38 Arneson qualifies this by insisting that persons face *effectively* equivalent options, correcting for inequalities in negotiating abilities for which people are not responsible and that do not balance out ("Equal Opportunity for Welfare," p. 88). I am not sure how he wants to accommodate the preferences one happens to have at the root end of the tree, presumably the age of maturity. But it is not the details of Arneson's construction that worry me above (though anyone might be worried about the information burden this picture carries with it!).
39 Rawls, "Social Unity," pp. 176–79.
40 Rawls, "Social Unity," pp. 179–80.
41 The example is adapted from Richard Brandt, *A Theory of the Good and the Right* (Oxford: Oxford University Press, 1979), p. 120.
42 Dworkin, "Equality of Resources," p. 302.
43 Cohen, "Currency of Egalitarian Justice," p. 926.
44 Cohen, "Currency of Egalitarian Justice," p. 927.
45 See T. M. Scanlon, "Preference and Urgency," *Journal of Philosophy* 72 (1975): 655–69; also see Daniels, *Just Health Care*, Ch. 2.
46 Cf. Cohen, "Currency of Egalitarian Justice," p. 933.
47 The point can be put in a different way, one that uses less of Rawls' construction. We might imagine that we have a number of "political values" which have to be balanced in arriving at what justice requires, all things considered. Thus there is some importance to holding people responsible for their ends – we certainly want to avoid the dissembling that not doing so might involve. Similarly, we do not want people to be disad-

vantaged by things not in their control. At the same time, we find value in autonomy, in people being able to pursue a life plan that includes the moral education of their children. When we balance all these values, we might well think that, all things considered, justice does not require us to compensate people for all their unchosen preferences: holding people responsible for their ends may prove more important. Though we have compromised with our egalitarian concern not to want people disadvantaged through no fault of their own, we are not here compromising with what justice requires: it requires the compromise. This point has a bearing on the comments in Section 4 as well.

48 Cohen would certainly agree with wanting to protect this underlying capacity, whatever else our diagreement.

49 Rawls' replies to Nozick on this issue elaborate the early form of this argument; cf. Rawls, "The Basic Structure as Subject," *American Philosophical Quarterly* 14 (1977): 159–65; Robert Nozick, *Anarchy, State, and Utopia* (New York: Basic Books, 1974).

50 This summary is based on Rawls, "The Domain of the Political and Overlapping Consensus," *New York University Law Review* 64 (May 1989): 234–35; 240ff.

51 We get what might be called "moral epistemology politicized"; Rawls discusses what objectivity means for moral and political constructivism in "Political Constructivism and Public Justification" (unpublished ms., 1988).

52 I still have reservations about the relationship and boundaries between justifications that are moral and those that are political.

Chapter 11

Determining "medical necessity" in mental health practice, with James E. Sabin

Managed care raises fundamental questions about the moral presuppositions of mental health insurance coverage. Which kinds of mental suffering create a legitimate claim for assistance from others through health insurance? When should individuals be responsible for correcting their own deficits of happiness or well-being, or for the disadvantages they suffer? And even if society concludes that an individual is entitled to assistance from others, when does this obligation fall to friends, families, or other social agencies, rather than to the health insurance system? This paper attempts to address these questions.

The concept of "medical necessity" is currently the major tool for allocating public and private insurance monies.[1] Medicare and Medicaid both determine coverage by reference to "medical necessity," and with regard to managed care, the Institute of Medicine concluded that "utilization review decision(s) invariably turn on whether a treatment of service is 'medically necessary.' "[2] To promote equitable access to mental health care, we must first understand how "medical necessity" actually functions in practice as a principle of allocation and gatekeeping.

Many insurance administrators believe that judgments about medical necessity in mental health are less precise than similar judgments in other areas of medicine. As a result they fear that if mental health services were given parity with other medical services – a primary objective for the American Psychiatric Association – insurance funds will be siphoned into a "bottomless pit."[3]

In previous work on home care and in vitro fertilization we have shown that determinations of medical necessity often rest on a range of moral considerations as well as clinical facts.[4] This paper reports the results of a study of difficult insurance coverage decisions brought to us by mental health clinicians and reviewers in a managed care setting.

We explored these cases with the involved personnel by applying elements of the Socratic approach – eliciting the clinician's (or reviewer's) considered views, varying crucial components of the case, and examining the effects on their reasoning about medical necessity.

This process revealed a recurrent conflict between what we call "hard-line" and "expansive" views of medical necessity. Although this conflict often surfaces as disagreement about medical facts and diagnosis, we believe that it frequently reflects unrecognized moral disagreement about the targets of clinical intervention and the ultimate goals of psychiatric treatment. In six case studies we examine the reasoning behind the determinations of medical necessity. In the discussion we present three models for defining medical necessity that can be discerned in the clinical reasoning, and propose what we regard as a defensible rationale for how the concept of medical necessity can be used in the administration of health insurance benefits.

DISTINGUISHING TREATMENT FROM ENHANCEMENT

Since 1 January 1991 the Harvard Community Health Plan (HCHP), a staff and group model HMO serving 550,000 members in New England, has offered unlimited outpatient coverage ("extended benefit") to patients with severe psychiatric and substance abuse disorders for medically necessary treatment, defined as case management, medication management, crisis intervention, and continuing care group. "Regular benefit" comprises other forms of treament for these patients and all treatment except medication management for those with less severe conditions, with an increased copayment after eight sessions and a full fee after twenty.[5] The following (disguised) cases are drawn from that insurance context.

> *Case 1: **The Shy Bipolar.** SB is the older of two children in a middle-class family. He is said to have been a happy, outgoing child until the second grade, when his father developed a depressive condition and his mother focused her attention on SB's father. SB became withdrawn and intensely shy. The school recommended psychological evaluation, which led to intermittent psychotherapy until the sixth grade.*
>
> *From high school to the end of his first year of college SB continued as a shy, rather isolated person who showed no adolescent rebelliousness. He did not date. At the end of his first year of college he was in a motor vehicle accident, suffering abdominal injuries that required multiple surgeries. During the year of his recuperation he developed a manic episode for which he was hospitalized. He stabilized on lithium and completed college.*

> *Throughout his twenties SB worked as a financial analyst. He lived at home with his parents, continued lithium, and participated in weekly or biweekly outpatient psychotherapy. A single effort to taper and stop the lithium led to signs of potential manic recurrence.*
>
> *In 1987 his employer changed health insurance and SB became a member of HCHP. At one point in the next four years SB and his doctor tried to taper the lithium due to what was thought to be lithium-induced lethargy. Hypomanic symptoms occurred within two months. Subsequently phenelzine was added to the lithium regimen and the lethargy improved.*
>
> *After the medications were stabilized, individual treatment focused on SB's social isolation. SB and his doctor identified a pattern of interpersonal sensitivity and defensive withdrawal, and SB accepted a referral for weekly group psychotherapy (not paid for by insurance) outside of the HMO. During the course of the next three-and-one-half years SB gradually extended his social range. He successfully moved into an apartment of his own. He began to participate in clubs and other social groups, and to date for the first time. His work performance, which had always been acceptable, improved so that he was promoted to a more senior position and received a substantial salary increase.*
>
> *HCHP has just adopted a new outpatient benefit. When HCHP put the new benefit structure into place, SB asked his doctor, "How much of the treatment should I be paying for under this new benefit?"*

Medication management for the Shy Bipolar is clearly medically necessary: he has a presumably organic illness diagnosable in *DSM-IV* terms as bipolar disorder. Lithium controls the manic symptoms and withdrawing it leads to recurrent mania. Phenelzine relieves the depressive lethargy. The Shy Bipolar's condition is fully analogous to heart failure, diabetes, or lupus, which require ongoing outpatient medication management, and which most standard insurance plans cover.

The Shy Bipolar's appointments were also used to define important psychosocial issues and develop strategies for approaching them, refer him to community resources and support participation, and review progress and revise plans as needed. Any psychiatrist who treats patients with major mental illness is familiar with this kind of psychodynamically informed case management. Insofar as the case management focuses on dysfunctions that arise from the bipolar illness, such as monitoring moods or coping with demoralization, the appointments are analogous to advice regarding exercise and nutrition for a patient with cardiac disease or diabetes. Under the terms of the HCHP extended benefit, the Shy Bipolar's clinician determined that the case management was medically necessary and would be covered without any arbitrary limit.

As the clinician reviewed the case with the authors, he came to believe that a strong argument could be made for covering group psychotherapy under the extended benefit in the same way as medication management and case management. In retrospect, the pattern of withdrawal, which started when the Shy Bipolar was in the second grade, could plausibly be regarded as the earliest manifestation of the bipolar disorder. The argument for coverage would be that he had been an outgoing child until the onset of the affective illness skewed his development. The manic episode and its aftermath interrupted any developmental readiness to outgrow the shyness during college years. Group therapy was prescribed to help him achieve the natural social potential that had been thwarted by the bipolar illness. Seen in this light, group psychotherapy is being prescribed to combat interpersonal deficits caused by the illness, much as medication combats the biologically based mood instability. However, as a way of guarding against "moral hazard," the HMO's extended benefit covered only continuing care group, designed for patients much more impaired than the Shy Bipolar, and not the kind of interpersonal group psychotherapy to which he was referred.

The following case further clarifies how clinicians distinguish between treatment of illness and enhancement of well-being:

Case 2: The Unhappy Husband. UH, an intelligent, professionally successful married father of two children, sought treatment because of severe unhappiness associated with marital distress. His wife suffered from an Axis II disorder that made her very difficult to live with. UH was committed to maintaining the marriage. A V code diagnosis – "Conditions not attributable to a mental disorder that are a focus of treatment" – was made. In twenty-six sessions of psychotherapy UH was able to clarify some of the pertinent dynamic issues in his marriage and developed a number of adaptive strategies for lessening his distress. The twenty-six sessions were highly productive. UH wished that his treatment would be covered by insurance, but he agreed that he was not suffering from an illness and that it was fair to expect him to pay.

The Unhappy Husband is probably suffering more than many of the HMO members being treated for illnesses, and psychotherapy definitely enhanced his well-being. What possible rationale could there be for not covering his treatment? The clinician's decision hinged on the question of what the Unhappy Husband is suffering from. By the criteria set forth in the then-current *DSM-III-R*, the Unhappy Husband does not have an illness. His suffering arises from the fact that although his wife's unchanging condition causes him great pain, his values preclude divorce. The clinician believed that under the prevailing agreements that govern insurance, individuals like the Unhappy Husband should be responsible for some or all of the cost of rectifying the unhappiness associated with an unfortunate existential situation. Paradoxically, if the Unhappy Husband expressed his suffering through somatic symptoms and presented to an internist rather than a mental health clinician, insurance would typically cover medical investigation and treatment, which would probably be less effective but costlier than psychotherapy. A 1989 survey of medium and large firms showed that only 2 percent of insured employees have coverage for outpatient mental health services equivalent to other medical services.[6]

If we surveyed the adult population, we would find many who suffer from shyness and social inhibition comparable to the Shy Bipolar in all but one detail – their shyness is not caused by an illness. The Shy Bipolar's clinician was ultimately prepared to authorize insurance coverage for group psychotherapy because he came to believe that shyness was a manifestation of the bipolar disorder, but was unable to do so because the HMO did not cover that form of psychotherapy under its extended benefit. How might clinicians reason about insurance coverage for normally shy people?

Clinicians who use a hard-line definition of medical necessity, as the Unhappy Husband's therapist did, would not approve insurance coverage of group therapy for people suffering from normal shyness. These clinicians would reason that social adaptation is arrayed along a normal distribution curve. Many people are shy and withdrawn. Others are unusually outgoing and adept at making relationships. While being outgoing and socially adept may be advantageous, hard-line clinicians believe that health insurance is not designed to rectify the normal distribution of social skills, however much competitive disadvantage and suffering the lack of these skills might entail.

"Expansive" clinicians may argue that normal shyness should be covered because the shyness stems from psychodynamic factors. Hardliners will respond, however, that while psychodynamic interpretations of shyness may provide valuable self-understanding and assist in changing the pattern of behavior, all behavior presumably reflects psychodynamic antecedents. The presence or absence of psychodynamic determinants does not in itself establish whether a *DSM-IV* mental disorder is present.

RESPONSIBILITY FOR TEMPERAMENT AND CHARACTER

Clinicians have particular difficulty agreeing about medical necessity when people suffer from what is colloquially called temperament or character – conditions that *DSM-III-R* classifies under Axis II. How do clinicians decide whether this kind of suffering creates a claim on insurance resources or whether it is the individual's responsibility to pay for treatment? The following two cases come from the practice of the same clinician, who was concerned about whether he could make a valid clinical justification for having taken a hard-line position in case 3 and an expansive position in case 4.

> **Case 3: The Cranky Victim.** *CV is a lonely, unhappy single man in his forties. He feels that he has been treated unfairly since childhood, when for reasons unclear to him he was frequently picked on in school. He acknowledges that he has acted in a demanding and irascible manner all of his adult life, and that these behaviors have contributed to an unhappy love life and tendency to lose friends. He believes, however, that his actions represent a natural response to the way the world has treated him. His brother, father, and an uncle are also irascible.*
>
> *Although a slow learner, CV completed high school and a vocational program in audiovisual technologies. Because he prefers to work independently, he does free-lance work, which barely provides adequate income.*
>
> *In the past CV has had several courses of psychotherapy. The most helpful was eighteen months of group treatment ten years ago. CV, however, preferred individual therapy. Even though it had not led to any identifiable changes, he felt happier while the therapy was going on and stated that individual therapy had helped him to understand himself better. Now a member of the HMO, CV requested individual treatment because of his ongoing unhappiness and isolation.*

The clinician did not authorize coverage for individual psychotherapy even though he believed that the Cranky Victim would feel happier and less alone while therapy was going on. The Cranky Victim's treatment history suggested that while group therapy had produced change, individual therapy had not. If the clinician were to authorize insurance coverage for any treatment, he would have chosen group (on the grounds of efficacy), not individual. The clinician diagnosed the condition as an interpersonal problem (V code), not a personality disorder, because although the Cranky Victim's behavior was "maladaptive" (in *DSM-III-R's* language) it was not "inflexible." The clinician believed that however intense the Cranky Victim's unhappiness might be, unless an illness caused it, health insurance should not cover treatment.

Clinicians, however, have experimented with antidepressants and mood stabilizers for non-FDA approved indications. Suppose the Cranky Victim were to undertake a trial with fluoxetine or carbamazepine with apparently positive results. Some might then say that he must have an illness because a medication was helping him.[7] It becomes unclear whether health insurance would pay for medication in these circumstances. If it would, why shouldn't it also pay for the psychotherapy that the Cranky Victim wants?

Furthermore, the Cranky Victim's father, uncle, and brother have similar irascibility, raising the possibility of a genetic basis for the traits that cause him such difficulty. It is easy to imagine that the Human Genome Project might ultimately identify genetic "defects" that underlie this kind of irascibility.[8] Would we then regard the Cranky Victim as the victim of his temperament rather than as responsible for it and for the consequences arising from it? The following case provides further insight into how this clinician reasoned about temperament, diagnosis, and insurance coverage.

> *Case 4: The Lost Administrator. LA is a thirty-five-year-old, single woman, successful in her work as an administrator and well-liked by her many friends. Although she appears confident and successful, she feels intensely "empty" and "lost." She is especially unhappy about her love life. LA has been involved with a series of men who have been attached to others or unwilling to make a commitment, and not drawn to men who might have been more reliable. Friends tell her, however, "You have everything you need to be happy. Why don't you let yourself enjoy your life for what it is?" In outpatient psychotherapy seven years earlier she had become increasingly frightened until she interrupted precipitously after eighteen months.*
>
> *LA is the third child and only daughter in a family of five. By the time of her birth her father was already suffering from severe diabetes. Throughout her childhood he experienced progressive complications including amputation, heart disease, kidney failure, and loss of vision. He died when she was sixteen. He was severely critical of her, and LA felt that her mother, who had been overwhelmed by his illness and financial burdens, was emotionally unavailable to her. LA's mother confirmed that LA had been a precociously responsible, undemanding child, and that she herself had indeed felt overwhelmed and unavailable during LA's growing up.*
>
> *LA's clinician made a V code diagnosis of interpersonal problem and an Axis I diagnosis of presumptive atypical depression. He recommended considering psychodynamic psychotherapy (individual and/or group) and a trial of antidepressant medication (which LA declined).*

The Lost Administrator was offered partially subsidized psychotherapy under the regular HCHP benefit, while the Cranky Victim was not. On what basis, if any, can their circumstances be distinguished?

The clinician could not say which of the two experienced more unhappiness. He recognized, however, that he felt decidedly more sympathy for the Lost Administrator than for the Cranky Victim and worried about how his reactions may have influenced his reasoning about medical necessity.

In blunt terms, the clinician believed that the Cranky Victim had a "bad attitude" and carried "a chip on his shoulder." Although the Cranky Victim suffered from the effects of his irascibility, he insisted that it was entirely justified by the way the world treated him. The clinician regarded the Cranky Victim as a person who was able to revise his attitudes and behavior but was unwilling to do so.

In contrast, the clinician saw the Lost Administrator as a victim of her temperament. Although her friends questioned whether she too suffered from a bad attitude and was refusing to take pleasure in a life that "has everything one needs to be happy," the clinician believed that she was indeed *trying* to find satisfaction in her life but was *unable* to do so, and not at all like the spoiled princess in the fable who refuses to be comfortable because she discerns a pea beneath her mattress.

In the course of discussion with the authors, the clinician came to fear that he had mixed moral and diagnostic reasoning in his thinking about the Cranky Victim and the Lost Administrator. He found himself uncertain as to whether his *DSM-III-R* diagnoses of the Cranky Victim (V code: interpersonal problem) and the Lost Administrator (Axis I: presumptive atypical depression) *explained* his judgment of medical necessity, or whether he had invoked the *DSM-III-R* diagnoses to *justify* his moral assessment that the Lost Administrator "deserved" treatment because she was trying to overcome her condition, whereas the Cranky Victim did not "deserve" treatment because he took no responsibility for himself and simply blamed others. Not all hard questions are definitively answerable, however, and the clinician remained perturbed.

CONTROVERSY ARISING FROM CLINICAL UNCERTAINTY

Case 5: The Abandoned Mother. Part I. AM is a divorced, fifty-year-old mother of two. In the previous year she had lost her job, moved to a new apartment, and her closest friend had left the area. Shortly before her initial mental health contact the daughter she had been closest to became engaged, and told AM that she would be staying with her future in-laws when she visited the area, not with AM.

AM became distraught and tearful. She was diagnosed as having an Adjustment Disorder with Depressed Mood. Coverage was provided under the regular benefit, with increased copayment after eight sessions and full fee after twenty. She did not develop rapport, however, with any of the three therapists she saw, and trials of imipramine, fluoxetine, and phenelzine produced no benefit. AM felt desperate and began to request hospitalization.

Eleven months after the treatment began, her situation was reviewed with a consultant. The consultant asked, "What is this patient suffering from? Does she have a form of major depression? Or is it life – is it being middle-aged, divorced, bereft of children, jobless, that makes her feel alone and angry?"

The consultant is posing a characteristic hard-line question. The Abandoned Mother's story is disturbing, but at this point in her course her condition did not clearly meet the *DSM-III-R* criteria for Major Depression or Dysthymia. If we apply a Depressive Disorder diagnosis to her ambiguous condition, we put the Abandoned Mother into the framework of illness, patient, doctor, medical treatment, and potential coverage of care under health insurance. If we call her condition "life," we are saying that although she is encountering painful circumstances and experiencing suffering, the paradigms of illness, patient, doctor, medical treatment, and insurance do not apply.

The concept of medical necessity forces us to pose questions in an either–or manner: treatment is or is not medically necessary. Clinical situations like the Abandoned Mother's, however, are often much more ambiguous. Further observations may help but do not always take away the uncertainty.

The Abandoned Mother: Part II. Following the consultation, AM continued outpatient therapy with yet another therapist. When her daughter again visited without staying with her, AM's suicidal preoccupations increased, and she spoke of plans to kill herself. She said she could not pay for outpatient treatment and again requested hospitalization. Those involved with insurance administration reviewed her case and changed the diagnosis to Depressive Disorder (atypical form) with significant suicidal risk, and authorized up to two half-hours of case management per week without escalating copayment ("extended benefit").

Although the Abandoned Mother's diagnosis and insurance status have now both been shifted, there is still room for controversy. The expansive clinician will say that her true condition has become clear over time – now we see that the Abandoned Mother is really suffering from Atypical Depression, not an Adjustment Reaction or an existential tantrum. But it remains possible to take a hard-line view and say that the Abandoned Mother has learned how insurance decisions are made and can now game the system to get the outcome she wants.

In case 5, controversy regarding medical necessity arose from uncertainty regarding the Abandoned Mother's diagnosis – whether she was suffering from an affective disorder or a hard time in her life. In the following case, the question of what constitutes medically necessary treatment arises from uncertainty about whether an effective treatment is available and if so what it is.

> *Case 6: The Abused Child. AC, six years old, moved with her mother to New England from another part of the country and became a member of the HMO. During the previous two years she had been repeatedly sexually abused by her stepfather, who had been prosecuted and was now in jail. AC's genitalia showed unmistakable signs of the abuse, but she was a remarkably happy-seeming child and was adjusting very well to her new environment.*

Whereas the Abandoned Mother was in a constant struggle over what she would get, neither the Abused Child nor her mother are making a demand on the HMO. While hard-liners can regard the Abandoned Mother as a person who refuses to take responsibility for adapting to relatively ordinary life experiences, the Abused Child is obviously not responsible for what happened to her. The HMO was fully ready to cover treatment for the Abused Child, but it was highly unclear whether at this point there was a treatment to offer, since her growth and development appeared to be proceeding well. The mental health clinician decided to offer attentive watching, and to follow the Abused Child closely with the pediatrician and the mother.

MORAL HAZARD

When the consultant in case 5 asked whether the Abandoned Mother was suffering from major depression or the vicissitudes of life, she was raising a question about what the insurance industry calls moral hazard as well as a question about diagnosis. Social programs that offer insurance protection against specified dangers create the hazard that individuals will alter their behavior so as to claim benefits, as by burning an insured property so as collect for loss, for example, or claiming to be unable to work so as to receive disability payments. Insurance underwriters fear that if mental health insurance becomes more available, individuals like the Abandoned Mother might claim to suffer from an illness when they are actually suffering from life, to obtain the attention and solace that psychotherapy, hospital care, and the sick role might provide.

If we too easily assimilate shyness (case 1), unfortunate existential situations (case 2), loneliness and irascibility (case 3), lack of satisfaction with ostensibly adequate opportunity (case 4), or life itself (case 5) to the category of disease and disability, we open a very wide door for health insurance claims. Quite apart from the obvious implications for the cost of insurance, mental health clinicians recognize the potential for doing unintentional harm to patients by ascribing a diagnostic label – the patient role, with its implication of pathology.[9] Thus although the insurance industry concern about moral hazard is primarily an actuarial concern with claim liability, guarding against moral hazard will sometimes protect individuals from iatrogenic harms of the sick role as well.

Potential insurers of mental health care are especially concerned with moral hazard because (1) many of the symptoms of mental illness are part of a continuum with everyday forms of distress; (2) diagnosis of some conditions – especially Axis II disorders – is controversial and uncertain;[10] (3) some forms of treatment – especially psychotherapy – seem similar to nonprofessional forms of human support and interaction; and (4) demand for mental health services has been shown to be highly responsive to the presence or absence of insurance coverage.[11] These factors create public concern that expanded coverage would lead to excessive utilization of care. When opponents of expanded mental health coverage apply disparaging terms like "rent-a-friend" to mental health treatment they are in part expressing a concern about moral hazard – that legitimate needs such as friendship will masquerade as needs for subsidized treatment, and the community paying for health insurance will incur expenditures it should not be liable for.

THREE MODELS UNDERLYING THE CONFLICT
OVER INSURANCE COVERAGE

We believe that these examples of front-line reasoning about insurance coverage reflect three different models – which we call "normal function," "capability," and "welfare" (see table 11.1) – for thinking about

Table 11.1. *Models of medical necessity*

Equal opportunity for	Target of clinical action	Ultimate goal of health care
1. Normal Function	Medically defined deviation	Decrease impact of disease or disability
2. Personal Capability	Unchosen constraint of personal capability	Enhance personal capability
3. Welfare	Unchosen constraint of potential for happiness	Enhance potential for happiness

medical necessity. Each model defines the ultimate goal of psychiatric care as helping the patient to come as close to equal opportunity in life as is possible, but the models answer the question, Equal opportunity for what?[12] in subtly different ways. Although the terms in which we formulate the three models come from moral philosophy, we believe that the models can help to illuminate practical controversies over current insurance coverage and provide guidance for future insurance design. In fact, failure to distinguish among these models may contribute to the difficulty advocates encounter in their efforts to promote nondiscriminatory insurance coverage for mental health services.

Normal function model

According to the normal function model, the central purpose of health care is to maintain, restore, or compensate for the restricted opportunity and loss of function caused by disease and disability.[13] Successful health care restores people to the range of capabilities they would have had without the pathological condition or prevents further deterioration.

The normal function model takes unequal distribution of human capabilities as a fact that health care will not change. Some people are socially adept. Others are shy in ways that cause suffering. The model prescribes compassion for those who are less fortunate in the natural lottery that distributes capabilities, but makes the health sector responsible for correcting only those conditions which – in *DSM-IV* terms – can be diagnosed as "a symptom of a dysfunction," that is, as mental disorders.

Health care is not the only agent of social responsibility. People suffering from lack of social skill can be ministered to by education, training, families, religious and community groups, and other social institutions. Treating illness and enhancing human capabilities may both be desirable social goals, but they should not be confused with one another. The normal function model holds that health-care insurance coverage should be restricted to disadvantages caused by disease and disability unless society explicitly decides to use it to mitigate other forms of disadvantage as well. Hard-line clinicians define medical necessity in accord with the normal function model.

Capability model

The capability model prescribes a broader role for health care. It holds that the distribution of personal capabilities like confidence, resilience, and sociability in the natural lottery should not be taken as a given. Health care should strive to give people equal personal capabilities, or at least give priority to those whose diminished capability (whatever the cause) puts them at a relative disadvantage.[14] The capability model makes no moral distinction between treatment of illness and enhancement of disadvantageous personal capabilities. It makes relative disadvantage in one's ability to function the morally relevant characteristic for determining insurance coverage. Consequently, if group therapy helps to alleviate significant disadvantages caused by normal shyness, or if fluoxetine gives "the introvert the social skills of a salesman,"[15] the capability model would hold that health insurance should provide coverage.

The normal function model asks health care to help people become *normal* competitors, free from disadvantages caused by disease or disability. The capability model, by contrast, would use health care to help people become *equal* competitors, free from disadvantageous lack of capabilities regardless of etiology. It makes a single *DSM-IV* criterion for diagnosing a mental disorder – "impairment in one or more areas of functioning" – its central focus, but unlike *DSM-IV* it does not require that the impairment be "a symptom of a dysfunction (underlying disorder)."

The kind of controversy that arises in psychiatry about insurance coverage for treatment of disadvantageous personal capabilities like shyness occurs in other areas of health insurance as well. A recent issue of *Growth, Genetics, & Hormones*, for example, was entirely devoted to the parallel issue of whether short children who are not deficient in growth hormone should be treated, and if so, if the treatment should be covered by insurance.[16] Expansive pediatric endocrinologists guided by the capability model have argued that because extreme shortness is a handicapping condition, insurance should provide the hormone to short children who have no endocrine abnormality.[17] Others who use the normal function model would limit insurance coverage to children with growth hormone deficiency.[18]

Welfare model

According to the welfare model, if people suffer because of attitudes or behavior patterns they did not choose to develop and are not independently able to alter or overcome, they should be eligible for insurance coverage. When the clinician in cases 3 and 4 distinguished between the Cranky Victim and the Lost Administrator on the basis of whether they were able and willing to change the attitudes and behavior that caused their suffering, he was unwittingly applying the welfare model.[19] The welfare model makes its central focus a different *DSM-IV* criterion for diagnosing a mental disorder – "present distress (a painful symptom)" – but like the capability model it diverges from *DSM-IV* and the normal function model in not requiring that the distress be a symptom of a mental disorder.

By training and temperament, mental health clinicians want to alleviate disadvantage, enhance personal capabilities, and reduce suffering. Offering treatment to the Shy Bipolar and not to the person who is normally shy but who suffers just as much, strains their moral commitments. Expansive clinicians are attracted to the capability model because it allows them to argue for extending insurance coverage to both. Similarly, to expansive clinicians, not offering insurance coverage to the Unhappy Husband, whose suffering was relieved by psychodynamic psychotherapy, is clinically unjustifiable and morally repugnant. The welfare model appeals to them because it supports claims for assistance based on personal suffering like that of the Unhappy Husband. The capability and welfare models provide expansive clinicians with a rationale for interpreting treatment of the conditions that *DSM-II* called "neuroses"[20] and Astrachan described as the "humanistic" tasks of psychiatry[21] as medically necessary.

PRACTICAL IMPLICATIONS FOR HEALTH INSURANCE

The era of laissez-faire with regard to health-care expenditure is by now a nostalgic memory. In the future, explicit priorities for allocation and (we predict) rationing will guide practice. A clear and well-grounded model of medical necessity will be crucial for the design of a just and practical insurance system. Which model should we choose?

To be useful, a model for defining medical necessity must pass three tests: Does it make distinctions the public and clinicians regard as fair? Can it be administered in the real world? and, Does it lead to results that society can afford? We believe that the normal function model meets these three criteria best.

First, all developed societies recognize treatment of illness as a primary societal imperative. An affluent society that refused to care for its sick would be regarded as grossly unfair. Thus it is not surprising that all three models agree that disadvantage and suffering caused by disease and disability have a special claim on collective resources. Second, although individual cases can pose difficult or insoluble diagnostic dilemmas, psychiatry has developed publicly accepted methods – currently embodied in *DSM-IV* – by which agreed-upon diagnoses can generally be established. Finally, while morally acceptable definitions of the scope of health care lead to costs that strain every society, the normal function model at least allows society to draw a plausible boundary around the potential scope of insurance coverage for mental health care.

Although the capability and welfare models capture basic moral insights, we believe that they cast too broad a net and pose severe problems for administration and cost. How are we to judge when the conditions for health insurance coverage have been met under these models? If individuals invoke the capability model and request treatment for incapacitating shyness, do we simply take their assessment of need at face value? If so, the insurer is subject to extensive moral hazard. If not, how are we to investigate the claim? Have shy people made reasonable efforts to overcome the condition – participating in social events, asking others for tips on socializing, taking public speaking classes, and so forth? Did they bring it on themselves, as by wishing to consort only with rich, beautiful, and famous people who intimidate them and elicit shyness? We have little idea of how to delve into questions like this. If the Cranky Victim invokes the welfare model and requests treatment on the grounds that he did not choose to be so irascible, similar problems arise. If we do not investigate, we create substantial risk of moral hazard. But if we do investigate, we are faced with a task for which we have few skills – reconstructing the history of the Cranky Victim's choices and assessing how responsible he is for creating and sustaining the attitudes and behaviors from which he suffers.

Public support for mental health insurance coverage, historically tenuous at best, might be compromised further if the public believed that third-party resources were subject to even more moral hazard than exists at present. If the public believed that mental health interventions replace reasonable efforts to modify one's attitudes and behaviors or to extend one's capacities through learning and practice, support would wane.

President Clinton's proposed "American Health Security Act" sets eligibility for insurance coverage of mental health and substance abuse treatment in accord with the normal function model. Coverage will be provided only if an individual "has, or has had during the 1-year period preceding the date of such treatment, a *diagnosable mental or substance abuse disorder*" (emphasis added).[22] If the health-care reform process ultimately interprets "medical necessity" in accord with the normal function model, insurers will need to clarify the implications of the model for clinicians and the public. Current insurance definitions of "medical necessity" often give no guidance as to which model should be used. The HMO at which this study was conducted defines "medically necessary" as "those medical services which are essential for the treatment of a Member's medical condition and are in accordance with generally accepted medical practice."[23] To place mental health services under the normal function model, this definition would change to something like "those mental health services which are essential for the treatment of a Member's mental health disorder as defined by *DSM-IV* in accordance with generally accepted mental health practice."

Insurance administrators are acutely aware that clinicians can always find ways to circumvent insurance restrictions. No model prevents the possibility of "gaming,"[24] and a recent survey showed that 68 percent of the physicians polled were willing to deceive third-party payers if they believed coverage criteria were unfair.[25] While clear criteria and monitoring systems make gaming more difficult, the most effective antidote to gaming is for clinicians and their patients to understand and endorse the rationale for the model used to determine coverage and to believe in the integrity of the system within which allocative decisions are made.[26]

A model for determining medical necessity allows us to determine what conditions are *eligible* for insurance coverage, but does not tell us how much of the total health-care budget should be devoted to mental health. A health plan, state, or nation might decide it could not afford to provide all treatment eligible for coverage, and that it needed to set priorities (or ration), as has recently occurred in Oregon.[27] Although some insurers deny coverage to Axis II conditions, all "mental disorders" are eligible for coverage under the normal function model. The Oregon priority setting process included borderline and schizotypal personality disorders in the proposed basic package, but antisocial personality disorder ranked below the cutoff point. To think rationally about *how* to finance, administer, and set priorities within mental health insurance, we must first be clear on what the insurance is *for*.

Whatever percentage of the health-care budget is devoted to mental health, we recommend that insurance cover three to six sessions for evaluation, so that clinicians working under the normal function model would be able to guide patients who are not suffering from a mental disorder toward potentially helpful alternatives. For the Unhappy Husband, the alternative was psychotherapy on a fee-for-service basis. For the Cranky Victim it might be courses in social skills or involvement in religious activities that could encourage a reframed view of his circumstances. In this way the clinician is not simply a *gatekeeper*, determining whether or not the person receives treatment covered by insurance, but a *caregiver*, who offers guidance and compassion if the person's suffering comes from causes other than mental disorder, and who is open to reviewing the initial diagnosis if new clinical facts emerge. Hard-line clinicians need not be hard-hearted.

Any model of medical necessity will ultimately have to be applied by clinicians at the front line.[28] We undertook this detailed study of how clinicians actually reason about medical necessity to see if current practice provides valuable guidance for future policy. We conclude that it does.

Conflict about mental health insurance coverage is rampant. Frequently the conflict between reviewer and clinician (or clinician and patient) is empirical: can a proposed intervention reasonably be anticipated to achieve the intended result? Even when the answer is yes, the parties often clash over the question of whether a less costly intervention might achieve a comparable result.[29] These conflicts over effectiveness may not currently be resolvable because of limited outcomes data, but they will ultimately yield to scientific progress.

When expansive and hard-line clinicians clash, however, their conflict is at least sometimes about the *ends* of health care, rather than about the *means* to achieve those ends. What may masquerade as a diagnostic conflict about what the patient *has* may in actuality reflect disagreement about what health care *should* be. Should it be restricted to limitations created by *DSM-IV* defined disorders in accord with the normal function model, or should it minister to other forms of limitation as well, as proposed by the capability and welfare models?

We recognize that the concepts of disease and disability have been subjected to extensive philosophical and sociological criticism. Our endorsement of the normal function model does not rest on a view of disease and disability as ultimately real in a metaphysical sense. We acknowledge that cases will continue to arise that seem arbitrary (like covering treatment for shyness caused by an illness but not for normal shyness) or painful (like not covering the kind of psychotherapy that helped the Unhappy Husband). Similarly, diagnostic categories will continue to change, and what is regarded as a mental disorder today may be seen as a cultural construct tomorrow.

Society, however, needs a publicly acceptable and administerable system for defining the boundaries of health insurance coverage. The conception of mental disorder embodied in *DSM-IV* provides a workable definition of these boundaries. *DSM-IV* is not free from error or bias. It is, however, the result of a highly public process open to scientific scrutiny, field testing, and repetitive criticism over time. The alternative to defining the boundaries of coverage by the normal function model and *DSM-IV* is not a more liberal system governed by the capability or welfare model, but one in which mental health benefits are arbitrarily capped, as occurs at present. As José Santiago has recently commented, "At stake is survival of services as a legitimate item in any reform effort."[30] We believe that the normal function model best ensures the survival of a robust mental health service sector.

Conflict about health insurance can occur at three levels. First, parties may differ about the goals of health care itself, as when expansive clinicians clash with hard-liners. Second, empirical conflicts may occur over how interventions (means) may relate to outcomes (ends). Finally, even with a well-clarified model for defining medical necessity, society will continue to struggle over how much medically necessary care it will provide.[31] All three levels of conflict pose major challenges. If we do not make clear distinctions among them, however, we will make no progress toward creating useful answers.

ACKNOWLEDGMENTS

The authors wish to thank the Robert Wood Johnson Foundation (grant no. 19450) and the Harvard Community Health Plan Foundation for their generous support.

REFERENCES

1. William M. Glazer, "Psychiatry and Medical Necessity," *Psychiatric Annals* 22 (1992): 362–66.
2. William A. Helvestine, "Legal Implications of Utilization Review," in *Controlling Costs and Changing Patient Care: The Role of Utilization Review*, ed. Bradford H. Gray and Marilyn J. Field (Washington, D.C.: National Academy Press, 1989), pp. 169–204, at 172.
3. Steven S. Sharfstein, "Third-Party Payers: To Pay or Not to Pay," *American Journal of Psychiatry* 135 (1978): 1185–88; Allen Beigel and Steven S. Sharfstein, "Mental Health Care Providers: Not the Only Cause or Only Cure for Rising Costs," *American Journal of Psychiatry* 141 (1984): 668–72; Richard B. Karel, "Tipper Gore's Former Staff Head Sheds Light on How Some Task Force Decisions Were Reached," *Psychiatric News* 28, no. 19 (1991): 10, 21.
4. James E. Sabin, Lachlan Forrow, and Norman Daniels, "Clarifying the Concept of Medical Necessity," in *Proceedings of the Group Health Institute* (Washington, D.C.: Group Health Association of America, 1991), pp. 693–707; Norman Daniels and James E. Sabin, "When Is Home Care Medically Necessary?" *Hastings Center Report* 21, no. 4 (1991): 37–8.
5. Helen S. Abrams, "Harvard Community Health Plan's Mental Health Redesign Project: A Managerial and Clinical Partnership," *Psychiatric Quarterly* 64 (1993): 13–31.
6. Patricia Scheidemandel, *The Coverage Catalog*, 3rd ed. (Washington, D.C.: American Psychiatric Association, office of Economic Affairs, 1993), p. 44.
7. M. Balint et al., *Treatment or Diagnosis: A Study of Repeat Prescriptions in General Practice* (London: Tavistock Publications, 1970).
8. Norman Daniels. "The Genome Project, Individual Differences, and Just Health Care," in *Justice and the Human Genome*, ed. Timothy S. Murphy and Marc A. Lappé (Berkeley and Los Angeles: University of California Press, 1994), pp. 110–32.
9. Thomas J. Scheff, ed. *Labelling Madness* (Englewood Cliffs, N.J.: Prentice Hall, 1975).

10. J. Christopher Perry, "Problems and Considerations in the Valid Assessment of Personality Disorders," *American Journal of Psychiatry* 149 (1992): 1645–53.
11. Willard G. Manning et al., *Effects of Mental Health Insurance: Evidence from the Health Insurance Experiment* (Santa Monica, Calif.: RAND, 1989).
12. Norman Daniels, "Equality of What: Welfare, Resources or Capabilities?" supplement, *Philosophy and Phenomenological Research* 19 (1990): 273–96.
13. Norman Daniels, *Just Health Care* (Cambridge: Cambridge University Press, 1985), ch. 2.
14. Amartya Sen, "Justice: Means versus Freedoms." *Philosophy and Public Affairs* 19 (1990): 111–21; see also Amartya Sen, *Inequality Reexamined* (Cambridge, Mass.: Harvard University Press, 1992).
15. Peter D. Kramer, *Listening to Prozac* (New York: Viking, 1993), p. xv.
16. Supplement 1, *Growth, Genetics, and Hormones* 8 (1992).
17. David B. Allen and Norman C. Fost, "Growth Hormone Therapy for Short Stature: Panacea or Pandora's Box?" *Journal of Pediatrics* 117 (1990): 16–21.
18. Norman Daniels, "Growth Hormone Therapy for Short Stature: Can We Support the Treatment/Enhancement Distinction?" supplement 1, *Growth, Genetics, & Hormones* 8 (1992): 46–8.
19. Richard J. Arneson, "Equality and Equal Opportunity for Welfare," *Philosophical Studies* 54 (1988): 79–95; G. A. Cohen, "On the Currency of Egalitarian Justice," *Ethics* 99 (1989): 906–44.
20. Ronald Bayer and Robert L. Spitzer, "Neurosis, Psychodynamics, and DSM-III," *Archives of General Psychiatry* 42 (1985): 187–96.
21. Boris M. Astrachan, Daniel J. Levinson, and David A. Adler, "The Impact of National Health Insurance on the Tasks and Practice of Psychiatry," *Archives of General Psychiatry* 33 (1976): 785–94.
22. *Health Security Act*, 151-183 O-93-1, Title I, Subtitle B, Sec. 1115(b)(1A) (Washington, D.C.: U.S. Government Printing Office), p. 46.
23. Subscriber's Agreement, Harvard Community Health Plan, Boston, Mass., October 1991.
24. E. Haavi Morreim, "Gaming the System: Dodging the Rules, Ruling the Dodgers," *Archives of Internal Medicine* 151 (1991): 443–47.
25. Dennis H. Novack et al., "Physicians' Attitudes towards Using Deception to Resolve Difficult Ethical Problems," *JAMA* 261 (1989): 2980–85.
26. Norman Daniels, "Why Saying No to Patients in the United States Is So Hard: Cost-Containment, Justice, and Provider Autonomy," *NEJM* 314 (1986): 1380–83.
27. David A. Pollack, David Pollichi, Bentson McFarland, Robert George, and Richard Angell, "Prioritization of Mental Health Services in Oregon," *Milbank Quarterly* 72 (fall 1994): 515–50; Philip J. Boyle and Daniel Callahan, "Minds and Hearts: Priorities in Mental Health Services," Special Supplement, *Hastings Center Report* 23, no. 5 (1993).
28. E. Haavi Morreim, *Balancing Act: The New Medical Ethics of Medicine's New Economics* (Dordrecht, the Netherlands: Kluwer Academic Publishers, 1991).

29. James E. Sabin, "The Therapeutic Alliance in Managed Care Mental Health Practice," *Journal of Psychotherapy Practice and Research* 1 (1992): 29–36.
30. José M. Santiago, "The Fate of Mental Health Services in Health Care Reform: II. Realistic Solutions." *Hospital and Community Psychiatry* 43 (1992): 1095–99, at 1098.
31. Hugh L Etang, ed. *Health Care Provision under Financial Constraints: A Decade of Change* (London: Royal Society of Medicine, 1990).

Postscript: More on capabilities and the goals of medicine

In "Determining 'Medical Necessity' in Mental Health Practice," James Sabin and I defended a distinction between treatments of disease and disability and enhancements of otherwise normal capabilities. Appealing to that distinction, we then defended, largely on policy grounds, a modest view of the goal of medicine (to keep people functioning normally) against a more expansive view (to eliminate any disadvantages in capabilities). I want here to add to that defense by suggesting that there is less theoretical support than there might at first seem to be for a more expansive role. Specifically, I claim that Sen's views about positive freedom or capabilities less directly support an expansive view than Sabin and I suggested in our discussion. These comments clarify some points that were on my mind but not developed in "Equality of What" (Chapter 10, especially toward the end of Section 2).

As I noted in Chapter 10 (see also Chapter 9), what might be called the *standard interpretation* of the requirements of equality of opportunity assumes that there is a background inequality in the distribution of capabilities. It is not a requirement of assuring equal opportunity on the standard interpretation that we eliminate this inequality in the distribution of capabilities. Applied to health care and construed as an account of the goals of medicine, the fair equality of opportunity principle thus ascribes to medicine the relatively modest task of keeping people functioning as close to normally as possible. In effect, as Sabin and I noted in Chapter 11 (see also Daniels 1992), health care, like compensatory education programs, aims to produce "normal competitors" but not necessarily "equal competitors." An unequal distribution of capabilities is left intact, once the distorting effects of past social practices and treatable disease and disability are addressed.

Why should we take the natural distribution of talents and skills as a baseline, as the standard view does? It might be thought that Rawls, for example, assumes this only because of the technological infeasibility of modifying that baseline. If that were true, then new, genetically based technologies might force us to modify that assumption. Would pursuit of equal opportunity then compel us to use medical technologies to modify the natural distribution of talents and skills? Would justice so compel us?

The answer to this question is not so straightforward as it seems, in part because Rawls is not making as simple a feasibility assumption as the one portrayed by this interpretation. A first and fundamental point to note is that our egalitarian concerns in general, and our concerns about equal opportunity in particular, form only part of our concerns about what justice requires. A theory of justice in general, or of justice for health care in particular, must combine concerns about equality with concerns about liberty; both of these must be reconciled with considerations about efficiency and the allocation of resources. Even if the fundamental intuition underlying our concerns about equality of opportunity pushed us toward thinking that we were obliged to take some steps toward the redistribution of capabilities such as talents and skills, rather than treating their "natural" distribution as a baseline, we must reconcile the pull of that concern with conflicting goals regarding liberty and efficiency. It may be better – even for those worst off with regard to talents and skills – to mitigate the effects of inequalities by redistributions of other important goods than to insist on "equalizing" the distribution of natural talents and skills (cf. Chapter 10).

Rawls' assumes that deliberators in his Original Position would make just such a reconciliation of competing concerns. His key assumption is that *some* unequal distribution of talents and skills can and must be taken as a baseline but that even given such inequality, the system as a whole can be made to work to the advantage even of those worst off with regard to marketable talents and skills. Rawls is quite explicit that environmental factors, ranging from culture within a family to educational and compensatory educational measures, will definitely affect the distribution of talents and skills. There is no reason to think that his account – or my extension of it to health care – would rule out our sometimes being obliged to use medical technologies to alter the distribution of talents and skills. What is made unlikely by Rawls' account – or my extension of it to health care – is that an individual who finds herself deficient in some normal (but not optimal) capability thereby has a claim, based on equality of opportunity, to assistance to rectify that (perceived) deficit.

In what follows I shall try to clarify this claim by examining further whether Sen's views about capabilities (described in Chapter 10) do support a much more expansive view of the role of medicine in the pursuit of equality of opportunity. A crucial point is one already made: a theory of justice requires integrating concerns for equality with concerns for liberty and efficiency. Sen's allegation that our egalitarian concerns really focus on capabilities, not resources or experiential states, or the claim that we explicate the goal of equal opportunity as the goal of achieving equality in capability sets, does not tell us what justice requires us to do.

In *Inequality Reexamined*, Sen (1992) comments that we must reconcile our concerns about efficiency with our concerns about equality in order to find out what justice requires. In other words, justice might not require us to pursue equality of capabilities after all. We might instead be required to permit some inequalities and act to mitigate their effects. Sen does not give us any discussion of how this reconciliation would take place in a theory of justice. Rawls, however, does: we take some natural distribution of talents and skills as a baseline – in fact, the normal distribution. Those with the least marketable capabilities will have lower prospects in life than those with more marketable capabilities, but Rawls mitigates the effects of this basic, residual inequality by requiring that inequalities in primary social goods like wealth and income be constrained so that the inequalities work to the advantage of those with the worst prospects in life. In this way, those with more marketable talents and skills must harness their advantages to maximizing the prospects of those who are worst off with regard to talents and skills.

In effect, Rawls divides responsibility for meeting our egalitarian concerns between two different principles (as noted in Chapter 10). The principle governing equality of opportunity leaves the normal distribution of capabilities in place, but the principles governing overall inequality in prospects in life mitigates the effects of doing so. If health care should be governed by a principle regulating fair equality of opportunity, then it too may leave the normal distribution of capabilities in place, concerning itself only with keeping people functioning as close to normally as possible. We would have to rely on other principles of justice governing our inequalities in life prospects to mitigate the effects of this pragmatic decision. The fact that Rawls appeals to the "moral arbitrariness" of the natural lottery for capabilities does not mean that the only reasonable way to address this problem within a comprehensive theory is to devote extensive resources toward equalizing capabilities. It may be that we can do better even by those worst off with regard to capabilities by leaving the distribution of capabilities mostly in place and mitigating the effects of doing so in other ways – at least that is his rationale. This dramatic restriction on the scope of what we can pursue in the name of equal opportunity – as compared to Sen's account – may not be what Sen has in mind, but then we need some clear idea of what restrictions are compatible with the overall demands of justice.

Even leaving aside the competing claims of liberty and equality, Sen's approach does not strictly speaking involve a pursuit of *equal* capability sets. Sen offers an approach to ranking differences in capabilities. How important a particular capability is will depend on the system of values – the plan of life or conception of the good – adopted by an individual. John may rank capability set *A* as better than capability set *B*, but Jane may make the opposite judgment because of her conception of the good. We may find some cases in which all can agree that set *C* is worse than sets *A* and *B*, but we may get no rankings for a broad range of capability sets. In fact, we are most likely to find that the clear-cut cases in which a set (say *C*) is ranked lower than others will be cases in which there is a significant departure from normal functioning – a disease or disability that has a significant impact on capabilities and thus on opportunities. In those cases, Sen's account will tend to agree with the standard model for thinking about our obligations to assist others with medical interventions, including genetic ones. But for a broad range of differences in capability sets, there may be "incommensurability" in the sense that these sets are ranked differently by people with different conceptions of what is good in life. Because of this widespread incommensurability, our egalitarian concerns do not commit us to pursuing equality of capabilities but only to assuring that individuals' capability sets are not distinctly worse than those enjoyed by others (see Cohen 1995, 278).

This qualification of the equal capability model has implications for the argument that equality of opportunity pushes us toward a much more expansive model of medical interventions. The model does commit us to assuring individuals that their capability sets are not clearly worse than those of others. As we noted, this suggests that significant diseases and disabilities will give rise to medical obligations. It may also be the case that when we find clear instances in which even "normal" individuals fall well short of enjoying the capability sets others rank as superior, we may have obligations to enhance their sets. Here, too, the equal capability account does not depart significantly from the standard rationale: the standard model allowed that we might have obligations, deriving from concerns about equality of opportunity, to provide enhancements in some cases. (I suggested that nontherapeutic abortions may actually be an example of this.) But what the equal capabilities model does not seem to imply, although we might have thought it would, is that whenever an individual lacks a capability that others enjoy, she has a claim on others for assistance in improving that capability. The shortfall in capabilities, from the individual's perspective, may not be viewed as a significant shortfall from the perspective of others with different plans of life.

We can better see the force of this qualification through an example. Suppose we are parents and we say to our friends, "Our son has some violin talent, but we cannot afford the best teacher for him. Without the best teacher, he will only be able to play in the Social Center Orchestra later in life, but with the best teacher, he will be able to play in the City Orchestra later in life. Other parents are able to secure the services of this teacher for their children, who have comparable potential. We – and our son – are at a disadvantage. Help us pay for the better teacher." If our friends were obliged to help us whenever our capability sets fall short of those enjoyed by others – at least by our own judgments – then our friends would seem to be hostage to the ways in which we value our capabilities.

Shifting the example to a social context and away from individual friendships does not really alter the point. We do not deny people equality of opportunity if we do not assist them in improving or developing every capability they want that some other people happen to have. If we thought equality of opportunity demanded that we assist people in these ways, we would make the principle hostage to expensive and demanding preferences individuals might have. Just as we do not owe it to our friends or others in general to contribute our resources to making them happy when they are unhappy because they have developed extravagant tastes, so too we do not owe it to others to improve any and every capability that they judge to be disadvantageous to them, given their plans of life.

This point has specific implications for those capabilities that bear on access to jobs and offices, as Cohen (1995, 286–87) has argued. Suppose Jill succeeds in getting a job as office manager when Jack does not because Jill is better at motivating others to work and at resolving disputes. Does Jack now have a complaint against us since his access to the job he wants is diminished because of a relative lack of the relevant interpersonal skills? I believe we reasonably reply to Jack that he is welcome to practice these skills and improve them – there are courses offered at the local community college – but there are many other jobs he is already well suited to perform, and the social and educational opportunities he has already enjoyed have equipped him to compete fairly for a broad array of jobs. We owe him nothing further in the name of "equal opportunity," though he is free to invest further in himself.

The equal capabilities model – whose name is now no longer quite accurate – seemed to support in a quite natural way a more expansive view of the role of medicine, or so Sabin and I suggested in Chapter 11. It seemed to push us toward any use of medicine, whether an enhancement or a treatment, that eliminated disadvantages in opportunity produced by inequalities in our capability sets. But the model falls short of its promise: it is not intended to tell us what justice requires, and therefore what we are obligated to do, in health care. That is because it only aims to clarify one component of our concerns for justice, our egalitarian concerns, and those egalitarian concerns must themselves be significantly modified in the context of an account of justice. The model also raised false expectations that we would have obligations to correct for every deficit – as judged by an individual – in a capability set. Where there are significant deficits, of the sort induced by serious disease and disability, we get results similar to those given by the standard model. But for a broad range of enhancements of normal capabilities, the equal capability model is actually much less demanding than it might have seemed.

REFERENCES

Cohen, Joshua. 1995. "Amartya Sen: *Inequality Reexamined,*" *Journal of Philosophy* 92:5(May):275–88.

Daniels, Norman. 1992. "Growth Hormone Therapy for Short Stature: Can We Support the Treatment/Enhancement Distinction?" *Growth: Genetics and Hormones* 8(Suppl. 1, May):46–8.

Sen, Amartya. 1992. *Inequality Reexamined.* Cambridge: Harvard University Press.

Chapter 12

The prudential life-span account of justice across generations

During the 1980s, the issue of intergenerational equity entered policy debates about the target of health and welfare resources. Not only did the issue surface in the United States, but it became an important theme in Europe and even in many developing countries (Daniels 1990). In large part, the concern is driven by demographics: we live in an aging world, partly as a result of increased life expectancy, but largely as a result of falling birth rates. As the age profile – the proportion of the population in each age group – changes, social needs change. For example, as society ages, proportionally fewer children need education, fewer young adults need job training, but more elderly need employment, income support, and health care, including long-term care. Where the change is rapid, concerns arise about the stability of transfer schemes, and tension rises not only between age groups but between birth cohorts. Changing needs find political expression, and the old and the young appear to compete for scarce public funds that meet basic human needs.

A divisive issue like intergenerational equity may be pushed aside in the heat of a presidential campaign, but it will resurface. Indeed, President Bush proposed using savings from capping growth in Medicaid and Medicare budgets to fund expanded health insurance coverage to the working poor and their families. Such a proposal would intensify a problem we already have: nursing homes are already being made less accessible to those on Medicaid in Georgia because of restrictions on reimbursement rates (Watson 1992). Similarly, competition between the old and the young is not far from the surface in Oregon. Oregon plans to fund expanded access to care for the working poor in part through implementing a health-care rationing plan for poor children and their adult caretakers on Medicaid. The Children's Defense Fund sharply criticized the plan because it did not include in the rationing plan Medicaid costs aimed at the elderly (Daniels 1991). In effect, the young, but not the old, were targets of rationing. In response, Oregon plans to extend its rationing plan to cover all Medicaid services, and some proponents of the Oregon plan hope to include Medicare services as well; the extension requires deciding how to rank the importance of medical services all across the life-span. Since universal access health-care insurance schemes in Canada and Europe must also face the problem of meeting the needs of old and young with limited resources, America's current focus on improving access to care will not push the issue of intergenerational justice aside for long.

Underlying the call for intergenerational equity lie two distinct problems of distributive justice. First, what is a just or fair distribution of social resources among the different *age groups* competing for them? The approach I will sketch to this problem, the Prudential Life-span Account (Daniels 1988), involves our imagining that we can prudently allocate a lifetime fair share of a particular resource, such as income support or health care, to all stages of our lives. Then, what counts as a prudent allocation between stages of a life will be our guide to what counts as a just distribution between age groups. But an institution that solves the age-group problem must also solve the second problem – the problem of *equity between birth cohorts*. What is fair treatment of different cohorts as they age and pass through transfer and savings schemes that solve the age-group problem?

It is important to distinguish these problems of distributive justice, because calls for intergenerational equity often confuse and conflate them. Some confusion is understandable, since the term "generation" is ambiguous. We can speak of the perennial struggle between the generations, meaning the conflict between age groups, or we may speak about the generation of the 1960s, meaning a particular cohort that was either born or came of age in that period. (I ignore yet another meaning, the obligation of present generations to preserve resources for more distant future generations, and concern myself only with contemporaneous generations.) Nevertheless, age groups and birth cohorts are different notions and give rise to distinct problems of distributive justice. Over time, an age group includes a succession of birth cohorts. Age groups do not age, but birth cohorts do. Since birth cohorts encounter unique conditions as they pass through life, there are important demographic, social, and economic differences between them. But the notion of an age group abstracts from the distinctiveness of birth cohorts and considers people solely by reference to their place in the life-span.

Not only are age groups and birth cohorts conceptually distinct, but distinct issues of justice concern them. Insisting, for example, that different birth cohorts should be treated equitably does not tell us just what transfers society ought to guarantee between the young and the old. Answering the age-group question, however, may teach us what to do for each birth cohort over time. Similarly, worries about age bias and age discrimination are largely concerns about justice between age groups, not birth cohorts. . . .

THE PRUDENTIAL LIFE-SPAN ACCOUNT

What is a just distribution of resources between the young and the old? The key to answering this question lies in the humbling fact that we all age. In contrast, we do not change sex or race. The relevance of these banal observations needs some explanation.

If we treat blacks and whites or men and women differently, then we produce an inequality between persons, and such inequalities raise questions about justice. For example, if we hire and fire on the basis of race or sex rather than talents and skills, then we create inequalities that are objectionable on the grounds of justice. If we treat the old and the young differently, however, we may or may not produce an inequality between persons. If we treat them differently just occasionally and arbitrarily, then we will be treating different persons unequally. But if we treat the young one way as a matter of policy and the old another, and we do so over their whole lives, then we treat all persons the same way. No inequality between persons is produced since each person is treated both ways in the course of a complete life. Thus the banal fact that we age means age is different from race or sex for purposes of distributive justice.

My account of justice between age groups builds on this basic point: Unequal treatment at different stages of life may be exactly what we want from institutions that operate over a lifetime. Since our needs vary at different stages of our lives, we want institutions to be responsive to these changes. For example, in many industrialized countries, we defer income from our working lives to our postwork retirement period through some combination of individual savings and employee or government pension or Social Security plan. In many such schemes there are no vested savings, but a direct transfer from the working young to the retired old. Viewed at a moment, it appears that "we," young workers, are taxed to benefit "them," the old. If the system is stable over the life-span, it appears that our needs for income vary through the different stages of life and we have designed a system that treats us appropriately – differently – at different ages.

The same point holds for health care. When we reach age sixty-five in the United States, we consume health-care resources at about 3.5 times the rate (in dollars) that we did prior to age sixty-five (Gibson and Fisher 1979). But we pay, as young working people, a combined health-care insurance premium – through private premiums, through employee contributions, and through Social Security taxes – which covers not just our actuarially fair costs, but the health-care costs of the elderly and of children as well. The point holds regardless of the difference between our mixed insurance scheme in the United States and the all-public scheme in Canada. Age groups are treated differently. The old pay less and get more, the young pay more and get less. If this system continues as we age, others will pay "inflated premiums" which will cover our higher costs when we are elderly. In effect the system allows us to defer the use of resources from stages in our lives when we need them less into ones in which we need them more. In general, budgeting these transfers prudently enables us to take from some parts of our lives in order to make our lives as a whole better.

We have learned two important lessons about the unequal treatment of different age groups. First, treating the young and old differently does not mean that persons are treated unequally over their life-span. Second, unequal treatment of the young and old may have effects which benefit everyone. These two points provide the central intuition behind what I call the prudential life-span account of justice between age groups: Prudent allocation among stages of our lives is our guide to what is just between the young and the old.

The life-span account involves a fundamental shift of perspective. We must not look at the problem as one of justice between distinct groups in competition with each other, for example, between working adults who pay high premiums and the frail elderly who consume so many services. Rather, we must see that each group represents a stage of our own lives. We must view the prudent allocation of resources through the stages of life as our guide to justice between groups. From the perspective of stable institutions operating over time, unequal treatment of people by age appears to be budgeting within a life. If we are concerned with net benefits within a life, we can appeal to a standard principle of individual rational choice: It is rational and prudent that a person take from one stage of his or her life to give to another in order to make his or her life as a whole better. If the transfers made by an income-support or health-care system are prudent, they improve individual well-being. Different individuals in such schemes are each made better off, even when the transfers involve unequal treatment of the young and the old. This means that neither old nor young have grounds for complaint that the system is unfair.

The contrast of age with race or sex should now be clear. When considered part of a prudent lifetime plan, differential treatment of people by age still involves treating them equally over their whole lives. There are no losers, since each person benefits. Differential treatment by sex or race always creates inequalities, benefiting some at the expense of others. Losers will have legitimate complaints about unfairness or injustice.

Before turning to the social use of this basic idea, it may help us to think about how an individual might design a lifetime health-care insurance policy. Suppose I am willing to spend only a certain amount of my lifetime resources insuring myself against health-care risks – health care, however important, is not the only good in my life. In any case, I accept the fact that the benefits I can buy with that lifetime premium will not meet every conceivable medical need I will have. Therefore, I must be willing to trade coverage for some needs at certain stages of my life for coverage at others. I also believe that I should give equal consideration to my interests at all points in my life. Unfortunately, if I know how old I am and think about things only from the perspective of what I consider important at that point in my life, then I risk biasing the design of my insurance package, for example, by underestimating the importance of things I will need much later in life. To compensate for this bias, I should pretend that I do not know how old I am and will have to live through all the trade-offs I impose at each stage of my life. For example, I know that if I give myself too much acute health care when I am dying, I do so at the expense of other services, e.g., long-term care services, that might improve my quality of life over a considerable period late in life. Similarly, if I save no benefits for old age, I doom myself to real misery.

Just as individuals set reasonable limits on their lifetime insurance premiums, prudent planners acting on behalf of society in general are limited by what counts as a "fair share" of health care. This share is not simply a dollar allotment per person. It consists of entitlements to services that are contingent on our having certain medical needs. Their problem is to find the distributive principle that allocates this fair share over the whole life-span. Their goal is a distribution that people in each age group would think is fair because they would all agree it makes their lives as a whole better than alternatives. To ensure that our planners avoid biasing the design in favor of their own age group, we shall force them to pretend that they do not know how old they are, and we require that they accept a distribution only if they are willing to live with what it does to them at each stage of their lives. Each stage of their own lives thus stands in as proxy for an age group, and they will age from conception to death in the system of trade-offs to which they agree.

Elsewhere (Daniels 1988, Ch. 3) I give a more detailed statement of these and some other qualifications on the concept of "prudent deliberation" appropriate for solving the age-group problem. I show that considerations of prudence require even further restrictions on the knowledge of the deliberators, making them even less like the standard "fully informed consumer" of economic theory. For example, they should judge their well-being by reference to all-purpose goods, like income and opportunity, rather than through the very specific lens of the "plan of life" they happen to have at a given stage of life. Otherwise the design of the lifetime allocation may be biased by a conception of what is good, which just happens to be held at a given point in life (see also Rawls 1971, 1982). . . .

Before we can understand what the Prudential Life-span Account tells us about health care, we must specify what principle of distributive justice governs the "lifetime fair share" of health care, and I shall do that shortly. But first I want to emphasize that the Prudential Life-span Account is quite general. It gives us a way of thinking about the distribution of many important goods, not just health care, as in the insurance example. For example, we are interested in income support at various stages of our life: how should we distribute such support over the life-span? The young and the old seem to be in competition here just as much as in the case of health care. The Prudential Life-span Account asks us to think about how planners who do not know their age would allocate a lifetime fair share of such entitlements to each stage of life. Here, too, the lifetime fair share is not some lump sum in dollars, but a range of contingent entitlements to support. These entitlements are specified relative to what justice in general permits in the way of economic inequalities between persons.

Prudent planners, operating under the constraints I have sketched before, would have to reason as follows about such entitlements to support. They cannot expand their lifetime income share by allocating it in certain ways, for example, by setting aside income early in life and investing it heavily in their own human capital or otherwise. Such investment strategies are already accommodated within the notion of a lifetime fair income share, or so I am supposing when I imagine them budgeting a fixed but fair lifetime share. (At the level of resources it is a zero-sum game, though resources can be allocated in ways that make their lives go better or worse overall.) These planners do not know how old they are, and they must allow for the fact that their preferences or views about what is good in life will change over the life-span. The prudent course of action would be to allocate their fair share in such a way that their standard of living would remain roughly equal over the life-span (call this the standard of living preservation principle). They would want institutions to facilitate income transfers over the life-span in such a way that individuals have available to themselves, at each stage of life, an adequate income to pursue whatever plan of life they may have at that stage of life. Of course, "adequate" is here relative to the individual's fair income share, as determined by the acceptable inequalities in the society. This principle has implications for income support in old age.

The Prudential Life-span Account also helps us think about the distribution of educational and job-training resources over the life-span. We are used to thinking of education as a process early in life, one that helps set the trajectory for the quality of later life. But as more and more people live longer in the context of rapidly changing technologies, and as societies age, we must think anew about the role of education throughout the life-span. We each have a stronger interest in retaining claims on educational and job-training resources during later stages of life than was the case in earlier generations. Restricting education to youth was more plausible when life expectancy was fifty years, but now that life expectancy is about seventy-five years, education later in life can vastly improve that second half of our adult lives that people a century ago rarely enjoyed. The shape of our lives has changed! Of course, education early in life remains crucial. But we must also shed the outdated view that education is just a matter for youth.

The generality of the Prudential Life-span Account is one of its virtues, offering us a unified account of how to distribute various goods across the life-span. Its strengths and weaknesses should be assessed independently of how I have applied it in the case of a particular good, like health care (see Daniels 1989b, 677–78, in response to a criticism by Jecker 1989). Before turning to my use of the approach in health care and in arguments about rationing health care by age, I want to consider some objections that have been raised to the prudential life-span account in general.

One objection to the Prudential Life-span Account is that its application can create some intergroup inequalities. This objection must be taken seriously because the rationale for adopting the prudential model for the age-group problem is that we can assume that intralife transfers will be an appropriate model for interage-group transfers, but if different demographic groups age differently, then the model breaks down. For example, raising the age of eligibility for income support benefits under Social Security, which arguably is a prudent and fair way to address both the age-group and birth-cohort problems, might leave African Americans, who have a lower life expectancy, worse off than whites or Asians. Similarly, a policy of rationing lifesaving medical services by age, which may be permissible under very special conditions of scarcity on my account, might have differential impact by class, race, or gender. Where such effects take place, they may constitute good reasons for not adopting such a rationing policy, or they might give us reasons to link the rationing to facts about group life expectancy. The general point is that the Prudential Life-span Account presupposes that solutions to the age-group problem will not disturb more general requirements of justice (see Daniels 1988).

Life-span, time, and equality

One interesting objection to my account is the charge that it presupposes an inadequate way of thinking about equality, namely the view that we are primarily concerned about equality over complete lives rather than between simultaneous segments of lives (McKerlie 1989a, b). Thus, I argued earlier that treating people differently at different ages does not always create an inequality that requires justification, judging from the perspective of their complete lives. In contrast, treating people differently by race or sex does create such inequalities. McKerlie, building on some suggestions of Parfit (1984, 149–58; 1986, 869–70), claims that the complete-lives view has some puzzling and perhaps unacceptable consequences. For example, suppose A's life has been worse than B's (say A had a poor childhood), but A is not scarred by his past. Complete-lives egalitarianism seems to imply we should favor A in the future to compensate for his past deficits, but it is not obvious our egalitarian intuitions agree. Similarly, according to McKerlie, complete-lives egalitarianism seems to leave us unable to complain about the following case. Our feudal society contains nobles and peasants who switch places every ten years. Over our whole lives, we are equally happy, but at each time slice significant inequalities exist. If no basic rights are violated by the arrangement, complete-lives egalitarianism seems unable to explain the aversion some egalitarians would have to the "switching places" case, which allows so much inequality between simultaneous segments of lives.

McKerlie objects to treating the complete-lives account as a sufficient account of our egalitarian concerns. My account, however, does not presuppose that it is a sufficient account, even though I invoke the complete-lives view for a limited purpose. My goal is to develop an account of how we should think about the design of social institutions that distribute goods over the whole of our lives. I set the problem up so that we considered only how *ex ante* we should want such distributive schemes to treat us at each stage of life. I then concluded that, because differential treatment by age does not then generate the same objectionable inequalities that sexist or racist treatment produce over complete lives, it does not face the crucial objection raised by those cases.

I am not, however, committed to thinking that just any inequality that then shows up between simultaneous segments of complete lives that are equally well-off is justifiable. My argument also requires that the differential treatment we permit between stages of life must work to make our lives go as well as possible, given fair constraints on lifetime shares of resources (generally, I am talking about resource inequalities between stages of life, not utility inequalities, as McKerlie generally does). Consequently, to accept an outcome like that involved in the "switching places" example involving nobles and peasants, we would have to believe that, compared to alternatives, such a scheme is a prudent way to allocate resources. That seems highly implausible. Given my limited purpose in designing institutions, rather than in thinking about all the egalitarian interventions we might imagine, my limited appeal to the complete-lives approach is not open to McKerlie's objection.

McKerlie considers an alternative to the "simultaneous segments" approach, namely one that is concerned with equality between corresponding segments of people's lives. That is, rather than complain that someone who is old is worse off than someone who is young, we should consider whether the person who is now old is worse off than the younger person will be when she or he is old. McKerlie rejects this alternative because he thinks his examples show that we are primarily troubled by inequalities between simultaneous segments of lives. I disagree. Assuming there is equality over complete lives, I am troubled less by inequality between corresponding segments than I am by inequalities between simultaneous segments. For example, I think the inequalities in salary and prestige that attach to academic ranks, which seem quite objectionable on a simultaneous segments view, may be rendered less objectionable when we see them as stages of a career that each academic goes through. If the unequal treatment by stage works to make each life go as well as possible, e.g., by providing incentives and rewards that help motivate and reward productivity through a career, then the corresponding segments view seems to correspond better to our intuitions than the simultaneous segments view.

It will help to consider McKerlie's argument in more detail. In his earlier work, McKerlie (1989a, b) suggested abandoning the standard concern for equality between complete lives in favor of a view that emphasized equality between simultaneous segments of lives. Imagine Alice and Betty, each living eighty years. Each has an alternating pattern of well-being in her life, with ten units in one decade, five in the next, but the patterns are reversed, as follows:

Decade	1	2	3	4	5	6	7	8
Alice	5	10	5	10	5	10	5	10
Betty	10	5	10	5	10	5	10	5

McKerlie's earlier view was that we should add the inequalities (five units) that show up in each decade. As a result, we would conclude there is objectionable inequality (forty units) between these lives. This inequality is simply ignored if we simply sum the well-being over each complete life: on that view, neither is better off and there is no inequality.

McKerlie (1989a, b) was just as concerned about the inequality between simultaneous segments that would show up in the case of Betty and Connie:

Decade	1	2	3	4	5	6	7	8	9
Betty	10	5	10	5	10	5	10	5	
Connie		10	5	10	5	10	5	10	5

Connie has the same pattern of well-being as Betty, but, because she is born ten years later, on McKerlie's view, there are thirty-five objectionable units of inequality in decades 2 through 8. If Connie had been born ten years earlier, no inequality would arise. McKerlie's view thus runs counter to a basic intuition: simply changing Connie's birth date, with no other effects on either life, should not make the situation more or less objectionable.

More recently, McKerlie (1993) adopts a more moderate position. Rather than rejecting the complete-lives view in favor of equality between simultaneous segments, he now proposes that we supplement our legitimate concerns about inequality over complete lives with a *further* concern about inequality between parts of lives. This further concern must be a "pure" concern about equality, not reducible to a concern about the bad effects of the inequality on the respective lives. Thus, even if there is no harm to Alice, Betty, or Connie from the out-of-synchrony patterns of well-being they enjoy, and even if they are equally well off over their whole lives, we should still be concerned about the inequality that emerges between simultaneous segments of their lives. We should, he says, be concerned about equality "for its own sake," ignoring our counterintuition about the irrelevance of Connie's birthday. Presumably, there will be circumstances when McKerlie would overturn equality over complete lives in order to favor the "further concern," but he does not tell us just how to rank these concerns under different conditions.

I agree with McKerlie that our concerns about distributive justice are not limited simply to concerns about equality over complete lives. The prudential life-span account of justice between age groups does impose important "further" constraints on how goods are distributed within our lives, between its parts or stages, even supposing equality (or otherwise fair distribution) between complete lives. (Remember that the prudential life-span account also presupposes "frame" principles that impose egalitarian limitations on other interpersonal matters of distribution, such as the fair equality of opportunity principle governing health care.) Specifically, we should permit distributions that treat us differently at different stages of life whenever such differential treatment works to make our lives go as well as possible. Our lifetime fair share of important goods need not be distributed equally to each stage of life, for doing that may well ignore the ways in which our needs for those goods vary at different stages of life. We should accept "unequal" treatment of stages of life if doing so is prudent (subject to the constraints on prudential reasoning I describe in Daniels 1988). For example, if our needs for certain kinds of health care or education vary at different stages of life, it would be imprudent to cap our access to such services with equal shares for each stage of life. That would mean some needs are unmet at some stages, while we have untapped resources at others.

The prudential life-span account would not automatically accept the inequalities involved in the Alice and Betty example. These inequalities do not work to make each life go as well as possible – or at least we cannot see from the example how that is happening. If, however, these patterns were necessary to make these lives go as well as possible, then my account is neutral between them.

A reminder about methodology is in order at this point. The account I have developed is aimed at solving a problem of *institutional* design: how should institutions that distribute important goods over the course of our lives be designed so that individuals in each age group are treated fairly? Specifically, I have in mind the complex transfer schemes that take goods from us at one stage of life (e.g., while we are productive workers) and give them to other individuals who are in other age groups (e.g., children or retirees). When are such transfer schemes fair to the individuals in each age group? Notice that I *do* conceive of this problem as an *interpersonal* problem of distributive justice, one that arises between individuals in different age groups. My account suggests that this interpersonal problem of justice between members of different groups has the same structure as – and thus reduces to – a problem of prudential allocation among stages of a life, at least when we can suppose that the transfer schemes are stable and operate over the course of whole lives. I thus reject McKerlie's attempt to show that my account is not about distributive justice between persons, and that I can only talk about justice between some notion of a *group* not reducible to its members. My claim is that the interpersonal problem is properly solved by solving the substitute problem about prudential allocation. In general, however, prudential allocation is not a solution to other problems of distributive justice.

The fact that my account is intended to apply to the design of institutions that distribute goods over a life-span also has a bearing on some of McKerlie's examples. For example, my account may not accommodate every intuition we have about how to respond to inequalities between individuals. Suppose John will live in poverty for the last ten years of his life while Jim will live his final ten years in very good circumstances. If Jim and John will end up equally well-off over their whole lives, does this mean we can divert no resources from Jim to John? My account is silent on this isolated issue about two individuals because it is aimed at answering a different question: How should we design transfer schemes that operate over the whole course of people's lives and that treat members of all age groups fairly? The answer is that we try to avoid transfer schemes that allocate resources so imprudently to John. . . .

McKerlie rests considerable weight on the example involving unequal power in a marriage. Suppose a marriage lasts four decades, and each partner takes turns dominating the other for two decades. He is surely right that we do not consider these equal partners or the marriage an ideal one. Alternating periods of tyranny is not the same as sharing power equally. Similarly, if each of us could vote for only two decades of our lives, and the rest of the time we were subject solely to the choices of others, we would not be satisfied that we had achieved the relevant sort of equality in citizenship rights. Rather, we would complain that for most of our lives we failed to enjoy democracy, and that someone or other always failed to enjoy democracy. With regard to some goods, including certain liberties we insist on equality at each stage of life. No plausible interpretation of the claim that we each have a right to select our representatives in government would put time constraints on the exercise of that right (except for the problem of competency or maturity). We are very much concerned about the negative effects of unequal power at every point in our marriages and in our political lives.

Does this show that we are always so bothered about inequality between parts of lives? Not in the general way McKerlie suggests. It depends on the good in question and the reasons for distributing it one way rather than another over the course of our lives. Suppose we could show that making more educational services (allocated from our lifetime fair share of such services) available to people early in their lives, rather than late in their lives, made their lives typically go better. We would probably not then think that the inequality in access to education between a child and a middle-aged adult was necessarily objectionable. (As I suggested earlier, the prudential life-span account actually emphasizes the importance of improving access to education at later stages of life, especially given increasing life expectancy.) In McKerlie's view the inequality in access to education between members of age groups is always objectionable – even if unequal access by age affects each person the same way as they age and even if the unequal access actually works to make each life better overall.

McKerlie thus ignores the fact that education works differently than voting rights or than power within a marriage. McKerlie has generalized from the wrong example. Why he has done so may have something to do with his (somewhat puzzling) belief that we have a "pure" interest in equality, aside from any of its effects.

I find one of McKerlie's criticisms very helpful. I have said (Daniels 1988) that I would give "priority" to the age-group problem over the problem of equity between cohorts. My real concern was that we could know what equity between birth cohorts required without having any solution to the age-group problem, and that each cohort had an interest in solving the age-group problem through intercohort transfer schemes. Therefore, I wanted to address the age-group problem first. But, as McKerlie notes, it is misleading to call this "priority." Since intercohort inequities would constitute unacceptable interpersonal inequalities, these must be accommodated by adjustments to the lifetime fair shares from which allocations that address the age-group problem are made.

LIFE-SPAN ALLOCATION OF HEALTH CARE

Consider now how the Prudential Life-span Account might be applied to the case of health care. I must explain how we should think about the notion of a "lifetime fair share" of health care, that is, explain what principle of distributive justice applies to the design of health care systems. I have argued elsewhere (Daniels 1985) that a central, unifying function of health care is to maintain and restore functioning that is typical or normal for our species. Health care derives its moral importance from the following fact: normal functioning has a central effect on the opportunity open to an individual. It helps guarantee individuals a fair chance to enjoy the normal opportunity range for their society. The normal opportunity range for a given society is the array of life plans reasonable persons in it are likely to construct for themselves. An individual's fair share of the normal opportunity range is the array of life plans he or she may reasonably choose, given his or her talents and skills. Disease and disability shrinks that share from what is fair; health care protects it. Health care lets a person enjoy that portion of the normal range to which his or her full range of skills and talents would give him or her access, assuming that these too are not impaired by special social disadvantages. The suggestion that emerges from this account is that we should use impairment of the normal opportunity range as a fairly crude measure of the relative moral importance of health-care needs at the macro level.

Because we have obligations to ensure people of fair equality of opportunity, we have social obligations to provide health-care services that protect and restore normal functioning. This account implies that there should be no financial, geographical, or discriminatory barriers to a level of care which promotes normal functioning, given reasonable or necessary limits on resources. We can guide hard public policy choices about which services are more important to provide by considering their relative impact on the normal opportunity range. Rights to health care are thus *system relative:* entitlements to services can only be specified within a system that works to protect opportunity as well as possible, given limited resources.

Our prudent planners solve the age-group problem if they can clarify what the right to health care means for each age group. To do this, they must agree to a principle for allocating their lifetime fair share to each stage of life. Remember, these planners do not know how old they are. This means that it is especially important for them to make sure social arrangements give them a chance to enjoy the fair share of the normal range of opportunities open to them at each stage of life. This protection of opportunity at each stage of life is particularly important, since they are planning for their whole lives and must keep in mind the importance of being able to revise their views about what is valuable in life as they age. But impairments of normal functioning by disease and disability clearly restrict the portion of the normal opportunity range open to individuals at any stage of their lives. Consequently, health-care services should be rationed throughout a life in a way that respects the importance of the age-relative normal opportunity range. In effect, all specific allocation decisions must be constrained by this principle.

It is important to consider some specific implications of this application of the prudential life-span account to health care. I can do so only briefly here.

Long-term care

Because the likelihood of needing long-term care increases with age, the aging of society raises urgent questions about the long-term care systems in many developed countries. Some experts suggest that long-term care "may well be the major health and social issue of the next four decades, polarizing society over the next 20 to 40 years" (Vogel and Palmer 1982, v). By 2040 there is likely to be a fivefold increase in the number of people age eighty-five and over in the United States and other European countries and similar increases in the numbers of very old who are nursing home residents or functionally dependent on the community (Soldo and Manton 1985, 286). These trends are present in many developing countries as well; in many of these cases, the absence of existing public long-term care systems magnifies the problem created by rapid changes in the economic and social structures that underlay care for the disabled elderly in the past.

It follows from my equality of opportunity account of justice in health care that long-term care is of comparable moral importance to acute care: they have the same function, protecting an individual's share of the normal opportunity range (Daniels 1985). Adding the perspective of the Prudential Life-span Account, two further points emerge. It may be prudent to trade some acute care services aimed at marginal extension of life for long-term care services that greatly improve quality of life over a longer period. Second, providing long-term care services that give relief to families, who provide the bulk of long-term care, provides a benefit at two stages of life. It helps both when we are providers of such care and when we are recipients of is. The suggestion that emerges from these considerations is that the U.S. system has undervalued the importance of long-term care and undersupplied crucial services that benefit us at various points in the life-span. Any redesign of our health-care insurance system should include reallocation of benefits reflecting these priorities.

In some universal access systems, like the Canadian and some European systems, long-term care services, including many social support and home services, are already incorporated in the benefit package. Rationing health care in these systems will require making explicit the way in which the importance of these services is measured against the importance of existing and forthcoming acute care technologies. We have not developed an adequate philosophical framework for thinking about how to make these judgments in any very specific manner (see Daniels 1993). I take this to be a crucial problem for the 1990s that bears on health-care rationing and the elderly. It is a problem that will have to be addressed by the Oregon Health Services Commission as it attempts to expand the ranking of services to include services for the elderly and disabled.

Rationing by age

In the United States, there is considerable concern that the increasing numbers of elderly will intensify the problem of rapidly rising health-care costs. Much of this rate of increase is due to the rapid dissemination of high-cost medical technologies, many of which are aimed at conditions that are prevalent among the elderly. In this context, there is a growing discussion about the need to ration beneficial medical treatments. In the United States, the greatest threat to health-care rights will come from the temptation to use ability to pay as a criterion for rationing, but there is a growing discussion of the relevance of age as a basis for rationing some high-cost medical technologies. Callahan (1987) has drawn considerable critical comment for his proposal that we consider rationing life-extending medical services explicitly by age. Less hypothetically, there is evidence that the British National Health Service already uses age as a basis for rationing some expensive technologies, such as renal dialysis (Aaron and Schwartz 1984), and in the United States, many transplants are not made available to people over age fifty-five. The explanation usually given, that the elderly will not fare as well as younger people, appears to have little in the way of controlled studies to support it.

Some critics of rationing by age consider it morally impermissible in exactly the way that rationing by race or sex would be. They consider age, as opposed to medical suitability, a "morally irrelevant" basis for distributing medical services. Others advocate a policy of rationing by age because they believe that the elderly have a duty to step aside and sacrifice for the young (Callahan 1987) or because they believe that it is fair for the elderly, who have had the opportunity to live a long time, to forgo services in favor of the young, who have had less opportunity to live (cf. Veatch 1988; Brock 1988; Kamm 1993).

The prudential life-span approach to the age-group problem provides a way to resolve this dispute (cf. Daniels 1988, Ch. 5). A policy will be fair to different age groups if prudent planners who do not know how old they are would choose it as a way of allocating a lifetime fair share of health care among the stages of life. Under very special conditions of resource scarcity, the following might happen: providing very expensive or very scarce life-extending services to those who have reached normal life expectancy can be accomplished only by reducing access by the young to those resources. That is, saving these resources by giving ourselves claim to them in our old age is possible only if we give ourselves reduced access to them in earlier stages of life. A central effect of this form of saving is that we increase our chances of living a longer-than-normal life-span at the cost of reducing our chances of reaching a normal life-span. Under some conditions, it would be prudent for planners to agree to ration such technologies by age, making them more available to the young than to the very old. More precisely, if we consider only information about life years saved and if rationing by age and rationing by lottery both yield the same life expectancy, it is not imprudent to prefer an increased chance of reaching that life expectancy through age rationing. If we add more information – e.g., that years later in life are more likely to contain disabilities or that years earlier in life are typically more important to carrying out central projects in life – then we can get the stronger result that age rationing is preferred to rationing by lottery.

Let's make this point more concrete by considering two rationing schemes. Scheme A (Age rationing) involves a direct appeal to an age criterion: No one over age seventy or seventy-five – taken to represent normal life-span – is eligible to receive any of several high-cost, life-extending technologies such as dialysis, transplant surgery, or extensive by-pass surgery. Because age rationing reduces utilization of each technology, there are resources available for developing them all, though under this scenario that development will be only for the young. Scheme L (Lottery) rejects age rationing and allocates life-extending technology solely by medical need. As a result, it can either develop just one such major technology, say dialysis, making it available to anyone who needs it, or it can develop several technologies, but then ration them by lottery.

Scheme A saves resources – defers their use until later in life – at a lower rate than Scheme L. Scheme L takes more from earlier stages so that later ones may benefit. Specifically, Scheme L involves reducing the chance that the young will reach a normal life-span because access to life-extending resources has been reduced. In return, Scheme L offers an increased chance of living a longer than normal span to those who do reach normal life-span. For instance, though this is an extreme example, Scheme A might offer a 1.0 probability of reaching age seventy-five (and dying right away), and Scheme L might give a .5 probability of reaching fifty and a .5 probability of reaching one hundred. Both yield the same expected life-span, but they do so differently. (Intuitions about science fiction cases are always of questionable utility, but for those who insist: Imagine there is a disease around which would kill everyone at age fifty, but a drug is available in short supply. We can give a half-dose to everyone, and they will then live to seventy-five and die. Or we can give a full dose to half the population by lottery at age fifty; lottery winners will live to age one hundred and die right away, but lottery losers will die right away at age fifty. The two scenarios produce equal average life-expectancies.)

Our prudent deliberators must choose between Schemes A and L (leave aside the science fiction example). I shall argue that prudent deliberators would probably prefer an age-rationing scheme to a lottery. The argument is complicated, however, by the vague way in which I have described conditions under which deliberators must choose, as anyone familiar with recent work in the theory of justice will have noted. I have left the description of these conditions vague because defending a particular construction is difficult and, for our purposes here, digressive. But the price I pay for sticking to the point is that I must now consider the way the argument might run under alternative constraints. Specifically, we must consider two alternative rules of rational choice that might be invoked to govern prudential reasoning about Schemes A and L.

One rule is the "maximin" rule (maximize the minimum), which tells us to make the worst outcome as good as it is possible to make it (which might mean to make it as unlikely to happen as possible). Maximin is appropriate to governing rational choices when real uncertainty – not just risk or probability – is a feature of the choice situation. That is, we cannot invoke likelihoods of outcomes, or even reasonably assume outcomes are equiprobable and assign numbers to them. Some might claim that maximin is also the appropriate rule when the worst outcomes are so grave that they cannot merely be weighed against better outcomes.

I have not described the choice as one in which the maximum rule is clearly the appropriate one. If it is the correct rule, then I think it is easy to show that Scheme A would be preferable to Scheme L. Suppose someone is inclined to like Scheme L because it seems to help us most later in life. This person thinks the life of the wise, revered elder is the best thing one could aim for, and does not mind taking some chances (if one could calculate them) to reach the Golden Age. Even such a person would have to admit that the worst outcome would be dying young. If we can assign no probabilities in our reasoning, for example, we can assign no probabilities to whether we are likely to die young or to live to the Golden Age, we are constrained by the maximum rule to minimize the likelihood of the worst outcome. This would force us to choose Scheme A.

I have not insisted on the maximum rule because I am not sure I want to insist that the "veil of ignorance" surrounding our prudent deliberators be so thick that they cannot predict the relevant estimates of the likelihood of longevity under the two schemes. After all, I want our deliberators to know enough about their social system so that they can make prudent judgments about the design of its health-care system. This means they must know something about its specific demography and the way it is affected by alternative arrangements of the health-care system. As a result, we might think it reasonable to adopt a more common rule of choice. This Standard Rule, as I shall call it, instructs prudent deliberators to maximize their expected net benefit or payoff when they face choices. It requires that they take into account not only the value of a payoff, but its likelihood or probability, and that they maximize the product of the two.

How would Schemes A and L fare under the Standard Rule? Suppose, for the moment, that we take as the payoff the number of years lived. The Standard Rule tells us to maximize the expected life-span. If our choice between Schemes A and L is a choice between schemes that each give equivalent expected life-spans – for example, the choice between a 1.0 probability of living to (and only to) seventy-five under Scheme A and, under Scheme L, a .5 probability of living only until fifty and .5 probability of living (only) to one hundred – then the Standard

Rule instructs the prudent deliberators to be indifferent. In the absence of a better scheme, there is a tie: Each must be deemed prudent and both are acceptable.

Even this tie is an interesting and important result. It tells us that age rationing cannot in general be ruled out on the grounds that it is imprudent. This means in turn that it cannot be ruled out under the conditions I have argued are appropriate for deciding what is just between age groups. Thus we cannot claim that age rationing is always unjust.

The argument I have just sketched for the Standard Rule seems too abstract, even for the situation I have described in which parties do not have knowledge of their conceptions of what is good in life. Even without the details of such knowledge, we still know enough about the frequencies of disease and disability as we age to know that years late in life, say after age seventy-five, are far more likely than earlier years to involve some forms of impairment. This knowledge suggests that it would be imprudent to count the expected payoff of years late in life quite as highly as the expected payoff of years more likely to be free of physical and mental impairment. To be sure, many people enjoy their later years relatively free of impairment – I am not drawing on a stereotype that all the old are frail and sick – and there is no suggestion here that age by itself gives us any basis for judging the value of these years less. Moreover, many people with impairments would admit to being no less happy than other people without impairments. Some people are happy and cope well, though others do not. Nevertheless, the prudent deliberators are estimating expected payoffs, which means they should take into account the frequencies of disability and disease. They then should discount the expected payoff of later years accordingly. Consequently, they would reject the idea that there is a tie between Schemes A and L, merely because life expectancies are equal. After considering disabilities, Scheme A would again seem more prudent.

We can think about the choice between Schemes A and L under the Standard Rule in a slightly different way, which may be an alternative or supplement to the above argument. Under some plans of life, the contribution of the last years to the overall meaningfulness of life might be very great. Still, such Golden Age plans are probably atypical. Most people are well aware of their mortality and construct plans in which the tasks and rewards of early and middle years are integral to their success. For them, later years can be wonderful, but they are gravy to the meat and potatoes of the rest of life. Without making the judgment that one plan of life is better than another or even, by itself, less prudent, deliberators, familiar with their society and culture but unaware of which conception of the good is theirs, would estimate it to be more likely that they will have typical plans than Golden Age plans. They might then select Scheme A over Scheme L because they want to increase their chances that they live through the middle stages of their lives: That is what will most ensure success of their probable plan of life.[1] Notice that if we want to block completely this type of probabilistic reasoning, then we start to push ourselves into a description of the problem of choice that makes the maximum rule seem more appropriate than the Standard Rule. Then the deliberators would choose Scheme A in any case.

My conclusion from these versions of the prudential argument is that there are conditions under which a health-care system that rationed life-extending resources by age would be the prudent choice and therefore the choice that constituted a just or fair distribution of resources between age groups. Specifically, faced solely with the alternative of rationing by age or rationing by lottery, prudent deliberators under special conditions of scarcity might find age rationing prudent and therefore morally permissible. Of course, other alternatives might be more prudent, but if the choice is restricted, then rationing by age would be fair to each person, treating them equally over their lives, and it would benefit each by maximizing chances of reaching normal life expectancy. This argument turns on no prior moral assumptions that life at one age is more *valuable* than life at another. It does not turn on the judgment that it is more important or valuable for society to save the young than the old or that society would benefit more from doing so. Instead it turns on the judgment each of us would in effect make, that we would each be better off (or not worse off) from an age-rationing scheme. Nor does it turn on prior moral views about the duties of the elderly to the young or vice versa.

One of the virtues of this argument is that it does not invoke moral judgments of any of these kinds. Contrast it, for example, with Brock's (1988) suggestion (similar to Veatch 1988) that the principle of equality of opportunity tells us directly that we should give everyone a better chance of reaching normal life expectancy through age rationing rather than give some people an extra opportunity to live much longer. I am reluctant, however, to appeal so directly to our intuitions about equality of opportunity. For example, if a young person has had "opportunity" enhanced through prior medical treatment, does she or he still have a greater claim than an old person who has never been so helped? Part of what is at issue is whether we should judge the equality of opportunity as ensured by the outcome (more equal chances at achieving normal life expectancy) or by a process (more equal chances through a lottery at receiving the life extending service). Our intuitions pull in different directions on this matter. My prudential argument, however, makes no such appeal to such intuitions.

Callahan's (1987) argument for rationing by age also turns crucially on claims about moral obligations that play no role in mine. The overall structure of Callahan's argument can be captured in the following three-step argument: (1) The only way life for the old is meaningful is if the old serve the young. (2) Therefore, the old ought to serve the young, e.g., by serving as moral exemplars who surrender claims on lifesaving services in favor of the young. (3) Consequently, the old can be compelled through age-rationing measures to carry out their obligations to the young.

This argument is both unsound and invalid. The first premise is false. There are many ways for the old to find meaning in life. Claude Pepper, for example, found meaning in old age by serving the old, not the young. In a culturally diverse society, we are likely to differ considerably in our views about what adds meaning to old age. But even if the first premise were true, the second step does not follow from it, nor the third from the second. From the fact that something makes my life meaningful, it does not follow that it is what I *ought* to do or seek. Many things might add meaning to my life, but I am not obliged to do them on either prudential or moral grounds. Moreover, many of the things I ought to do are not things that society should compel me to do, which is the force of the conclusion of the argument.

Whereas Callahan puts his argument to use as a rationale for a general policy, I do *not* advocate age rationing as a policy. My argument supports age rationing only under very limited conditions and only when there is no more prudent alternative. Alternative strategies for allocating resources, one more fine-tuned to the conditions of patients and the likely outcomes of treating them, would probably be judged preferable to rationing by age. In contrast, there is considerable unclarity as to just what role scarcity and cost containment play in Callahan's argument. He prefaces his discussion with concerns about rising health-care costs and claims about scarcity, but the argument itself (as sketched above) does not appeal to scarcity. Nor does Callahan show just what the savings would be if his policy were adopted (Schwartz and Aaron 1988 argue there would be very minor savings at best).

Before turning to the issue of equity between birth cohorts, I want to note that the prudential life-span account, like most other theories, falls short of telling us just how to ration services over the life-span (as McKerlie 1989a and Emanuel 1991 note). Given limited resources, we must sometimes choose to protect the normal opportunity range better at one stage of life than another or for some groups rather than others. This problem is quite general: all principles of distributive justice lack content until they are embodied in institutions that ration scarce resources needed to satisfy the principles. The principles alone do not tell us how to ration. Are there other moral constraints, or is this merely a political process? This is a crucial, but remarkably unexplored area of philosophical inquiry (see Daniels 1993).

EQUITY BETWEEN BIRTH COHORTS

In the United States, many people have pointed to the fact that benefit ratios – the overall ratio of benefits to contributions – have been falling for successive cohorts entering the Social Security system, and there is considerable concern that these ratios will continue to fall. In Europe, there is concern about the financial stability of income transfer schemes into the next century, since there will be proportionally fewer employed workers to support retirees. Some of the shrillest proponents of intergenerational equity in the United States call for dismantling the Social Security system and forcing each cohort to rely on its own resources for income support (and health insurance) in old age. The claim seems to be that fairness requires each cohort to depend on its own individual retirement accounts. A special form, then, of the problem of equity between birth cohorts is the question, what inequalities in benefit ratios are fair or equitable? More generally, what inequalities in the treatment of different cohorts are just or fair as these cohorts pass through institutions intended to meet the requirements of justice between age groups?

Since each birth cohort ages, it has an interest in securing institutions that solve the age-group problem effectively. Unfortunately, institutions or transfer schemes that solve the age-group problem operate under considerable uncertainty. There is uncertainty about population and economic growth rates, as well as about technological change, which further affects productivity. Errors are likely to abound, and inequalities in benefit ratios between cohorts will arise as a result. Despite these sources of error, institutions that solve the age-group problem must remain stable over time. They must be able to weather the political struggle that results if errors are allowed to produce unjustifiable or unacceptable inequalities in benefit ratios. Such institutions will be able to survive the struggle among coexisting birth cohorts only if each feels it has a stake in preserving them. Each will feel it has such a commitment only if it believes these institutions work to its benefit within the limits of fairness. Such commitment will be sustained, then, only if the practical target of our policy is to aim for *approximate equality* in benefit ratios.

One objection to this suggestion is that it ignores the fact that some cohorts may be wiser or more prudent than others and may therefore contribute more to productivity. Since many believe that people should be rewarded for their contributions, they insist that benefit ratios should reflect *desert*. Specifically, they urge that each cohort should depend on its own savings. But this appeal to desert would require disentangling the many sources of change that contribute to rising or falling economic fortune. It would not justify simply relying on individual or cohort savings, for they result from many factors other than moral desert.

Since it is hard to see how a stable system could incorporate such factors in its scheme of benefits, it seems reasonable for cohorts to aim for approximate equality in benefit ratios and to seek other ways of persuading each other to act prudently over time. Each cohort, after all, has an interest in securing stable institutions that solve the age-group problem. Cohorts must therefore cooperate to achieve such stability. But cooperation will require some *sharing of risks* across cohorts. In general, the burdens of economic declines and of living through unfavorable retiree/employee ratios must be shared, as must the benefits of economic growth and favorable retiree/employee ratios. This suggests again that approximate equality in benefit ratios should be the practical target of public policy, if not a hard and fast rule.

My solution to the birth-cohort problem is open to another important objection. Birth cohorts, some argue, cannot be trusted to abide by a transfer scheme that ideally solves the age-group problem through intercohort transfers, because, as they age, they will use their increasing political power to revise the scheme in favor of their old age, benefiting heavily at both ends of the life-span. Thomson (1989) suggests that a particular cohort has been greedy in just these ways in New Zealand, and that similar distortions have occurred in transfer schemes elsewhere. His argument is compatible with the view that this behavior is just the result of the special circumstances or opportunities that faced a particular cohort. But a stronger version of this objection insists that the pattern is general or inevitable. For example, some public choice theorists (e.g., Epstein 1988) have argued that large-scale, stage-managed transfer schemes are sitting ducks for the self-interested behavior of aging cohorts, as their political power increases.

We should notice that not all cohorts behave in this way. More important, it is not obvious what the alternative is. If we avoid schemes that depend on intercohort transfers of the sort that take place in the U.S. Social Security system, then we still have to answer the question, how can social institutions facilitate adequate types and rates of savings? That is, we are back to the age-group problem, but we must now solve it by relying only on the resources of one cohort. Moreover, we are ruling out an important advantage offered by a system which involves intercohort transfers, namely that it tends to share risks more widely over time. Rather, we should take advantage of the fact that an equitable form of risk sharing would be much more desirable than the results of "privatizing" the age-group problem for each cohort. (See Buchanan in Cohen 1993, however, for a view emphasizing the importance of not allowing intercohort transfer schemes to interfere with the general rate of savings in a society.)

Objections to unequal benefit ratios should not lead us to eliminate intercohort transfer schemes, at least not on the grounds that "equality" will then result. Making each cohort solely responsible for its own well-being over the life-span will by no means ensure that different cohorts will fare equally well. Inequalities will come about because of uneven economic growth rates. It is not at all obvious that inequalities of benefit ratios in intercohort schemes will generate more intolerable forms and degrees of inequality than the inequalities that result when each cohort must depend on its own resources and good luck. Cooperation may be a better strategy than "go-it-alone," and the problem becomes one of institutional design and of securing a long-term commitment to schemes that are fair.

Several strategies are available for adjusting benefits so that we can achieve approximate equality in benefit ratios despite demographic shifts and other sources of uncertainty and error. One strategy is to build a cushion of unexpended benefits while the ratio of workers to retirees is still relatively high. This strategy has been adopted in some recent financing reforms of the U.S. Social Security system, though there is always a risk that these benefits will be a target of convenience of politicians seeking to relieve budget deficits.

A second strategy is more basic, for it involves rethinking some of the policies toward retirement that have dominated developed welfare systems in recent decades. Many current policies provide considerable incentives for older workers to withdraw from the work force well before any disability actually makes such withdrawal necessary. It is also quite difficult for older workers to find flexible, part-time employment that can reduce the need for drawing on income support benefits. Underlying these incentives and policies are both economic and moral considerations. Pushing older workers out of the work force in periods of unemployment, when there are large numbers of young workers seeking employment opportunities, may have seemed an acceptable way to ration jobs by age, or it may have seemed an appropriate way to make room for better-educated and potentially more productive workers in technologically advancing economies. These economic considerations may have been reinforced by the view that the elderly want to enjoy more leisure time. These underlying considerations should be reassessed.

Health status for the elderly remains quite good well into the mid-seventies. Millions of elderly who would be happier with some form of meaningful work, at least on a part-time basis, find themselves facing forced withdrawal from the work force. At the same time, many European economies face a shortage of workers in the next few decades. Under these conditions, it may well be wise to consider revising the existing benefits and incentives that lead workers to withdraw from the work force early. The new shape of a life, with many vigorous and healthy years extending well beyond standard retirement age, means that we must revise our antiquated conception of the typical course of life.

In the United States, compulsory retirement ages have been raised or eliminated, at least for large categories of employment, and this may encourage some reassessment of the employability of older workers. It may not be enough, however, simply to eliminate legal or quasi-legal barriers to the employment of willing, elderly workers. Rather, we may have to encourage the emergence of flexible employment practices that accommodate the needs of older workers. Such practices may become an increasingly important way of ensuring the welfare rights of an aging population.

CONCLUSION

I have offered a rather abstract and general description of two problems of distributive justice highlighted by the aging of society. Solving them gives us a way to clarify the content of welfare rights and to resolve disputes about intergenerational equity. It would be easy in this paper to lose sight of the most important aspect of my approach: I offer a unifying vision. We all pass through institutions that distribute goods over our life-span. If these institutions are prudently designed, we each benefit throughout our lives. It is only prudent to treat ourselves differently at different stages of life, as our needs change. What is prudent with respect to different stages of a life determines what is fair between age groups. Prudence here guides justice. If as policymakers, planners, and the general public we can all keep our eye on this unifying vision and if we can ignore the divisive talk about competition between age groups and birth cohorts, then our target will be policies that benefit all of us over our whole lives. Establishing such policies would mean doing justice to the old and the young. If such policies are stable and benefit successive cohorts in comparable ways, then we have gone far toward ensuring justice across generations.

ACKNOWLEDGMENT

This paper is based in part on material contained in my *Am I My Parents' Keeper? An Essay on Justice between the Young and the Old*

(Daniels 1988), and I thank the publishers for permission to draw on that material here. I also wish to acknowledge the generous support of the National Endowment for the Humanities (Grant RH-20197) and the National Library of Medicine (1RO1LM05005).

NOTE

1 Allen Buchanan has suggested to me that there is another important reason why rationally prudent individuals would discount later years. *Fecundity* of benefits is one important factor to take into account in calculating expected benefit. But if this is so, then, other things being equal, a later year is worth less than an earlier one because whatever opportunities for generating further benefits from activities pursued in a later year are less than those generated at an earlier year. The same reasoning is what leads economists to discount future dollars; they are worth less because there is less time to invest them and hence they are less fecund, a point which has nothing to do with inflation.

REFERENCES

Aaron, H., and Schwartz, W. 1984. *The Painful Prescription*. Washington, D.C.: Brookings Institution.
Brock, D. 1988. "Ethical Issues in Recipient Selection for Organ Transplantation." In D. Matthieu, ed., *Organ Substitution Technology: Ethical, Legal, and Public Policy Issues*, pp. 86–99. Boulder, CO: Westview.
Callahan, D. 1987. *Setting Limits: Medical Goals in an Aging Society*. New York: Simon & Schuster.
Cohen, Lee M., ed., 1993. *Justice Across Generations: What Does It Mean?* Washington, D.C.: American Association of Retired Persons.
Daniels, N. 1985. *Just Health Care*. Cambridge: Cambridge University Press.
Daniels, N. 1988. *Am I My Parents' Keeper? An Essay on Justice between the Young and the Old*. New York: Oxford University Press.
Daniels, N. 1989a. "The Biomedical Model and Just Health Care: A Reply to Jecker," *Journal of Medicine and Philosophy* 14:6:677–80.
Daniels, N. 1989b. "Justice and Transfers between Generations." In Paul Johnson, Christoph Conrad, and David Thomson, eds., *Workers versus Pensioners: Intergenerational Justice in an Aging World*, pp. 57–79. Manchester: Manchester University Press.
Daniels, N. 1990. "Human Rights, Population Aging, and Intergenerational Equity," In *Population and Human Rights: Proceedings of the Expert Group Meeting on Population and Human Rights, Geneva, 306 April 1989*. ST/ESA/ Series R/107, pp. 207–27. New York: United Nations.
Daniels, N. 1991. "Is the Oregon Rationing Plan Fair?" *JAMA* 265:17:2232–35.
Daniels, N. 1993. "Rationing Fairly: Programmatic Considerations," *Bioethics* 7:2–3:224–33.
Emanuel, E. J. 1991. *The Ends of Human Life: Medical Ethics in a Liberal Polity*. Cambridge, MA: Harvard University Press.

Epstein, R. A. 1988. "Justice Across the Generations." Paper presented at the Conference on Intergenerational Justice, University of Texas, Austin.

Gibson, R. M., and Fisher, C. R. 1979. "Age Differences in Health Care Spending, Fiscal Year 1977," *Social Security Bulletin* 42:1:3–16.

Jecker, N. 1989. "Towards a Theory of Age-Group Justice," *Journal of Medicine and Philosophy* 14:6:655–76.

Kamm, F. 1993. *Mortality and Morality*. Vol. 1. Oxford: Oxford University Press.

McKerlie, Dennis, 1989a. "Equality and Time," *Ethics* 99:475–91.

McKerlie, Dennis. 1989b. "Justice between Age Groups: A Comment on Norman Daniels," *Journal of Applied Philosophy* 6:227–34.

McKerlie, Dennis. 1993. "Justice between Neighboring Generations." In Lee M. Cohen, ed., *Justice across Generations: What Does It Mean?* pp. 215–26. Washington, D.C.: Public Policy Institute, AARP.

Parfit, Derek. 1984. *Reasons and Persons*. Oxford: Oxford University Press.

Parfit, Derek. 1986. "Comments," *Ethics* 96:832–72.

Rawls, John. 1971. *A Theory of Justice*. Cambridge. MA: Harvard University Press.

Rawls, John. 1982. "Social Unity and the Primary Goods." In A. K. Sen and B. Williams, eds., *Utilitarianism and Beyond*, pp. 159–85. Cambridge: Cambridge University Press.

Schwartz, W., and H. Aaron. 1988. "A Tough Choice on Health Care Costs," *New York Times* (6 April):A23.

Soldo, G. J., and K. G. Manton. 1985. "Changes in the Health Status and Service Needs of the Oldest Old: Current Patterns and Future Trends," *Milbank Memorial Fund Quarterly* 63:2:286–323.

Thomson, D. 1989. "The Welfare State and Generational Conflicts: Winners and Losers." In Paul Johnson, Christoph Conrad, and David Thomson, eds., *Workers versus Pensioners: Intergenerational Justice in an Aging World*, pp. 33–56. Manchester: Manchester University Press.

Veatch, R. 1988. "Justice and the Economics of Terminal Illness," *Hastings Center Report* 18:4:33–40.

Vogel, R. J., and H. C. Palmer, eds. 1982. *Long-Term Care: Perspectives from Research and Demonstrations*. Washington, D.C.: Health Care Financing Administration, U.S. Department of Health and Human Services.

Watson, T. 1992. "New Worry for Those Growing Old," *Boston Globe* 241(21 February):3.

Chapter 13

Problems with prudence

CHALLENGES TO THE CLASSICAL MODEL

The Prudential Life-span Account rests on two assumptions which I have treated so far as uncontroversial. The first assumption is that there is an important difference between distributive problems that cross the boundaries between persons, on the one hand, and problems that involve allocation within a life (between the stages of a life), on the other. The elaborate "frame" I constructed to isolate the age-group problem from interpersonal transfers of goods is motivated by the view that persons are basic entities for purposes of the theory of justice. For example, taking goods from one person to benefit another requires justification. More generally, deciding which inequalities between persons are justifiable is the central issue in distributive justice. By showing that the problem of distribution between the young and the old, which appears to be interpersonal, can be reduced to a problem of intrapersonal, prudential allocation, I try to replace a more complex and problematic issue with a less problematic one. If the boundaries between persons are not so important, or if similar problems arise for distributions within a life as between them, then the motivation for my strategy is undermined.

The second assumption that I have treated as uncontroversial is this: Rationality requires that we show equal concern for all parts of our (future) lives. Parfit (1984, 313) refers to this assumption as the Requirement of Equal Concern. I used this assumption in Chapter 3 of Daniels (1988), to justify the restrictions placed on prudent deliberators, and in later chapters it affected the reasoning of prudent deliberators choosing how to distribute health care and income support over the life-span. If rationality does not require that we be equally concerned about all parts of our future, then my arguments will have to be qualified and my account will turn out to be based on stronger presuppositions than it now appears to have.

These two assumptions are quite standard in moral philosophy. The assumption about the importance of the boundaries between persons appears in diverse normative theories, ranging from Nozick's (1974) libertarianism to Rawls' (1971) justice as fairness. It also motivates, at least in part, the appeal of contractarian approaches to the foundations of ethics, for contracts respect the distinctness of persons. Assuming the Requirement of Equal Concern is no less standard, both in philosophy and in economic theory. Nevertheless, both of these assumptions have come under powerful criticism in Parfit's (1984) brilliant and provocative work, *Reasons and Persons*. My task is to provide some defense of these assumptions and to offer qualifications, where necessary, in the face of Parfit's arguments.

RATIONALITY AND THE REQUIREMENT OF EQUAL CONCERN

We might begin by noting some features of the classical theory of individual rationality, which Parfit calls the Self-Interest Theory, or SI. The central claim of this theory is

(S1) For each person, there is one supremely rational ultimate aim: that his life go, for him, as well as possible. (Parfit 1984, 4)

Other claims of the theory are

(S2) What each of us has most reason to do is whatever would be best for himself, and
(S3) It is irrational for anyone to do what he believes will be worse for himself, and
(S4) What it would be rational for anyone to do is what will bring him the greatest expected benefit. (Parfit 1984, 8)

SI involves other claims, but they are not relevant to the argument here. In his subsequent discussion of SI (in Part Three of his book), Parfit says it is also committed to

The Requirement of Equal Concern: A rational person should be *equally* concerned about *all* the parts of his future.

The Requirement of Equal Concern, we may take him to mean, is implicit in the other claims of SI. For example, the greatest expected benefit (in S4) is aggregated over the whole life. In some classical formulations of the theory, such as Sidgwick's (1907) and Rawls' (1971), the Requirement of Equal Concern is explicit.

Parfit considers a variety of arguments against SI. In Part One of his book, he considers arguments that SI is self-defeating. In Part Two, he argues that SI occupies an untenable and arbitrary position in between morality and an alternative account of individual rationality, namely, the (Critical) Present Aim Theory. Morality is neutral about time and persons. It takes interests and desires into account regardless of whose life they involve and regardless of when they occur within a life. In contrast, the Present Aim Theory is biased in favor of one's own present aims, and so is nonneutral with regard to both time and persons. The Self-Interest Theory is neutral about time but biased about persons. Parfit argues that this in-between position is untenable because there is no consistent basis for being neutral with regard to time but not persons. These are important arguments, which have been discussed elsewhere (see Kagan 1986). If we think that the way in which experience involves persons through time gives some reason to be neutral about one but not the other, then these arguments will not be persuasive. I want to concentrate in any case on Parfit's ultimate challenge to the importance of persons.

In what follows, I shall consider only those of Parfit's arguments against SI that rest on claims about personal identity. Parfit suggests that it is uncritical, commonsense acceptance of a Non-Reductionist View, for example, the belief in a Cartesian ego or mental substance, which leads us to think that rationality implies the Requirement of Equal Concern. On such a view, since the ego or mental substance is what makes each of us the person we are over time, then we think we must be equally concerned about what happens to "it" at all points. There is what Parfit calls a "further fact" over and above the psychological continuities. In contrast, on Parfit's Reductionist View, the facts relevant to deciding whether we are the same person over time are facts about the connectedness and continuity of mental events (and perhaps some facts about their causes). If these are the underlying facts, however, then the metaphysical basis for the Requirement of Equal Concern may be removed. Since psychological connectedness and continuity can vary in degree, the door may be open for us to care more about some parts of our lives than others. To understand Parfit's claims, we must look more closely at his terminology and arguments.

Parfit (1984, 211) says that on the Reductionist View, "each person's existence just consists in the existence of a brain and body, and the occurrence of a series of interrelated physical and mental events." The central features of the position are

(1) that the fact of a person's identity over time just consists in the holding of certain more particular facts,
(2) that these facts can be described without either presupposing the identity of this person, or explicity claiming that the experience in this person's life are had by this person, or even explicitly claiming

that this person exists. These facts can be described in an *impersonal* way.

If we reject either or both of (1) or (2), we get a Non-Reductionist View. A Non-Reductionist holds that "personal identity over time does not just consist in physical and/or psychological continuity. It is a separate, further fact," for example, a fact about the persistence of a purely mental entity such as the Cartesian ego (Parfit 1984, 210).

Through a series of thought experiments, involving teletransporting replicas of persons to distant places (in the way Mr. Spock may be "beamed" down to a planet in *Star Trek*), or replacing parts of one person's brain with parts of another, Parfit argues that only two kinds of facts can and should underlie our judgments about personal identity. Suppose we want to know whether two "person stages," A and B, are stages of the same person. If A and B share desires, beliefs, and intentions, or if B remembers having an experience A had, or if B carries out A's intentions, then A and B have *direct psychological connections*. If enough direct connections hold between B and A they are *strongly connected*. When overlapping chains of strong connectedness hold between person stages, then they have *psychological continuity*. Parfit's main arguments in Part Three are intended to show that only facts about psychological connectedness and continuity are relevant to answering questions about personal identity. I shall return later to consider some further points about the concept of personal identity and Parfit's metaphysics, but for now let us consider how Parfit uses these metaphysical conclusions.

Parfit first argues that, if one is a Reductionist, an Extreme View is not irrational. On this Extreme View, first suggested in Butler's criticism of Locke and echoed in Sidgwick (cf. Parfit 1984, 307), we seem to have no reason to be concerned about later stages of ourselves if no further fact, beyond connectedness and continuity, links us to them. If personal identity does not involve a deep further fact, namely, about a persistent Cartesian ego or mental substance, it is a less deep fact or involves less (Parfit 1984, 312). We may then have no more reason to care about later stages of ourselves than we do about other persons.

But a Moderate View is also not irrational, and it is this view which most interests us. Parfit argues that we should each then reason as follows: My reasons for caring about my future, if I care at all, must depend on my concerns about my connectedness and continuity (with or without normal causes) with my later stages. But then, it may be rational to care less about parts of my future with which I am less strongly connected. That is, I can "discount" or care less about the well-being of person stages less strongly connected to me than I do about those with which I am more strongly connected. On this view, it is not the mere *temporal* remoteness of future stages that leads to my caring less. Here there is no disagreement with the classical self-interest theorist who condemns what economists call "pure time preferences." Parfit argues that since connectedness is a relation that holds to a lesser degree with future stages, then it is defensible to believe it has a different degree of importance. Therefore it is not irrational for me to discount the well-being of my future person stages according to their degree of connectedness with me now.

This conclusion, Parfit argues, is incompatible with the Self-Interest Theory, since it seems to involve a rejection of the Requirement of Equal Concern. Instead of being required to care equally about all parts of my future, I may care less about parts of it to which I am less connected. Parfit says we are not rationally *required* to have this discount rate, only that it is not irrational to have it.[1] Revising the Self-Interest Theory to include a discount based on degree of connectedness would destroy the central claims of the theory, however. Parfit (1984, 317) says "it would break the link between the Self-Interest Theory and what is in one's own best interests." That is, it contradicts S3, the claim that it is irrational for anyone to do what he believes will be worse for him. "If it is not irrational to care less about some parts of one's future," Parfit (1984, 317) concludes, "it may not be irrational to do what one believes will be worse for oneself. It may not be irrational to act, knowingly, against one's own self-interest."

Parfit's argument is more puzzling on close examination than it first appears to be. There may be something close to an equivocation involved in it. What are one's "own best interests" or "one's own self-interest"?[2] Are the future interests I am discounting really my own interests? To make his point, Parfit requires that these interests be one's own. These discounted interests of future person stages must count as interests of the person doing the discounting. If I discount them, they must still be *mine* to discount. Though they are really mine, I care about them less.

If, however, personal identity is determined by the fact that there exists between two-person stages an appropriate degree of connectedness and/or continuity (with the right kind of cause), that is, "Relation R" holds (as Parfit 1984, 215 refers to it), then perhaps this later stage, whose interest I am discounting, is not fully or completely part of me. Its interests are not really or fully (or to an adequate degree) *mine*. But then, if I care less about *those* interests, I am not caring less about *my* interests. Consequently, I am not necessarily doing what is worse for myself if I ignore what are not completely or really my interests in any case. That is, if personal identity is a matter of degree, resting solely on facts about psychological connectedness and continuity, then the following is true: If I discount the interests of relatively unconnected stages of myself, I am in the relevant sense still attending only to those interests which are really mine.[3]

On this reading of Parfit's claims, I make personal identity depend on degree of connectedness and continuity, in the same way I make my concern so dependent. But this means I have not really rejected the Requirement of Equal Concern. I still show my dominant concern for all and only what is me – that is all I care about. The Revised Self-Interest Theory, which includes the discount rate for connectedness, only appears to be discounting *my* future well-being. Actually, it is just identifying (*isolating*, more precisely) what counts as *my* future well-being. The dispute between the Classical and the Revised Theories, it turns out, is only a dispute about what counts as my future, not a dispute about whether it is *rational* to be concerned about all parts of my future. (Both formulations of the dispute raise problems for my account of how to solve the age-group problem, for both make it harder to justify certain transfers from the young; that is why I must return to the claims about the importance of personal identity.)

In suggesting that Parfit may be equivocating about personal identity here, I may be too contentious (or even mistaken). In any case, I shall return later . . . to discuss further Parfit's views about personal identity. In the remainder of this section I want to consider a less contentious way to express my concerns about Parfit's argument for a discount rate based on the degree of connectedness. I shall be concerned more with what counts as a person's *interests* and less with what counts as the *same person's* interests.

Suppose we formulate corresponding principles of individual rational action for the Classical and the Revised Theories. For the Classical Theory the principle would presumably be: Act so as to maximize personal expected utility over your lifetime. We can think of an individual as having a utility function. Such a function has as its inputs or "arguments" the individual's resources, talents, skills, preferences, and values, and it has as its output particular values of the quantity utility. The Classical Action Principle implies the Requirement of Equal Concern for the following reason: We do not discount *utilities* or well-being merely because of the time at which the utility occurs or because of the degree of psychological connectedness of the person having the utility with other stages of himself. We discount only for the reduced *probability* of future utilities (this is what "expected utility" means).

What does the corresponding action principle for the Revised Self-Interest Theory look like? To answer this question, we must first understand how to discount *classical utilities*. A discount rate based on psychological connectedness may be thought of as a more complex utility function than the one used in the Classical Theory. On this view, we first calculate utility as in the Classical Theory: We then take that result as an argument in a new utility function which includes the discount rate. (Let us ignore the fact that psychological connectedness is not a uniform function over time.) The values (or outputs) of this function will be discounted utility. This discounted utility represents well-being from the perspective of an individual Discounter prospectively assessing the outcomes *he cares about*. The discount rate thus works the way an additional set of preferences would, were they added into the original (Classical) utility function. We can even think of discounted utility as plain utility or well-being *from the point of view of a Discounter*. It is what that Discounter takes to be relevant to his well-being.

Having done the necessary discounting, we are ready to state a principle of rational action for the Revised Theory. A likely candidate is this: Act so as to maximize personal expected discounted utility over your lifetime. Suppose a Discounter adopts this principle. He now can comply with the basic insight of the Classical Theory, that it is irrational for anyone to do what he believes will be worse for him. It would certainly be worse for a Discounter to maximize utility over his life-span rather than discounted utility, since what he prospectively cares about is discounted utility. Indeed, if his utility function includes a discount rate for psychological connectedness – this is what he *cares* about – it would be imprudent for him to maximize utility rather than discounted utility. The Discounter who prospectively acts rationally will make things *worse* for himself only if we take his *interests* or well-being to be captured by utility and not discounted utility. [Note the contrast with my more contentious point. Earlier I complained that net personal expected utility does not capture the *Discounter's* interests because some of that utility does not belong to person stages which are (fully? actually? completely?) part of *him*. Here the point is that utility does not measure *interests* for the Discounter: only *discounted utility* does.]

The Discounter may seem to be acting in accord with his own best interests only because we have interpreted discounted utility in a particular way. We have treated discounted utility as if *it*, rather than utility, were actually a measure of well-being from the perspective of the Discounter. Perhaps the Discounter should think of discounted utility not as the relevant measure of utility, but as a *distortion* of utility, a distortion induced by the peculiarly curved lens of the discount rate. For him discounted utility is "utility as it matters to me now." He knows (or should realize) that well-being for less-connected stages of himself will really be less if he maximizes his discounted utility. It is just that he cares less about the fact that less-connected stages of himself will be worse off than they would be if he cared about utility and not just discounted utility.

But this attitude is not to be confused with short-sightedness, which it would be if the Classical Theory were true. If he really believes the discount rate is reasonable, the Discounter will think of the distortion as a *correction*. What is valuable to him (prospectively) is not his utility but his discounted utility. His principle of action is: Act so as to maximize expected discounted utility over your life-span. In acting on this principle, he will knowingly be acting against his self-interest as measured by expected utility over his life-span. But since he (prospectively) cares only about discounted utility, he will not be knowingly acting against what in fact he takes to be his own best interests. He will still not be knowingly doing what he thinks is worse for himself.

Parfit's (1984, 317) claim is that the Revised Theory, which includes a discount rate for connectedness, "breaks the link between the Self-Interest Theory and what is in one's own best interests." My earlier complaint was that this claim is false if we redefine personal identity, and thus what counts as *"one's own* best interests." My second complaint is that if we construe "interests" as a Discounter must, then he will *not* be doing what he believes is worse for himself when he discounts (later) utility. From his perspective, it is not utility, but discounted utility, that defines his lifetime *interests*. (Remember that interests cannot be defined entirely independently of the person's aims and preferences; cf. note 2.)

This interpretation of what is involved in the Revised Self-Interest Theory also involves accusing Parfit of an equivocation. This time the equivocation is on the notion of the same person's *interests* rather than on the notion of the *same person's* interests. Though I believe this equivocation is important, in what follows I shall drop, for the sake of argument, these complaints about equivocation. Instead, I want to point out some problems that arise for Discounters on the assumption that they really are ignoring some of their own interests.

Suppose our Discounter plans his life at an early time E and then ages in the normal way. He now finds himself living at a later stage L of his life which is less connected with E, and his utility level is lower than it would have been had his plan not prospectively discounted utility. From the standpoint of L, E now seems to be the stage of life whose utility the Discounter would prefer to discount. Could he now (at L) retrospectively plan his life, he would discount utility at E, saving more resources for use at L. At L, the Discounter now cares about his utility at L. Looking through the lens of his discount rate, he is not discounting his utility at L, but only his utility at other, less connected points in his life. How he used to care about his utility at L, when he discounted it at E, is not how he cares about it now. Similarly, how he now cares about the utility he had at E is not how he cared about it at E. But the Discounter cannot remake history.

Nor, does it seem, can he learn much from it. At L, he might bemoan his low utility at L, wishing perhaps that his earlier self had not been a Discounter, though he cannot criticize himself for any irrationality unless he is ready to conclude that discounting is irrational. As an inveterate Discounter, however, he has to plan the rest of his life in a way that virtually guarantees that later in life he will again regret his current plans just as he now regrets his earlier ones. Here we have broken the link between acting rationally and improving one's strategies for planning by learning from cases in which we do not do well.

A small point about regret. Parfit (1984, 187) remarks that someone who has a bias toward the near future may regret having had the bias in the past, but that gives him no reason to regret still having it. He still has no reason to care that a future, less-connected stage of himself will suffer in the future. We might note, however, that the Discounter may regret his imprudence more than the Classical Non-Discounter. The imprudent Non-Discounter can at least look back at all the utility enjoyed early in life through a lens that does not discount the earlier utility. He can say, "At least I had it good then!" But the Discounter, looking back at an earlier time, when he was not well connected to his current self, will not care that he enjoyed himself so much then. He cannot console himself by recalling or imagining the full value of his earlier personal utility.

I do not want to beg any questions. The Discounter does well if, at E, he acts successfully to maximize personal expected discounted utility, even if this means that at L he is not as well-off as he would be had he earlier maximized personal utility. At L, however, the Discounter is no longer discounting his utility at L. Judged at L, the results of his "successful" plan at E leave him not only with lower utility but with lower discounted utility. The function that takes utility and the discount rate as its arguments and has discounted utility as its values is one the Discounter uses to assess his well-being *as he ages*. His former successes are responsible for his current dissatisfactions. But if he adheres to the distorting lens of his discount rate, he cannot improve on his dissatisfying outcomes – as judged by himself when those outcomes are realized. Since he prospectively cares less about those later outcomes, which affect less-connected stages of himself, he adheres to his discount rate. But when he eventually becomes that stage of himself, he will be dissatisfied with the results.

When we look at the graph of a continuous function through a magnifying glass, the segment in focus seems discontinuous with the rest of the line. It is on a new scale. We can move the glass along the line, and the effect is not a new, continuous function, but relocation of the discontinuity. A Discounter looks at his well-being through such a magnifying glass. As he ages, the utility he cares about, discounted utility, will lead to different assessments of his well-being for *the same point* in his life. At E, his discounted utility for point L will be a different value from what his discounted utility for L will be at L.[4]

This analogy suggests that adopting a discount rate based on connectedness introduces problems similar to the problems that arise from time-indexed desires. When Brandt (1979) discusses this issue, he concludes that desire–satisfaction accounts of well-being are unacceptable because there is no whole-life perspective from which one can consistently construct a plan of life that maximizes desire–satisfaction. Instead, he suggests that an "enjoyment" account of happiness can avoid this sort of incoherence. The Discounter avows, as a matter of principle, as it were, that the perspective from which to plan a life is one's present interests, including one's preferred discount rate. But such a person must make assessments of his well-being at many points in his life and he must make new plans as well. He gives himself no concept – such as utility – on the basis of which he can arrive at uniform evaluations of his well-being for the same point in his life. From different points in his life, the Discounter will assign the same point in his life different values of discounted utility. In this sense, there is no way for evaluations and plans to cohere over a lifetime.

When we give up the Requirement of Equal Concern and adopt, instead, a discount rate for utilities based on psychological connectedness, we are abandoning the requirement that there be a uniform way of assessing the well-being of a given point or stage in a life. By making that assessment relative to the point in life at which the assessment is made, we lose the possibility that evaluations and plans will cohere over a lifetime. (It converts the problem of interpersonal comparisons of utility into an intrapersonal problem.) This may seem only a way of spelling out the implications of Reductionism. It may seem only a redescription of what happens when we decide that Relation R (including connectedness) is what matters, not personal identity. But I am inclined to think such *relativity* in assessment, which leaves us without a kind of coherence, may count as an argument against a discount rate of this type. Perhaps we have found a consideration which shows that the fact of reduced connectedness is not enough reason for concluding that connectedness is less important (cf. Parfit 1984, 314).

One last point concerns where Parfit's criticisms of the Classical Theory leave him strategically, given his adherence to some form of

Consequentialism (perhaps Utilitarianism). When the Discounter assesses his well-being for purposes of action, either prospectively or retrospectively, he uses discounted utility, not utility. He is thus committed to the following kind of relativism: He will assign different values to his well-being at a given stage depending on how connected he is to that stage at the time he makes the assessment. The measure of well-being for him is thus *local*. The utilitarian, in contrast, places great importance on the fact that his principle of action (Act so as to maximize total expected utility) uses a *universal* measure of well-being for purposes of guiding action. Parfit's strategy for attacking the Self-Interest theorist was to show he was arbitrary in splitting his own utility off from everyone else's, caring only about personal utility and discounting the utility of others. The self-interest theorist tries to adhere to an untenable middle ground that partially, but not completely, localizes utility assessment. The Discounter, in contrast, fully localizes it (at least with respect to connectedness, if not with respect to time). In this sense he is less arbitrary.

But now it seems that an even greater *gulf* has emerged between the concerns of rationality (to do what is best for oneself, using a local measure of well-being), and the concerns of Consequentialism or Utilitarianism, which are committed to universal measures of well-being. What seemed initially plausible (to me, at least) about the Classical Theory was that it appeared to be committed to a nonlocal measure of well-being (no discounting of utilities by time or connectedness). In this regard it resembled Utilitarianism. Both theories could accept that the principle of individual rational action was one requiring the maximization of personal expected utility, a temporally nonlocal measure of well-being. To get from individual rationality to morality it was not necessary to introduce or justify the idea of nonlocality for measures of well-being. It was necessary only to justify the move from one nonlocal measure to another, and this move could be understood as the move from rationality to morality (no wonder it was hard!).

But now the move from rationality to morality is also the move from locality to universality of measures of well-being, which is why the gulf between the two seems so much larger. Parfit pushes individual rationality much further away from morality than we thought it was. We might have thought that one attractive feature of utilitarianism was the nonlocality of its measure of well-being, and that this was attractive because it had some connection to how it was rational to carry out assessments of personal well-being. But now all (!) that can be said for utility is that such universality is appropriate from a moral point of view.

PERSONAL IDENTITY AND THE BOUNDARY
BETWEEN PERSONS

In Part Three of his book, Parfit argues that personal identity is a less deep metaphysical fact than our commonsense beliefs presuppose it is. Because it is a less deep fact, it may be less important, for example, to moral theory or to the theory of individual rationality. Of greatest concern to us, the boundaries between persons may not be as morally important as we make them out to be in the theory of distributive justice. As Parfit (1984, 339) puts it,

> If some unity is less deep, so is the corresponding disunity. The fact that we live different lives is the fact that we are not the same person. If the fact of personal identity is less deep, so is the fact of non-identity. There are not two different facts here, one of which is less deep on the Reductionist View, while the other remains as deep. There is merely one fact, and this fact's denial. The separateness of persons is the denial that we are all the same person. If the fact of personal identity is less deep, so is this fact's denial.

Consider the implications of this claim for the problem of imposing burdens on one person to benefit someone else. The attempt to balance the gains of one against the losses of another is ruled out by some people, and it is minimally viewed as needing a special justification by others. In general, the claim that the gains outweigh the losses, which would satisfy a utilitarian, will not satisfy those who think the boundaries between persons should be more strictly protected and harder to cross. One way to formulate respect for the boundary would be what Parfit (1984, 337) calls the *Claim about Compensation*: Someone's burden cannot be *compensated* by benefits to someone else.

Parfit says we cannot deny the Claim about Compensation. Nevertheless, becoming Reductionists by abandoning the Non-Reductionist View can have two effects on the Claim about Compensation. In becoming Reductionists, Parfit argues, we come to believe that personal identity is not what matters in metaphysics or morals. Rather, psychological connectedness and continuity are what matter. Consequently, if certain parts of our lives are not well connected, we should treat them, in some respects, like different lives. This belief suggests we might extend the *scope* of the Claim about Compensation. It should apply within lives and not just between them. For example, we might think burdens imposed on the child are not compensated by gains to the adult.

The second effect of becoming a Reductionist may be that we change the *weight* we give the Claim about Compensation. If the unity of persons is less, so is their separateness. But if separateness involves less, it also has less moral significance. So the Claim about Compensation may be given less moral weight, perhaps none at all. Doing this may support the utilitarian view that we need no special justification to aggregate benefits and burdens across persons.

These conclusions clearly threaten a central assumption of the Prudential Life-span Account. I have assumed that the boundary between persons *is* morally significant and that it is always problematic how we are to aggregate or balance benefits and burdens across those boundaries. Consequently, I sought the theoretical advantage that would result from reducing the interpersonal problem of justice between age groups to an intrapersonal problem of prudent allocation over the lifespan. In what follows, I cannot respond to Parfit's extended argument in favor of Reductionism and against Non-Reductionism in any detail. Instead, I shall suggest that there is an alternative way to view the results of some of his arguments against a Non-Reductionist View. On this alternative view, persons and personal identity may indeed "matter," though not for the reasons that underlie a Non-Reductionist View. My argument here draws on my earlier work (see Daniels 1979; for a similar critique of Parfit see White 1989).

I must first review at least the outline of Parfit's attack on the Non-Reductionist View. On a Non-Reductionist View, a person is a separately existing entity, distinct from his brain and body. The classical example is the Cartesian ego. On a Reductionist view, a person's existence consists in the existence of a brain and body, and the occurrence of interrelated physical and mental events. On this view a person is distinct from his brain and body but is not a separately existing entity. Parfit (1984, 211) compares persons to nations, as Hume did. A nation's existence involves the existence of its citizens, living together in certain ways, on its territory, and a nation is distinct from its citizens and territory; but a nation is not a separately existing entity.

These different views of the metaphysics of persons not surprisingly give rise to different views of personal identity. The Non-Reductionist views personal identity as an all-or-nothing, determinate matter of fact. It is a separate fact beyond the facts about physical and psychological continuity. The fact of personal identity holds in every case completely or not at all. The Reductionist believes personal identity involves only physical and psychological continuity, facts which can be described in an impersonal way. To the Reductionist, personal identity may not be determinable in certain cases: There may be no fact of the matter. Moreover, personal identity is not what matters – or should not be what matters – when we think about our relationship to future person stages. Only the facts about connectedness and continuity matter to our survival and how we should view its importance to us.

Parfit brings two main lines of evidence to bear against the Non-Reductionist View. One line draws on actual cases of people with split brains (severed corpora callosa) who experience two unified streams of consciousness. Since "ownership" by a person cannot explain the unity of these streams of consciousness, Parfit (1984, 245ff.) argues, we have evidence for the Reductionist View.

The other line of evidence rests on thought experiments and explores our beliefs about personal identity in cases we do not, and perhaps cannot, actually encounter. The Non-Reductionist believes that personal identity must always be a fact of the matter when we consider a relationship between two person stages. Parfit challenges this belief by imagining thought experiments in which there is no fact of the matter about whether the same person exists through certain transformations. The question, Is this the same person? becomes empty in certain cases, a consequence that cannot obtain if the Non-Reductionist View is true. For example, Parfit (1984, 236) imagines a neurosurgeon gradually replacing bits of his brain with bits of Greta Garbo's. Early in the operation, Parfit remains Parfit. At the end, he has become Garbo. In the middle, there is a spectrum of cases in which there is no answer to the question about personal identity. Consequently, we cannot accept the Non-Reductionist View since it implies there is always a fact of the matter.

A further implication of the Non-Reductionist View, which it shares with common sense, is that personal identity is what matters to us when we contemplate the future. When we think about a future pain, personal identity seems to be what matters. Whether it is *my* pain rather than the experience of someone just like me seems to make all the difference to my concern about it. Parfit wants to undermine this belief that personal identity is what matters.

Suppose I know that at some point in the near future there will be a person stage B which resembles what I am like in important ways. B has access to many of my memories and can act on many of the intentions I now form. B is psychologically connected and continuous with me. In Parfit's (1984, 215) terms, Relation R holds between me and B, and we may suppose it holds only between me and B (and there are no competitors to B). Parfit argues that I now know all the relevant facts for deciding whether a severe pain that B will experience should make me anxious. But the facts that matter here have to do only with Relation R.

The situation is different for the Non-Reductionist, who thinks that not all the facts are in when I know about Relation R. A Non-Reductionist might still want to ask a further question: Is B's pain *mine*? Am I the self or subject who will experience the pain? The Non-Reductionist believes there is some deep, further fact that underlies our answer to these questions. For example, is there a Cartesian ego which B shares with me?

Parfit uses thought experiments to bring the contrast between the two views into sharp relief and to permit us to "test" the contrasting accounts. For example, suppose I have use of Mr. Spock's teletransporter. I step into it. It dissolves me into particles which are dispersed, but it transports information about those particles sufficient to reconstitute an exact replica of me on Mars (or next door). Is the replica me? If it experiences pain, is it my pain? Or have I died and does someone else, who is exactly like me, now live? Should teletransportation be described as death or transportation?

We might think we could just ask the replica. But this will not do. Suppose the teletransporter malfunctions and deposits two replicas elsewhere, or leaves me intact and deposits a replica somewhere else. Both survivors in this case will think they are me. On Parfit's view, in this case, I may be survived by both replicas, but I shall be identical with neither, since identity is a one-to-one relationship. But if the machine does not malfunction, then I have no deeper reason or further fact to think the one replica or survivor is identical with me than I do to think either of the two survivors is. The only facts that count in determining survivorship are facts about connectedness and continuity (Relation R), and these are the only facts that remain to determine any meaningful notion of personal identity. The deep further fact the Non-Reductionist requires is just not available.

I believe we can reject the Non-Reductionist position without accepting Parfit's claim that our concepts of persons and personal identity are reducible to only those facts about connectedness and continuity with which he is concerned. These facts may constrain what count as acceptable concepts of persons – our concepts of persons and personal identity must be compatible with facts about connectedness and continuity. But other facts may contribute to the concepts of persons that we do and should employ. There is another version of Reductionism which is compatible with the claim that personal identity matters. If this is true, we can accept Parfit's critique of the Non-Reductionist without accepting his conclusions about the lack of depth or importance of the boundary between persons. There is space here only to sketch the alternative view.

First, it might be important to note that facts about the degree of connectedness or continuity among the stages of a person – the strength of Relation R – may themselves depend on facts about how persons think about themselves over time and on facts about how other persons think about us over time. What kinds of intentions I form, for example, will affect the relations of connectedness and continuity. But what intentions I form may depend on how connected and continuous

I want the stages of my life to be. Similarly, I may make a special effort to preserve certain kinds of memories or to erase others. These actions will affect Relation R over time. This is not to suggest that the facts underlying Relation R are all under my control, but to some extent some of them surely are. Even if the facts underlying Relation R are all that matter, they are not fixed as metaphysical bedrock; they are plastic. I can make myself into a more or less connected person over time, depending on what importance I attach to doing so. The importance of the degree of connectedness is not itself determined by the facts of connectedness – at least I may be able to make the facts conform to some prior importance I attach to having them obtain.

Nor should we think of my decisions to affect connectedness in these ways as arbitrary. They may rest on important facts about me and my relations to others. Some projects, which I may consider of great importance, may be realizable only in the long run. To undertake them would require that I think of myself as committed over the long run. I may have to form certain intentions and engage those around me to treat me as having those intentions, if I am to succeed. Success will depend on my cooperation with myself and others over time. In this way, what is valuable to me may determine who I must become.

For my own purposes, I require the cooperation of others in shaping my life, including its degree of connectedness and continuity. But social purposes will also require that I treat myself and that others treat me as having a certain degree of connectedness and continuity over time. If others are to work cooperatively with me, and we are to share the benefits of cooperative activities, then we may attribute great importance to promoting continuity and connectedness within the lives of persons. We will want to hold people accountable – both legally and morally – to commitments and responsibilities over time. Social structures that promote our viewing ourselves as the same person over time may thus be necessary for us to live together in certain productive ways. If this is true, then these facts may require us to attach importance to personal identity which does not derive from the facts of connectedness and continuity themselves. We may even idealize (fictionalize?) how connected and continuous persons are in order to carry on certain activities which require those fictions. Nevertheless, those idealizations may define what persons are, or at least what our beliefs about them have to be, if we are to plan our lives effectively and cooperate with others successfully.

Metaphysics may be the bedrock, but it underdetermines what kinds of structures – including persons – we can and *ought* to build on it. The "ought to" here may be prudential, capturing what rational or reasonable persons should do. Or it may be moral. Parfit's claim that only Relation R matters and that personal identity does not would have to be rejected. The position I am sketching, which implies what I have elsewhere (Daniels 1979) called the "plasticity" of persons, can be thought of as a Reductionist position. At least it does not depend on the belief that persons are separate entities, like Cartesian egos. But persons – their identity and survival – are not reducible merely to some given set of facts about connectedness and continuity, as Parfit has proposed. I am not interested here, however, in insisting that this account is properly described as Reductionist. I insist only that one can thus give a better account of how we do and should view persons than Parfit's. White (1989) has made a similar point using the terminology of "supervenience." The identity of a person is a fact that *supervenes* not just on a base of facts about connectedness and continuity but on a base that includes facts about the ways in which others view and treat us.

If my sketch of an alternative account is preferable to Parfit's, then the central assumption about the boundaries between persons that motivates my Prudential Life-span Account is defensible. We need not believe in Cartesian egos, or defend them against Parfit, to think that the boundaries between persons are an important fact of deep moral significance. This account also has implications for my discussion of discounting for connectedness (see page 290ff.). Parfit argued that it was not irrational for me to think that my concern about my future well-being could be discounted according to my degree of connectedness with my future person stage, since connectedness is what really matters. But we have reasons to think personal identity important in ways that go beyond the facts about connectedness. Indeed, we might want to alter facts about connectedness in accordance with what we think important. People will then have good reasons not to discount for connectedness. Some of my earlier concerns in this chapter bear on these reasons.

In short, as I have attempted to demonstrate, both assumptions underlying the Prudential Life-span Account can be defended against arguments of the sort Parfit offers. This does not prove that these classical assumptions are firm ground on which to build, but at least my construction does not rest on what we know to be sand.

NOTES

1 I am not sure why we are not required to have the rate on the view that the sole grounds for caring about our future is our concern about connectedness and continuity.
2 Parfit's argument does not turn on a particular equivocation about "interests." Suppose interests were defined independently of a person's preferences or what he cares about, and that we took prudence to involve the

maximal satisfaction of interests over a life-span. Then if rational action involved the attempt to satisfy one's preferences or aims, it would indeed be problematic whether prudence was required by rationality. This argument does not turn on any points about personal identity and is not Parfit's.

3   Of course, as Parfit (1984, 206) notes, strong connectedness cannot be a criterion of personal identity because it is not transitive.

4   Whether the Discounter is committed to what have been called inconsistent time preferences (see Elster 1984) is an interesting question. Discount rates that give absolute priority to stages very strongly connected with the current stage, but that give equal and smaller rates to less-connected stages, will generate inconsistent time preferences. I ignore this complication for Parfit here.

REFERENCES

Brandt, R. 1979. *A Theory of the Good and the Right*. Oxford: Oxford University Press.

Daniels, N. 1979. "Moral Theory and the Plasticity of Persons," *Monist* 62:3:265–87.

Daniels, N. 1988. *Am I My Parents' Keeper? An Essay on Justice between the Young and the Old*. New York: Oxford University Press.

Elster, J. 1984. *Ulysses and the Sirens*. 2nd ed. Cambridge: Cambridge University Press.

Kagan, S. 1986. "The Present-Aim Theory of Rationality," *Ethics* 96:4:746–59.

Nozick, R. 1974. *Anarchy, State, and Utopia*. New York: Basic Books.

Parfit, D. 1984. *Reasons and Persons*. Oxford: Oxford University Press.

Sidgwick, H. 1907. *The Methods of Ethics*. London: Macmillan.

Rawls, J. 1971. *A Theory of Justice*. Cambridge, MA: Harvard University Press.

White, S. 1989. "Metapsychological Relativism and the Self," *Journal of Philosophy* 86:298–323.

Chapter 14

Merit and meritocracy

I

Sometimes a person has abilities and interests which enable him or her to fill a given job, position, or office – hereafter, I shall use only "job" – better than other available persons. In what sense do such abilities and interests constitute a basis for claiming the more capable person merits the job? Does the fact that someone possesses special abilities and interests which are needed for the superior performance of a job of considerable social importance and prestige allow that person a legitimate claim to greater rewards for the job? I shall explore some of the issues associated with these questions by analyzing the notion of a meritocracy, a social order built around a particular notion of merit. I hope that examination of such a hypothetical social order will allow me to assess the broader implications of this particular notion of merit for a theory of distributive justice.

I am not concerned with certain classical meritocracies, that is, with certain views of aristocracy according to which social class was thought to imply differences in merit or ability with positions and rewards conferred accordingly.[1] Rather, I take as my model variants of the type of meritocracy portrayed by Michael Young who, in his now classic satire or fantasy, *The Rise of the Meritocracy*, anticipated many features of a social ideal adopted by more recent writers.[2] Young imagines a worldwide society in the twenty-first century in which all assignments of jobs and rewards are based on merit. The system (a pervasive extension of the British Civil Service, he remarks) is feasible because great advances in testing for intelligence and ability allow accurate predictions of performance and permit appropriate educational tracking. All social barriers to the development of such abilities – social class, family background (but not the family), race, and religion – are prevented from influencing decisions on education or career. Basic wages for different jobs are equal in order to avoid tiresome debates about the basis for inequalities in compensation. Nevertheless, vast inequalities of benefits and other rewards accompany jobs. These rewards are justified because they either provide incentives or ensure efficient working conditions. Overall, rewards are proportional to merit. Merit is construed as *ability plus effort*.

Though Young's meritocracy can be viewed as the inspirational model behind my remarks, I shall not discuss the details of his construction, except for his notion of merit. Instead, I would like to sketch a theory of meritocracy – or, rather, of meritocracies, since there are many variants – which generalizes some of Young's ideas. We will see that a number of social theories share what might be called a "meritocratic core," though they differ on other critical features of distributive justice. My analysis of the principles underlying this core reveals, I believe, that claims of merit, in the restricted sense of that term relevant to meritocracies, are derived from considerations of efficiency or productivity and will not support stronger notions of desert.

II

I take a meritocracy to be a society whose basic institutions are governed by a partial theory of distributive justice consisting of principles of the following types:

(1) A principle of job placement that awards jobs to individuals on the basis of merit;
(2) A principle specifying the conditions of opportunity under which the job placement principle is applied;
(3) A principle specifying reward schedules for jobs.

It is obvious that such principles constitute only a partial theory of distributive justice: they say nothing, for example, about liberty or its distribution, or about many other questions. But I shall concentrate on just this much here since most meritocrats do. There is, I shall argue, a preferred principle for job placement and one for opportunity to which most meritocrats would agree. But meritocrats will still vary widely on reward principles. My schema allows us to separate problems common to what meritocrats generally share from problems that arise from reward schedules.

Most meritocrats share certain empirical assumptions which give rise to a principle of job placement. First, they assume that different jobs require different sets of human abilities and different personality traits, including motivation, if they are to be performed with maximum competence. Certain motor skills or mental skills are more critical for some jobs than others. Second, meritocrats assume that people differ in the constellation of abilities and personality traits they possess. Some people possess more developed motor skills, some more developed mental skills, than others. Usually, this second assumption is not couched solely in terms of actual skills possessed. Rather, it is assumed people differ in their natively determined capacity to develop a given level of a certain skill. Often the ambiguous word "ability" does double duty here, hedging bets between claims about inequalities of skills and claims about inequalities of capacity. In any case, most meritocrats believe it is obvious that people differ in levels of skill and it is at least probable that they differ in the capacity to acquire levels of skills.[3]

From these two assumptions meritocrats infer that some arrays of assignments of individuals to jobs will be more productive than others. That is, if we take care to match people with the jobs they are best able to perform, then we will have produced a relatively productive array of job assignments. Actually, we are unlikely to find just one particular array of job assignments that is more productive than any other. But it seems likely, given these empirical assumptions, that there is an equivalence class of maximally productive arrays of job assignments for any fixed set of jobs and individuals.

A warning is needed about the notion of productivity. It must be accepted as an intuitively applicable notion for a wide range of jobs, positions, or offices for which no standard measurement of productivity exists. For such jobs, economists often take market-determined wage levels to indicate average productivity. But such a device is not satisfactory for many reasons. So I shall assume we can talk meaningfully about the productivity of doctors, teachers, lawyers, hairdressers, and so on, even though no single quantitative measure seems acceptable. Meritocrats and nonmeritocrats alike operate with intuitively acceptable, if imprecise, notions of competent or productive job performance.

The principle I believe would be preferred for job placement makes use of the equivalence class of maximally productive arrays of job assignments. This Productive Job Assignment Principle (PJAP) says that job assignments should be made by selecting a member from this equivalence class; if no assignment of available applicants to open jobs is a member of the maximal equivalence class (because, say, some jobs are already held), select an assignment from the next most productive equivalence class, and so on. Such a principle seems desirable because, in the absence of arguments showing that justice or other considerations of right demand some array other than a maximally productive one, there is good reason to seek productivity in social arrangements. I want to leave it an open question how a meritocrat would respond to a claim that justice demanded – as compensation for past services or past injuries – that someone not selected by the PJAP nevertheless be given a particular job. Some such claims would seem to be weighty enough to justify overriding the presumption in favor of productivity considerations that underlies selecting the PJAP in the first place. But more on this point shortly.

If the PJAP is adopted, then the notion of individual merit can be applied in the following restricted way. An individual may claim to merit one job more than another job, or to merit one job more than another person does, if and only if his occupying that job is an assignment that is part of an array of assignments selected by the PJAP. The claim of merit or relative merit is dependent for its basis on the rationale for the PJAP. Merit does not derive from having the abilities themselves, but only from the fact that abilities can play a certain social role. We focus on the relevant abilities because of their utility, not because there is something intrinsically meritorious about having them. Clearly the particular notion of merit I am concerned with here should not be confused with the more general concept of desert; it should also not be confused with certain ordinary uses of "merit" which are similar to the broader notion of desert. I am concerned with merit as it plays a role in the types of meritocracies I am analyzing.

To see why the PJAP is the preferred principle, consider the following case.[4] Jack and Jill both want jobs *A* and *B* and each much prefers *A* to *B*. Jill can do either *A* or *B* better than Jack. But the situation *S* in which Jill performs *B* and Jack *A* is more productive than Jack doing *B* and Jill *A* (*S'*), even when we include the effects on productivity of Jill's lesser satisfaction. The PJAP selects *S*, not *S'*, because it is attuned to macroproductivity, not microproductivity, considerations. It says, "Select people for jobs so that *overall* job performance is maximized."

It might be felt that the "real" meritocrat would balk at such a macroprinciple. The "real" meritocrat, it might be argued, is one who thinks a person should get a job if he or she is the best available person for *that* job. We might formulate such a view as the microproductivity principle that, for any job *J*, we should select the applicant who can most productively perform *J* from among those desiring *J* more than any other job. The microprinciple would select *S'* not *S*.

Given the rationale for treating job-related abilities as the basis for merit claims in the first place, namely that it is socially desirable to enhance productivity where possible, I think that the macroprinciple seems preferable. There is something anomalous about basing a merit claim, given our restricted notion of merit, on claims about microproductivity considerations while at the same time ignoring macroproductivity considerations. We seem to need an explanation why the latter considerations would not overrule the former ones. Alternatively, we might try to divorce the merit claim from all productivity considerations, but this approach makes it completely mysterious why job-related abilities are made the basis of merit in the first place.[5]

I suppose one reason some may think the micromerit principle is preferable to the PJAP is that it seems *unfair* to Jill that she gets the job she wants less even though she can do the job Jack gets better than he can. But what is the sense of unfairness here based on? After all, under this arrangement, Jack has the job he prefers and overall productivity is enhanced. If Jill had her way, Jack would not have his, and macroproductivity would suffer as well. It is also important to note that *B* is a job Jill wants, though not as much as she wants *A*. The PJAP does not force people into jobs they do not want at all.

I believe the sense of unfairness here derives from particular, inessential features of our economic system. In many hiring or job placement situations in our society, we make no effort to calculate macroproductivity from job assignments. We assume that macro-productivity is always directly proportional to microproductivity as calculated by relative ability to do a given job considered in isolation. So in most hiring that is done on a merit basis (and of course most is not), we tend to use the microprinciple. From the microproductivity point of view conditioned by such a habitual practice, it does look as though the macro-PJAP makes Jill pay a price we ordinarily might not make her pay.

But if this explanation does *account for* the sense of unfairness some feel, it does not justify it in a relevant way. Our task is not just to describe the intuitions we have, influenced as they are by existing economic arrangements. Rather, where we have some reason to think the intuitions are just a by-product of existing institutions, where our task is to find principles to establish institutions we think more just than existing ones, then we may be forced to modify or abandon some of our habitual intuitions. If the PJAP appears on theoretical grounds to be a more plausible principle governing the institution of job place-ment, then our attachment to microproductivity considerations may seem unjustifiable. Moreover, if an individual's sense of fairness were molded by institutions which took macroproductivity into account, not just microproductivity, then our data on unfairness might disappear. If Jill (and others) knew the PJAP and not the microprinciple were deter-mining job placement, no legitimate expectations of hers (or ours) would be unsatisfied if she were selected for *B* rather than *A*.

I have been trying to show that it is appropriate to use the macro-PJAP rather than the alternative microproductivity principle, since the rationale for worrying about job-related abilities at all is their overall connection to productivity. For purposes of my exposition, however, I do not have to rule out some version of the microprinciple wherever it is construed as a rough, practical guide to the application of the macroprinciple. That is, given societies (like ours) in which there is no provision for a more scientific method of calculating maximally productive job arrays, in which most hiring or placement for positions is done on a decentralized, job-by-job basis, then the microprinciple may be the best rule of thumb. Such a compromise in practice is not, however, a compromise with the rationale behind the PJAP. It is important to note, however, that the PJAP seems to presuppose a more sophisticated theory of productivity measurement and may also commit us to more elaborate, centralized hiring than the microprinciple. Since my task here is to analyze where a particular notion of merit leads us, I need not evaluate these last considerations to determine the ultimate desirability of the PJAP or the microprinciple.

In any case, keeping in mind the compromise just proposed, I will assume that meritocrats can agree on the macro-PJAP. But it must be clear what this assumption implies: an individual merits a job if his or her placement in that job is part of an array of maximally productive job assignments. Such a merit claim does not presuppose that any kind of desert claim is present other than what can be derived from productivity considerations. Our obligation to honor a merit claim so derived is only as strong as the prima facie obligation to encourage productivity.

Some may feel that the truncated notion of merit emerging from my analysis must be an incorrect one because it omits any appeal to a stronger notion of desert. They are inclined to assert that if Jill has the greater ability, then Jill *deserves* the job. But the force of my argument is to leave us wondering whether there is a plausible basis for such a desert claim at all, given that our selection of certain abilities as relevant for job placement was based on their connection to productivity. One possible basis is the view that such desert claims derive from a purported "right to self-fulfillment": Jill has a right to be maximally self-fulfilled, and exercising her best abilities in a suitable job is necessary for such self-fulfillment. It is worth noting, however, the lack of any uniform connection between a person's sense of fulfillment and the exercise of his (objectively) best abilities. I may be more fulfilled not doing what I am best at, even more fulfilled than someone who is better at doing the same job. And it would not do at all to say that my right to self-fulfillment should provide a basis for desert only when I would be exercising my objectively best (most productive) abilities. But this would be the only way to grant Jill and deny Jack a desert claim to job *A*, assuming that (subjectively) each would judge *A* more self-fulfilling. I conclude that ability-based merit claims of the type I have picked out do not support claims to "deserve" particular placements.

Before considering the two remaining types of principles regulating meritocracies, I would like to comment briefly on the relevance of merit claims as I have described them to the contemporary issue of affirmative action and preferential hiring. Opponents of the preferential hiring of competent minority members or women sometimes argue that not choosing the most competent job applicant, as measured by some relevant test score or by standard professional criteria, is a violation of the presumed rights of the most competent applicant. Of course, this argument is only one of many and I do not think it is the most powerful, but I am concerned here only with it.[6]

Suppose I am right that the proper way to analyze a merit claim for a job based on possession of certain abilities is to derive the claim from a macroproductivity principle such as the PJAP. Then several difficulties face the opponent of preferential hiring who appeals to a merit claim. For one thing, it becomes much harder to argue that a higher test score or higher standing on relevant professional criteria automatically gives one a stronger claim to a job or position than someone else who can perform it competently but not quite as well. Even assuming valid criteria, such scores would automatically establish a merit claim only on a microprinciple, such as the one we thought less desirable. If we adopt a macroproductivity principle, such as the PJAP, then the strength of my claim to a particular job is not determined by my "pretested" competency for that job. Other macroproductivity factors count. Indeed, if we consider some of the macroproductivity considerations that might result from a better mix of races and sexes in certain positions, it becomes plausible that microproductivity considerations alone would be misleading. A better mix of race and sex in such professions as the law, teaching, and medicine might well pay dividends in terms of services rendered to those who would not otherwise get them, inspiration to long-suppressed motivation, the overcoming of racial and sexual stereotypes which are unproductive in other ways, and so on. But the proponent of affirmative action should beware that the appeal to the PJAP does not backfire. Suppose, for example, productivity is reduced because of sexist or racist opposition to what otherwise would be a meritocratic placement. Then the PJAP might play a conservative role, capitulating to existing biases. (We might have to appeal to considerations of justice to block such applications of the PJAP.)

I think there is an even more important effect of accepting the analysis of merit I have proposed. Whether my claim to merit a particular job more than another depends on the PJAP or on a microprinciple, it nevertheless depends for its justification only on efficiency or productivity. If considerations of right or justice demand that we override such efficiency considerations – for example, to satisfy a concern for equality in the distribution of certain social goods or to compensate for past injustice or to reward for past service – then we are not faced with a case of pitting claims of right against other claims of right. Rather, we pit considerations of productivity against considerations of justice. Many will feel less concerned about such compromises of productivity than they would if a claim to merit a job was really a claim of right, a claim of justice. If a claim to merit a job is a real desert claim supporting a right claim, if it is derived from considerations other than productivity alone, then it might seem far more problematic why such a claim is given less weight than the other principle of justice appealed to in overriding it. At least, a more clear-cut argument would seem to be needed to establish priorities among such claims of justice than would be needed to temper productivity considerations by appeal to principles of justice. I am not implying that we should never temper demands of justice by appeal to efficiency considerations. Rather, I am pointing out the apparent shift in the weight of the objection to preferential hiring when one moves from the assertion, "An appeal to just deserts backs my claim to have a right to that job," to the assertion, "An appeal to productivity supports my claim to have that job."

Of course, my argument here does not take into account the role of expectations in actual situations. One could argue that people who claim a right to a given job on the basis of their better qualifications are doing so because they have been led to form specific expectations about how society distributes social goods, such as desirable positions.[7] When institutions are presumed to and do lead people to form certain expectations, and then society "changes the rules of the game," some sort of compact or contract may be violated. But such an argument from expectations can become woefully conservative if it turns out that the principles governing those institutions and the expectations they generate are not acceptable principles of justice.

A further objection is that a productivity consideration such as that underlying the PJAP *can* become the basis for a claim of right or an entitlement claim if, for example, the PJAP would be adopted as a principle of justice. Suppose, for example, that Rawlsian contractors in an original position would agree to adopt meritocratic job placement principles and conditions of opportunity as part of a preferred conception of justice. (I think this choice is in fact made by Rawls' contractors.) Then the PJAP, although supported by arguments based on productivity considerations, would give rise to entitlements. I have no quarrel with this objection if it is appropriately qualified. My argument above can provide the appropriate qualifications. Such contractors should not choose the PJAP without first choosing relevant compensatory and retributive principles which take priority over entitlements derived from the PJAP. I need not argue that merit claims can never be construed as entitlements; I need only show that they are entitlements only if they are not superseded by stronger ones.

One last objection is worth noting. It may well be argued that for certain jobs, productivity considerations alone may give rise to claims of right by those most competent to perform them. Suppose it could be shown that recipients of certain services or products – perhaps, for example, patients or students – have a right to the highest quality service or product possible. Then it might be argued that those most capable of providing the service or product have a right to the relevant jobs. At least it might be shown that there is a duty to give such persons the jobs. If the details of such an argument could be satisfactorily provided, it might force an important qualification of the PJAP; it might force us to use the microprinciple for assignments to certain jobs. Alternatively, such cases might be handled simply by giving extra weight to the satisfaction of student or patient interests and rights in the calculation of macroproductivity. The difficulty of deciding which way to handle these cases derives from the unfortunate imprecision of the broad notion of productivity (macroproductivity) I have appealed to; nor can I remedy the imprecision in any simple way here.

<h3 style="text-align:center">III</h3>

I would like to return now to discuss the remaining types of principles meritocrats share. Although there may be some exceptions, I believe that most meritocrats would view fair, rather than just formal, equality of opportunity as the appropriate precondition for application of the PJAP. Formal equality of opportunity obtains when there are no legal or quasi-legal barriers to people having equal access (based on merit) to positions and offices or to the means (education and training) needed to qualify one for access to such jobs. Fair equality of opportunity requires not only that negative legal or quasi-legal constraints on equality of opportunity be eliminated, but also that positive steps must be taken to provide equality of access – and the means to achieve such equality of access – to those with inferior initial competitive positions resulting from family background or other biological or social accidents.

If we make the empirical assumption that conditions of fair opportunity maximize the availability of human talents which would otherwise be wasted under conditions of merely formal opportunity, then considerations of productivity alone carry us some way toward the preference for fair opportunity. Fair, not formal, opportunity is likely to yield the optimal equivalence class of maximally productive job assignment arrays. Of course efficiency considerations alone may *not* always point to

310

fair rather than formal opportunity. If a tremendous superfluity of available abilities resulted from formal opportunity alone, then in order to produce increases in the maximally productive class of job assignments, more might have to be invested in fair opportunity than is justified by the size of those increases. Similarly, if early, arbitrary selection of some individuals for special training for certain jobs was maximally efficient, other nonutilitarian arguments might be needed before fair opportunity would be preferred. Rawls, for example, does not rest his argument for fair opportunity on grounds of efficiency alone. Rather, he argues that people will feel they do not have fair access to the centrally important social good of self-realization if formal, rather than fair, opportunity is instituted.[8] In any case, I will assume that meritocrats generally treat fair, not formal, opportunity as the precondition for applying the PJAP. Little in my argument hangs on this assumption.

Thus far I have said nothing about the rewards and burdens that accompany different jobs. The PJAP, as I have presented it, is defined without reference to any particular schedule of rewards and burdens. So far, although an individual may claim to merit a job when his having it satisfies the PJAP, there is no sense given to his meriting any particular set of rewards or burdens. I have deliberately dissociated the meritocratic basis for job assignment from the process of determining the schedule of benefits and burdens associated with different jobs or positions.[9]

I think it is possible for meritocrats to differ on the reward schedules they join to the system structured by the PJAP and fair equality of opportunity. Consider the following six meritocracies which differ only in their reward schedules:

(1) Unbridled meritocracy. The reward schedule allows whatever rewards those who attain positions of power and prestige can acquire for themselves.
(2) Desert meritocracy. The reward schedule allows rewards proportional to the contribution of the jobs (but not constrained by efficiency considerations as in meritocracy 3); alternatively, the desert basis might have nothing to do with productivity – it might be moral worthiness, for example.
(3) Utilitarian meritocracy. The reward schedule allows inequalities that act to maximize average or total utility.
(4) Maximin meritocracy. The reward schedule allows inequalities that act to maximize the index of primary social goods of those who are worst off.
(5) Strict egalitarian meritocracy. No inequalities in reward are allowed.

(6) Socialist meritocracy. The reward schedule allows no inequalities in the satisfaction of (basic?) needs.

My list allows for meritocracies which no one may explicitly have supported. And, for the sake of brevity, it does not include all possible favorites. But the main point should be clear, namely, I do not consider it an essential feature of a meritocracy that efficiency is the sole principle governing selection of reward schedules, but I do believe that an appeal to productivity in job assignment is always involved in meritocracy through the PJAP.

A number of qualifying remarks are in order. First, unless certain empirical conditions obtain, meritocracy may prove to be a theory which greatly underdetermines social structure on just the points it was intended to determine. If application of the PJAP is to determine job placement effectively, then the equivalence class of maximally productive jobs would have to be fairly small. I am inclined to believe, however, that the equivalence class of maximally efficient arrays of job assignments will be quite large under real conditions of fair equality of opportunity. With adequate education and training, most people might competently perform almost any job, or at least a very large range of jobs. At the least, relevant abilities will turn out to be far less scarce a resource than most meritocrats think. If I am right, then the claims that individuals can make vis-à-vis one another – for example, that one merits a job more than another – would be substantially weakened. We would lack principles sufficient to justify claims to be placed in a given job since our candidate for a necessary and sufficient condition turns out to be far from sufficient under these empirical conditions.

Second, other empirical difficulties face application of the PJAP. This principle presupposes that we have very good ways of predicting which constellation of abilities and personality traits will lead to successful – that is, productive – performance of a given job. But many of our current efforts in those directions are woefully inadequate. Much is often made, for example, of the fact that IQ scores correlate fairly with job status; the average doctor has a higher IQ score than the average carpenter, and so on. But what is not so often noted is that IQ scores correlate miserably with level of success at a given job. So the argument that knowledge of IQ gives us a good estimate of how well someone will do at a given job is unfounded.[10] All this point means is that we are far from having available to us the measuring and predicting instruments needed to operate a thoroughly meritocratic society such as the one Young describes, since we cannot meet the conditions necessary for applying the PJAP.

Third, my analysis of meritocracy seems to allow too many types of theories in under that name. For example, Rawls explicitly argues that his Second Principle does not lead to the type of meritocracy advocated by Young because natural abilities are viewed as social, not just individual assets, and inequalities act to help the worst-off members of the society.[11] But if Rawls, or at least someone much like him who subscribes to type (4) meritocracy, is stuck with the label "meritocrat" on my schema, still, he is not thereby committed to any of the undesirable features of the meritocracies attacked in *A Theory of Justice*. At the same time, the label captures the fact that he shares with other meritocrats certain common principles.

A final, most important qualification: My analysis might seem to imply that we know how to apply the PJAP independently of fixing a reward schedule. But such independence is unlikely. Different reward schedules would presumably affect the motivations of individuals who contemplate entering certain jobs. Just this point is at the heart of Rawls' view that material incentives will be necessary if we are to procure the greatest talent possible for certain burdensome jobs. So it seems we cannot fix on an equivalence class of maximally productive job assignments, which we need for application of the PJAP, until we know something of the reward structure. But this fact does not alter my main point: we can distinguish the PJAP from the reward principles, and what all meritocrats share is appeal to the PJAP and fair equality of opportunity, however else they may differ in their use of reward schedules.[12]

If we keep our attention on the shared features of meritocracy, we can see why many varied theorists have found something attractive in it. Indeed, insisting that job placement be meritocratic under conditions of fair equality of opportunity leads to serious criticism of existing institutions. However, these shared principles always operate against a background determined by the reward schedule. And in our society, the reward schedule is rarely itself the target of challenge by meritocrats. Meritocracy becomes controversial when we begin to see the consequences of meritocratic job placement operating in a context of certain reward schedules.

The meritocracies I listed earlier include three types of reward schedules. Inegalitarian meritocracies (unbridled, desert according to contribution, and utilitarian) allow significant inequalities in rewards with no special constraints to protect those with the worst jobs. Egalitarian meritocracies either allow no significant inequalities or allow inequalities not based on the social functions of the jobs but rather on the needs or other deserts of the job holder. The maximin meritocracy allows inequalities but constrains them in ways that act to benefit those whose abilities tend to lead to low-reward jobs. Inegalitarian meritocracies may be open to a criticism that egalitarian or maximin meritocracies avoid.[13]

Suppose that the abilities and traits that qualify a person for high-reward jobs are primarily the result of natural and social contingencies over which he has little control. We might suppose that even the agent's choices about which abilities he wants to develop are made within a range heavily determined by factors beyond his control. Then it seems one's qualifications for meritocratic job placement are largely the result of happy or unhappy accident, and one has done little to *deserve* them. It is just this fact which made it so hard to establish a desert claim, which connects abilities to jobs, stronger than the weak merit claim I derived from productivity considerations. So it seems that the meritocrat is committed, given his concern for productivity, to distributing at least some social goods, the jobs themselves, in accordance with a morally arbitrary distribution of abilities and traits.

Suppose further, however, that a reward schedule allows significant inequalities of reward to be associated with different jobs. Then, the fortuitous possession of certain natural abilities and traits makes one the beneficiary of significant social rewards as well. Such a double reward for undeserved abilities and traits seems to ramify morally arbitrary facts into ones of great social significance. This objection, of course, is the basis for Rawls' attack on nonmaximin meritocracies.[14] Egalitarian meritocracies avoid the criticism. And maximin meritocracies dodge its main force since they moderate the effects of fortuitous distributions of talents. For anyone who feels the power of this argument against moral arbitrariness (and not everyone does, notably Nozick),[15] the price the meritocrat must pay is the adoption of egalitarian – or fairly egalitarian (maximin) – reward schedules.

Unfortunately, many proponents of meritocracy have been so concerned with combating the lesser evil of nonmeritocratic job placement that they have left unchallenged the greater evil of highly inegalitarian reward schedules. One even suspects that an elitist infatuation for such inegalitarian reward schedules lurks behind their ardor for meritocratic job placement. In any case, they often ignore the distinction between principles governing placement and those governing reward and the fact that quite different rationales are involved in justifying two such different types of principles.

NOTES

This paper grew out of remarks I made as commentator on Alan Soble's "Meritocracy and Rawls' Second Principle" presented at the Western Division APA Meetings, New Orleans, April 1976. I have benefited from discussion with Hugo Bedau and John Troyer, as well as from comments on versions of this paper read at Tufts, Brown, Calgary, Georgetown, and the Society for Philosophy and Public Policy Symposium at the Pacific Division APA Meetings, Spring 1977.

1 It is an interesting question, which I cannot pursue here, whether such meritocracies are not just as concerned with productivity as the modern versions I do discuss, though their social goals and the means of achieving them differ.

2 Michael Young, *Rise of the Meritocracy* (London: Thames and Hudson, 1958).

3 Some meritocrats assume (see Richard Herrnstein, *IQ in the Meritocracy*, Boston: Atlantic, Little Brown, 1973) that there is some one scale of capacity differences, usually taken to be IQ, which suffices to rank-order people for job eligibility across the whole spectrum of jobs. I do not think such a uniquely hierarchical view is presupposed by the meritocratic core principles I describe. For critical discussion of IQ as a basis for such scale, see my "IQ, Heritability, and Human Nature," in *PSA 1974*, ed. R. S. Cohen et al., in *Boston Studies in the Philosophy of Science*, XXXII (Dordrecht: Reidel, 1976), pp. 143–180; J. Cronin, N. Daniels et al., "Race, Class & Intelligence," *International Journal of Mental Health* 2, no. 4 (1975): 46–132; N. J. Block and G. Dworkin, *The IQ Controversy* (New York: Pantheon, 1976), Part IV; and S. Bowles and H. Gintis, *Schooling in Capitalist America* (New York: Basic Books, 1976), ch. 4.

4 John Troyer urged me to consider the implications of this case.

5 Yet another alternative, which I am not concerned to refute here, is that personal traits or achievements other than those related to job competence should be the basis for claims of desert or merit for job placement.

6 More powerful objections are based on the inappropriateness of compensating (perhaps the wrong) individuals for injuries done to others in a group, or on the injustice of using racial or sex quotas at all, or on the injustice of making a small group of nonminority males pay the brunt of the compensation for past injustice. I cannot consider these objections here.

7 Alan Goldman suggests such an argument in "Affirmative Action," *Philosophy & Public Affairs* 5, no. 2 (Winter 1976): 191.

8 John Rawls, *A Theory of Justice* (Cambridge, Mass.: Harvard University Press, 1971), p. 84.

9 Thomas Nagel makes a related point when he says, "Certain abilities may be relevant to filling a job from the point of view of efficiency, but they are not relevant from the point of view of justice, because they provide no indication that one deserves the rewards that go with holding that job. The qualities, experience, and attainments that make success in a certain position likely do not in themselves merit the rewards that happen to attach to occupancy of that position in a competitive economy." See "Equal Treatment and Compensatory Discrimination," *Philosophy & Public Affairs* 2, no. 4 (Summer 1973): 352.

10 There is much evidence that IQ plays little direct causal role in determining job level and social status. Much of its influence is artifactual, the effect of such tests being used for educational tracking and job placement.

11 Rawls, *A Theory of Justice*, p. 106ff.

12 Two further objections might be raised here. John Troyer has suggested the

first: Why would someone who rejects productivity considerations in his reward schedule, adopting instead a strong desert-based reward schedule, subscribe to the PJAP? The answer is, I think, that people might consistently want to know that their rewards will be based on, say, moral worthiness or industriousness and still believe that access to jobs should be determined by merit, as earlier defined, because it is important to secure proper performance. A second objection is that not all the principles of reward I have described can be readily construed as governing a society's basic institutions or structure, as Rawls would have it. This objection has weight, but how much depends on the clarity of the notion of "basic structure." For worries about this clarity, see Hugo Adam Bedau, "Social Justice and Social Institutions," *Midwest Studies in Philosophy* 3 (February 1978).

13 The following discussion of moral arbitrariness, in particular the debate between John Rawls and Robert Nozick on the question, is pursued at greater length in a different version of this paper in *Justice and Economic Distribution*, ed. John Arthur and William Shaw (Englewood Cliffs, N.J.: Prentice-Hall, 1978).

14 Rawls, *A Theory of Justice*, p. 106ff.

15 Robert Nozick, *Anarchy, State & Utopia* (New York: Basic Books, 1974), ch. 7.

Chapter 15

Rationing fairly: Programmatic considerations

Despite its necessity, rationing raises troublesome questions about fairness. We ration in situations in which losers, as well as winners, have plausible claims to have their needs met. When we knowingly and deliberately refrain from meeting some legitimate needs, we had better have justification for the distributive choices we make. Not surprisingly, health planners and legislators appeal to bioethicists for help, asking what justice requires here. Can we help them? I think we are not ready to yet, and I will support this claim by noting four general rationing problems that we remain unsure how to solve, illustrating how they plague Oregon's rationing plan.

Before turning to the four problems, I want to make several preliminary remarks. First, philosophers (including me) have traditionally underestimated the importance of rationing, thinking of it as a peripheral, not central, problem. Since we simply cannot afford, for example, to educate, treat medically, or protect legally people in all the ways their needs for these goods require or the accepted distributive principles seem to demand, rationing is clearly pervasive, not peripheral.

Rationing decisions share three key features. First, the goods we often must provide – legal services, health care, educational benefits – are not divisible without loss of benefit, unlike money. We thus cannot avoid unequal or "lumpy" distributions. Meeting the educational, health-care, or legal needs of some people, for example, will mean that the requirements of others will go unsatisfied. Second, when we ration, we deny benefits to some individuals who can plausibly claim they are owed them in principle. They can cite an accepted principle of distributive justice that governs their situation and should protect them. Third, the general distributive principles appealed to by claimants as well as by rationers do not by themselves provide adequate reasons for choosing among claimants: they are too schematic. This point was driven

317

Justice and justification

home to me by the way in which my "fair equality of opportunity" account of just health care (Daniels 1985, 1988) fails to yield specific solutions to the rationing problems I shall survey. Finally, even the best work in the general theory of justice has not squarely faced the problems raised by the indeterminacy of distributive principles. Rawls (1971), for example, suggests that the problem of fleshing out the content of principles of distributive justice is ultimately procedural, falling to the legislature. Perhaps, but the claim that we must in general turn to a fair democratic procedure should not be an assumption, but the conclusion, either of a general argument or of a failed search for appropriate moral constraints on rationing. If however, there are substantive principles governing rationing, then the theory of justice is incomplete in a way we have not noticed. This point cuts across the debates between proponents of "local justice" (Walzer 1983; Elster 1992) and "global justice" (Rawls 1971; Gauthier 1986), and between liberalism and communitarianism (cf. Emanuel 1991; Daniels 1992).

FOUR UNSOLVED RATIONING PROBLEMS:
ILLUSTRATIONS FROM OREGON

The fair chances/best outcomes problem

Before seeing how the fair chances/best outcomes problem arises in Oregon's macrorationing plan, consider its more familiar microrationing form: Which of several equally needy individuals should get a scarce resource, such as a heart transplant? Suppose, for example, that Alice and Betty are the same age, have waited on queue the same time, and that each will live only one week without a transplant. With the transplant, however, Alice is expected to live two years and Betty twenty. Who should get the transplant (cf. Kamm 1989)? Giving priority to producing best outcomes, a priority built into some point systems for awarding organs, would mean that Betty gets the organ and Alice dies (assuming persistent scarcity of organs, as Brock 1988 notes). But Alice might complain, "Why should I give up my only chance at survival – and two years of survival is not insignificant – just because Betty has a chance to live longer? It is not fair that I give up everything that is valuable to me just so Betty can have more of what is valuable to her." Alice demands a lottery that gives her an equal chance with Betty.

Some people agree with Alice's complaint and agree with her demand for a lottery. Few would agree with her, however, if she had very little chance at survival; more would agree if her outcomes were only somewhat worse than Betty's. Still, at the level of intuitions, there is much disagreement about when and how much to favor best outcomes.

Brock (1988), like Broome (1987), proposes breaking this deadlock by giving Alice and Betty chances proportional to the benefits they can get (e.g., by assigning Alice one side of a ten-sided die). Kamm (1989, 1993) notes that Brock's proposal must be amended once we allow differences in urgency or need among patients. She favors assigning multiplicative weights to the degree of need or urgency. Then, the neediest might end up with no chance to receive a transplant if their outcomes were very poor, but, compared to Brock's "proportional chances" proposal, they would have greater opportunity to get an organ if their outcomes were reasonably high.[1] Both Brock's and Kamm's suggestions seem ad hoc. That there is some force to each of Alice's and Betty's demands does not, as Brock would have it, mean the force is clearly equal; similarly, assigning weights to more factors, as Kamm does, seems to add an element of precision lacking in our intuitions about these cases. Our intuitions may fall short of giving us clear, orderly principles here.

We might try to break the deadlock at the level of intuitions by appealing to more theoretical considerations. For example, we might respond to Alice that she already has lost a "natural" lottery; she might have been the one with twenty years expected survival, but it turned out to be Betty instead. After the fact, however, Alice is unlikely to agree that there has already been a fair "natural" lottery, even assuming that there were no prior differences in access to care and so on: To undercut Alice's demand for a new lottery, we would have to persuade her that the proper perspective for everyone to adopt is *ex ante*, not *ex post*, information about her condition (cf. Menzel 1989). But what should Alice know about herself *ex ante*? If Alice knows about her family history of heart disease, she might well not favor giving complete priority to best outcomes. Perhaps Alice should agree it is reasonable to adopt a more radical *ex ante* position, one that denies her all information about herself, a thick "veil of ignorance." Controversy persists. Behind such a veil, some would argue that it would be irrational to forego the greater expected payoff that would result from giving priority to best outcomes.[2] Citing Rawls' adoption of a maximin strategy, Kamm (1993) argues against such "gambling" behind the veil. Alternatively, she appeals to Scanlon (1982): If Alice would "reasonably regret" losing to Betty, then she should not be held to a scheme that favors best outcomes. Unclear about our intuitions, we are also stymied by a controversy at the deepest theoretical levels.

The best outcomes problem arises in macrorationing as well. Consider HHS Secretary Louis Sullivan's (1992) recent refusal to grant a Medicaid waiver to Oregon's rationing plan. Sullivan's main criticism of the Oregon plan is that in preferring treatments that provide greater net benefits the plan discriminates against the disabled.[3] The clearest

Justice and justification

example of such discrimination would be this: Two groups of patients are in need of a treatment that can give them a net benefit of a given magnitude; because one group has a disability, e.g., difficulty walking, that would not be affected by the treatment, we deny them the treatment. Neither Sullivan nor the NLC give an example, even hypothetical, of how this situation could arise in the Oregon scheme. The denial of coverage for aggressive treatment of very low birthweight (<500 gr) neonates, which they do cite as an example of discrimination, is not an appropriate example, because the denial is premised on the lack of benefit produced by aggressive treatment of such neonates.

Consider an example suggestive of the Oregon scheme. Suppose two treatments, T1 and T2, can benefit different groups of patients, G1 and G2 as follows. T1 preserves life for G1s (or provides some other major benefit), but it does not restore a particular function, such as walking, to G1s. T2 not only preserves life for G2s (or provides some other major benefit), but it also enables them to walk again. The Oregon Health Service Commission ranks T2 as a more important service than T1 because it produces a greater net benefit (I ignore the OTA 1991 argument that net benefit is not a major contributor to rank). Sullivan says that it is discriminatory to deny G1s T1, even though a single person would clearly consider relative benefit in deciding between T1 and T2.

The Sullivan/NLCMDD objection can, with charity, be interpreted as a version of Alice's complaint that favoring best outcomes denies her a fair chance at a benefit. Interpreted this way, the Sullivan/NLCMDD objection is that we cannot rule out giving G1s any chance at the benefit treatment would bring them simply because G2s would benefit more from the use of our limited resources. In effect, they seem to be saying we should give no weight to best outcomes. As I noted earlier, this extreme position does not seem to match our intuitions in the microrationing case. But neither does the alternative extreme position, that we must always give priority to better outcomes. The point is that a rationing approach that ranks services by net benefit, whether it turns out to be Oregon's scheme or simply Hadorn's (1991) alternative proposal, thus carries with it unsolved moral issues. To justify ranking by net benefit we must be prepared to address those underlying issues.

The priorities problem

Oregon's (intended) methodology of ranking by net benefit also ignores the moral issues I group here as the priorities problem. Suppose that two treatment/condition pairs give equal net benefits. (Remember, this does not generally mean they produce the same health outcomes, only the same net benefits). Then the OHSC should rank them equal in importance. But now suppose that people with C_1 are more seriously impaired by their disease or disability than people with C_2. Though T_1 and T_2 produce equivalent net gains in benefit, people with C_2 will end up better off than people with C_1, since they started out better off. Nothing in the method of ranking treatment/condition pairs by net benefit responds to this difference between C_1s and C_2s. Nevertheless, most of us would judge it more important to give services to C_1s than it is to give them to C_2s under these conditions. We feel at least some inclination to help those worse off than those better off. For example, if C_1s after treatment were no better off than C_2s before treatment, we are more strongly inclined to give priority to the worst off. Our concern to respect that priority might decline if the effect of treating C_1s but not C_2s is that C_1s end up better off than C_2s. How troubled we would be by this outcome might depend on how great the new inequality turned out to be, or on how significant the residual impairment of C_2s was.

Suppose now that there is greater net benefit from giving T_2 to C_2s than there is from giving T_1 to C_1s. If C_1s are sufficiently worse off to start with than C_2s, and if C_1s end up worse off or not significantly better off than C_2s, then our concern about priorities may compel us to forego the greater net benefit that results from giving T_2 to C_2s. But how much priority we give to the worst off still remains unclear. If we can only give a very modest improvement to the worst off, but we must forego a very significant improvement to those initially better off, then we may overrule our concern for the worst off. Our intuitions do not pull us toward a strict priority for the worst off.

Just what the structure of our concern about priority is, however, remains unclear. The unsolved priorities problem not only affects a methodology that ranks by net benefit or by net QALYs. It affects cost/benefit and cost/effectiveness rankings, including Eddy's (1991a) "willingness to pay" methodology. So too does the aggregation problem, to which I now briefly turn.

The aggregation problem

In June of 1990, the Oregon Health Services Commission released a list of treatment/condition pairs ranked by a cost/benefit calculation. Critics were quick to seize on rankings that seemed completely counterintuitive. For example, as Hadorn noted (1991), toothcapping was ranked higher than appendectomy. The reason was simple: an appendectomy cost about $4,000, many times the cost of capping a tooth. Simply aggregating the net medical benefit of many capped teeth yielded a net benefit greater than that produced by one appendectomy.

Eddy (1991b) points out that our intuitions in these cases are largely based on comparing treatment/condition pairs for their importance on a one:one basis. One appendectomy is more important than one toothcapping because it saves a life rather than merely reduces pain and preserves dental function. But our intuitions are much less developed when it comes to making one:many comparisons (though we can establish indifference curves that capture trades we are willing to make; cf. Nord 1993). When does saving more lives through one technology mean we should forego saving fewer through another? The complex debate about whether "numbers count" has a bearing on rationing problems. How many legs should we be willing to forego saving in order to save one life? How many eyes? How many teeth? Can we aggregate *any* small benefits, or only those that are in some clear way significant, when we want to weight these benefits against clearly significant benefits (e.g., saving a life) to a few? Kamm (1987, 1993) argues persuasively that we should not favor saving one life and curing a sore throat over saving a different life, because curing a sore throat is not a "competitor" with saving a life. She also argues that benefits that someone is morally not required to sacrifice in order to save another's life also have significant standing and can be aggregated. If we are not required to sacrifice an arm in order to save someone's life, then we can aggregate arms saved and weigh them against lives saved. She suggests that our judgments about aggregation differ if we are in contexts where saving lives rather than inducing harms (positive vs. negative duties) is at issue.

Kamm shows that we are not straightforward aggregators of all benefits and that our moral views are both complex and difficult to explicate in terms of well-ordered principles. These views are not compatible with the straightforward aggregation (sum ranking) that is presupposed by the dominant methodologies derived from welfare economics. Yet we do permit, indeed require, some forms of aggregation. Our philosophical task is to specify which principles governing aggregation have the strongest justification. If it appears there is no plausible, principled account of aggregation, then we have strong reason to rely instead on fair procedures and an obligation to give an account of such procedures (see Postscript).

The democracy problem

When Sullivan rejected Oregon's application for a Medicaid waiver, he complained that the methodology for assessing net medical benefit drew on biased or discriminatory public attitudes toward disabilities. Adapting Kaplan's (Kaplan and Anderson 1990) "quality of well-being" scale for use in measuring the benefit of medical treatments, Oregon surveyed residents, asking them to judge on a scale of 0 (death) to 100 (perfect health) what the impact would be of having to live the rest of one's life with some physical or mental impairment or symptom; for example, wearing eyeglasses was rated 95 out of 100, for a weighting of −0.05. Many of these judgments seem downright bizarre, whether or not they reflect bias. For example, having to wear eyeglasses was rated slightly worse than the −0.046 weighting assigned to not being able to drive a car or use public transportation or the −0.049 assigned to having to stay at a hospital or nursing home. Other weightings clearly reflected cultural attitudes and possible bias: having trouble with drugs or alcohol was given the second most negative weighting (−0.455) of all conditions, much worse than, for example, having a bad burn over large areas of one's body (−0.372) or being so impaired that one needs help to eat or go to the bathroom (−0.106). Having to use a walker or wheelchair under one's own control was weighted as much worse (−0.373) than having losses of consciousness from seizures, blackouts, or coma (−0.114).

Claiming that people who experience a disabling condition, like being unable to walk, tend to give less negative ratings to them than people who have experienced them, Sullivan argued Oregon was likely to underestimate the benefit of a treatment that left people with such disabilities. Excluding such treatments would thus be the result of public bias.[4] His complaint carries over to other methodologies, e.g., Eddy's (1991a) willingness-to-pay approach and the use of QALYs in cost-effectiveness or cost-benefit analyses.

Sullivan's complaint raises an interesting question: Whose judgments about the effects of a condition should be used? Those who do not have a disabling condition may suffer from cultural biases, over-estimating the impact of disability. But those who have the condition may rate it as less serious because they have modified their preferences, goals, and values in order to make a "healthy adjustment" to their condition. Their overall dissatisfaction − tapped by these methodologies − may not reflect the impact that would be captured by a measure more directly attuned to the range of capabilities they retain. Still, insisting on the more objective measure has a high political cost and may even seem paternalistic.

Sullivan simply assumes that we must give priority to the judgments made by those experiencing the condition, but that is not so obvious. Clearly, there is something attractive about the idea, embedded in all these methodologies, of assessing the relative impact of conditions on people by asking them what they think about that impact (cf. Menzel

1992). Should we give people what they actually want? Or should we give them what they should want, correcting for various defects in their judgment? What corrections to expressed preferences are plausible?

The democracy problem arises at another level in procedures that purport to be directly democratic. The Oregon plan called for the OHSC to respect "community values" in its ranking of services. Because prevention and family planning services were frequently discussed in community meetings, the OHSC assigned the categories including those services very high ranking. Consequently, in Oregon, vasectomies are ranked more important that hip replacements. Remember the priority and aggregation problems: it would seem more important to restore mobility to someone who cannot walk than to improve the convenience of birth control through vasectomy in several people. But, assuming that the Commissioners properly interpreted the wishes of Oregonians, that is not what Oregonians wanted the rankings to be. Should we treat this as error? Or must we abide by whatever the democratic process yields?

Thus far I have characterized the problem of democracy as a problem of error: a fair democratic process, or a methodology that rests in part on expressions of preferences, leads to judgments that deviate from either intuitive or theoretically based judgements about the relative importance of certain health outcomes or services. The problem is how much weight to give the intuitive or theoretically based judgments as opposed to the expressed preferences. The point should be put in another way as well. Should we in the end think of the democratic process as a matter of pure procedural justice? If so, then we have no way to correct the judgment made through that process, for what it determines to be fair is what counts as fair. Or should we really consider the democratic process as an impure and imperfect form of procedural justice? Then it is one that can be corrected by appeal to some prior notion of what constitutes a fair outcome of rationing. I suggest that we do not yet know the answer to this question, and we will not be able to answer it until we work harder at providing a theory of rationing.

CONCLUSION

I conclude with a plea against provincialism. The four problems I illustrated have their analogues in the rationing of goods other than health care. To flesh out a principle that says "people are equal before the law" will involve decisions about how to allocate legal services among all people who can make plausible claims to need them by citing that principle. Similarly, to give content to a principle that assures equal educational opportunity will involve decisions about resource allocation very much like those involved in rationing health care. Being provincial about health-care rationing will prevent us from seeing the relationships among these rationing problems. Conversely, a rationing theory will have greater force if it derives from consideration of common types of problems that are independent of the kinds of goods whose distribution is in question. I am suggesting that exploring a theory of rationing in this way is a prolegomenon to serious work in "applied ethics."

ACKNOWLEDGEMENT

This work was generously supported by the National Endowment for the Humanities (RH20917) and the National Library of Medicine (1R01LM05005). I also wish to thank Tufts University and Harvard's Program in Ethics and the Professions for Sabbatical support.

NOTES

1 Kamm (1989, 1993) distinguishes urgency, that is, how imminent death would be without a transplant, from need. Need should, in her view, reflect how important living longer is to an individual; specifically, living longer may be more important to someone who has lived a short life than it is to someone who has lived a longer life, so there may be a decreasing marginal utility of living longer.
2 I argued as such in a Battelle project on heart transplantation in the early 1980s; others have made similar arguments.
3 I am taking Sullivan's criticism at face value, though I suspect the rejection of the Medicaid waiver was motivated by political considerations, not incompatibility with the ADA (cf. Hadorn 1992; Capron 1992; Menzel 1992).
4 The OTA (1991) notes that men gave dismenorhea a greater negative weight than women. The effect of this weighting is that greater net benefit, and thus higher rank, accrues to treating dismenorhea if we include the judgments of men than if we counted only the judgments of women.

REFERENCES

Brock, Dan. 1988. "Ethical Issues in Recipient Selection for Organ Transplantation." In D. Mathieu, ed., *Organ Substitution Technology: Ethical, Legal, and Public Policy Issues*, pp. 86–99. Boulder: Westview.
Broome, John. 1987. "Fairness and the Random Distribution of Goods" (unpublished manuscript).
Capron, Alexander. 1992. "Oregon's Disability: Principles or Politics? *Hasting Center Report* 22:6(November–December):18–20.

Daniels, Norman. 1985. *Just Health Care*. Cambridge: Cambridge University Press.

Daniels, Norman. 1988. *Am I My Parents' Keeper? An Essay on Justice between the Young and the Old*. New York: Oxford University Press.

Daniels, Norman. 1992. "Liberalism and Medical Ethics" *Hasting Center Report*. 22:6(November–December):41–3.

Eddy, D. 1991a. "Rationing by Patient Choice," *JAMA* 265:1(January 2):105–8.

Eddy, D. 1991b. "Oregon's Methods: Did Cost-Effectiveness Analysis Fail?" *JAMA* 266:15(October 16):2135–41.

Elster, John. 1992. *Local Justice: How Institutions Allocate Scarce Goods and Necessary Burdens*. New York: Russel Sage.

Emanuel, Ezekial. 1991. *The Ends of Human Life: Medical Ethics in a Liberal Polity*. Cambridge, MA: Harvard University Press.

Gauthier, D. 1986. *Morals by Agreement*. Oxford: Oxford University Press.

Hadorn, David. 1991. "Setting Health Care Priorities in Oregon: Cost-Effectiveness Meets the Rule of Rescue," *JAMA* 265:2218–25.

Hadorn, David. 1992. "The Problem of Discrimination in Health Care Priority Setting," *JAMA* 268:11(16 September):1454–9.

Kamm, Frances. 1987. "Choosing between People: Commonsense Morality and Doctors' Choices" *Bioethics* 1:255–71.

Kamm, Frances. 1989. "The Report of the US Task Force on Organ Transplantation: Criticisms and Alternatives," *Mount Sinai Journal of Medicine* 56:207–20.

Kamm, Frances. 1993. *Morality and Mortality*. Vol. 1. Oxford: Oxford University Press.

Kaplan, R. M., and Anderson, J. P. 1990. "The General Health Policy Model: An Integrated Approach." In B. Spilker, ed., *Quality of Life Assessments in Clinical Trials*. New York: Raven Press.

Menzel, Paul. 1989. *Strong Medicine*. New York: Oxford University Press.

Menzel, Paul. 1992. "Oregon's Denial: Disabilities and Quality of Life" *Hastings Center Report* 22:6(November–December):21–5.

National Legal Center for the Medically Dependent and Disabled. 1991. Letter to Representative Christopher H. Smith.

Nord, Eric. 1993. "The Relevance of Health State after Treatment in Prioritising between Different Patients." *Journal of Medical Ethics* 19:1(March):37–42.

Office of Technology Assessment (OTA). 1991. *Evaluation of the Oregon Medicaid Proposal*. U.S. Congress.

Oregon Health Services Commission. 1991. *Prioritization of Health Services: A Report to the Governor and Legislature*.

Rawls, John. 1971. *A Theory of Justice*. Cambridge, MA: Harvard University Press.

Scanlon, Thomas. 1982. "Contractualism and Utilitarianism." In Amartya Sen and Bernard Williams, eds., *Utilitarianism and Beyond*, pp. 103–28. Cambridge: Cambridge University Press.

Sullivan, Louis. 1992. Press Release (August 3, 1992). Health and Human Services Press Office.

Walzer, Michael. 1983. *Spheres of Justice*. New York: Basic Books.

Postscript: Fair procedures and just rationing

These comments explore briefly a key problem we must face if we accept the argument of "Rationing Fairly." That argument can be summarized briefly as follows:

(1) General principles of distributive justice are too indeterminate to provide us with clear solutions to a cluster of key rationing problems.
(2) We do not have a substantive theory of rationing that can provide bridge principles between institutional design and more general principles of justice; there may be such a theory, but it is not available to us.
(3) We must solve the problems of institutional design in real time.
(4) In the absence of (available) substantive principles for resolving these problems, we must rely on a fair procedure. The basic idea is that the outcome of a fair procedure will then count as fair, even if we cannot cite a substantive distributive principle by reference to which the outcome is fair.

The problem we must face is to describe what counts as a fair procedure for resolving moral disagreements about rationing. Specifically, since many will insist that a fair procedure contain democratic features, we must explain why a fair democratic procedure is an appropriate way to settle a moral problem about rationing. I here only suggest, in a preliminary way, a way around these justificatory worries. More work would have to be done to see just how much practical force the line of justification affords.

Let us suppose that we have two ways of addressing one of the unsolved rationing problems I earlier described, the priorities problem. Suppose, for the sake of specificity, that one-third of the population is willing to give significant priority to the sickest patients, but that two-thirds of the population is not. (We might, for example, find this out through a sophisticated polling method, for example, relying on Nord's (1993) use of indifference curves.) The difference shows up in this way. The minority is willing to trade away much more significant benefits to people who are less sick in order to obtain some benefits for the sickest. The majority is willing to trade away much less in benefits for those who are better off to start with. The population is divided then in the pattern of concern it shows for the sickest patients. We can then imagine that we could use these two positions as distinct criteria for ranking various kinds of treatments that might be applied to the very sick or the mildly sick. Each position yields a different ranking of services, a different rationing strategy. Which criterion should we use, if either? How should we decide?

I want to begin by examining several things that seem problematic about using a democratic procedure, say one resting on a majority vote of a fairly selected committee or commission, to decide this issue. First, consider the analogy to Brian Barry's (1979) discussion of the presuppositions underlying the acceptability of majority rule. He imagines five people confined to a railroad car that has no posted rule about smoking. Under what conditions should a majority vote be used to determine such a rule? For such a vote to give a determinate answer, we might imagine they are making only one choice with two alternatives. A more complex set of choices would outstrip the power of a majority vote to yield answers that reflected in a plausible way the initial preferences. He also notes that the constituency is itself not open to doubt: all travelers are voters. But finally, he notes that no vital or fundamental interest of a party must be at stake. Otherwise simple voting might be too risky for a loss. Barry's example warns against the tyranny of a majority and reminds us of the procedural and substantive constraints, including constitutional restrictions, we impose on majority rule to get distributively fair outcomes out of democratic processes.

Our rationing case may seem to raise some of the worries about a fundamental or vital interest. A simple majority vote reflecting the "two-third versus one-third" division in my supposition would leave the sickest patients feeling that their vital interests had been compromised. Of course, if we adopted the minority position, we can also imagine that the many mildly ill would also complain that fundamental interests of theirs are compromised as well, since they must give up an even greater restoration of functioning in order to provide some benefit to the sickest. The real difficulty here, of course, is that we cannot cite a basic principle that tells us how to protect the fundamental interests at stake here specifically enough: that is why we were appealing to the democratic process in the first place. Despite Barry's caution, then, that we should worry about the adequacy of a simple voting procedure when fundamental interests are at issue, we may be in a position where we can find no more principled way to worry about those interests.

Barry's caution warns us about an important limitation we face when we think of formal democratic procedures, as social choice theorists may, as a kind of market mechanism for aggregating preferences. There is a more general worry about this perspective on what a democratic procedure is all about that is raised by the rationing examples. How are we to think about the view of the one-third that wants to give more weight to the sickest patients? Is this just a "preference," a kind of taste or desire that might be satisfied, like a taste for a good piece of smoked salmon? Is a dispute about giving weight to the sickest just like a dispute about which preference is "best" between smoked salmon and caviar? I believe not.

We expect reasons that play a role in moral justification to be given for the different weights. Even if the moral reasons given by the minority and majority in this example do not persuade each other, our presumption in this case is that we have not simply been driven back to a matter of a difference in taste, for salmon or caviar. Presumably, the difference may rest in complex views about the kinds of suffering involved, or they may rest on complex differences in comprehensive moral views that the various groups hold. We need not be skeptics or nihilists to recognize the irreducibility of this difference, at least in real time. We can still hanker for an account of why we should settle *by mere vote* what looks like a matter of principle or a matter of the weight of moral reasons. ("Voting might does not make right.") Yet, we standardly rely on democratic procedures to arrive at policies that in effect favor one position rather than another on matters of value, since such disagreements are common. The point here is that the justification for relying on the democratic process cannot simply be the account that derives from the view of democracy as a market. So too in our case.

We might drop the idea that the democratic procedure is a way of reflecting and aggregating private interests (as in the social choice perspective) and still look for a justification of the fair procedure in terms of its *outcome*. We might hope the justification will take the form of showing that a democratic, open procedure is most likely to arrive at rational agreement on the "right answer," at least over time. I believe this would be very difficult to show, despite, for example, Habermas' best efforts. And, in any case, we must get acceptable and justifiable outcomes in real time, not at the limit of timeless rational discourse.

The strategy of justification I shall pursue derives directly from Beitz's (1989) informal contractarian view, which he calls "complex proceduralism." We have interests that derive from being actors or participants in fair procedures and from being the objects of such procedures. The terms of participation should be ones we can imagine everyone agreeing to, given their interests in both roles. This account is egalitarian because it can be justified to everyone. Specifically, the terms of participation in fair procedures are such that no one can reasonably refuse to accept them in light of those interests. Beitz divides these "regulative" interests into *recognition, equitable treatment*, and *deliberative responsibility*. The account does not pick out optimal or unique procedures but shows instead that a particular one cannot be reasonably rejected and so can be considered among the ones that are fair. The strategy for thinking about justification of a particular procedure is to consider whether it can reasonably be rejected given these regulative interests.

The regulative interests bear on our roles as participants and objects of procedures. Our interest in recognition bears on the interest each of us can be presumed to have in our public role as participant. Being openly excluded from the role of actor or participant is a basic denial of moral status; being effectively excluded by various discriminatory practices is also intolerable and could not be made acceptable to those who are so denied recognition.

Our interest in equitable treatment primarily concerns our role as objects of public policy, people who are affected by it. We would insist on some substantive constraints on how procedures are likely to affect us, namely, that they not violate basic principles of justice. This of course means that we must have some prior conception of what those must be; here Beitz includes both procedural and substantive constraints of the sort we might find in constitutions. The point of our interest in equitable treatment is not to allow procedures to "be placed unfairly in jeopardy." (Barry's concern about vital interests in the railroad car example fits here.)

Finally, we have an interest in deliberative responsibility. We want procedures that "foster a process of public reflection in which citizens can form political views in full awareness of the grounds as well as the content of the (possibly competing) concerns of others" (Beitz 1989, 113). We have an interest in accepting institutions that "embody a common (and commonly acknowledged) commitment to the resolution of political issues on the basis of public deliberation that is adequately informed, open to the expression of a wide range of competing views, and carried out under conditions in which these views can be responsibly assessed . . . Citizens conceived as participants in public decisions . . . will wish to regard their judgments as the most reasonable ones possible under the circumstances" (Beitz 1989, 114). Of course, as Beitz points out, our interests in the openness and the quality of the process may be in conflict.

Suppose then that a democratic process for addressing the rationing questions I described had these features: (1) the commission responsible was either elected or appointed by duly constituted authorities and was fairly representative of the community as a whole; (2) the commission must be familiar with the effects of the choices on all relevant categories of patients; (3) it must (publicly) hear arguments or testimony from various groups or individuals about these effects and their interests in the situation; (4) the committee must subject preliminary proposals about its choices to public review and discussion; (5) within some reasonable time period, the committee is accountable for voting on a recommended rationing policy. How does such a procedure fare on this strategy?

Can people reasonably reject it on grounds that it fails to satisfy the regulative interests? I think not. I want to emphasize the degree to which we are relying on a democratic procedure to resolve what is an openly moral issue. We might agree it does not resolve the issue, at least from the point of view of moral reasoning, but it resolves it from the point of view of the need to formulate policy and to act on it. In thinking about our regulative interests, then, the justification will emphasize points about our reliance as moral agents on a procedure that aims at morally acceptable outcomes.

The described procedure appears to satisfy our recognition interests, but the details need more careful examination than I can offer. I described the procedure as "fairly representative" of everyone and so have not specifically addressed questions that might be raised, such as, Must the group actually include representatives of the sickest or most disabled groups? My goal here is not to resolve these issues but simply to set them in a framework where their relevance to justification is clear.

Our interest in "equitable treatment" might seem crucial, especially in light of the worries Barry raised. But the point here is that the kinds of general principles of justice we might ordinarily cite as giving content to the substantive worries about equitable treatment do not help us specifically. For example, even if fair equality of opportunity is a constitutional constraint, it does not tell us what to do about the priority problem, other than to reject a view that no priority should be given to the sickest. We also have some worries about the effects of "persistent minorities." Here too, I will leave this as an issue for discussion, not resolution by my comments.

Our final interest is in "deliberative responsibility." Since the procedure must stand in for us as moral agents, it must foster the sense that relevant considerations have been addressed as well as it is reasonable for them to be given time and other resource constraints. The process would not force us to address issues appropriately if it did not leave room for considering all relevant views and information or if it did not leave room for reassessment. Openness is necessary, and procedural provision for improving quality through the invitation of experts is desirable. We may not be happy about having to resolve a question of policy with moral implications simply by vote, but if the deliberative process is as open as possible to moral considerations, we may have to settle for an outcome that rests on voting. The point is to try to make the process bring out the best in its participants by way of moral deliberation.

Part of what is so discomforting about relying on a democratic process here is that we appeal to it to address moral uncertainty. But how we address moral uncertainty in the individual case is also discomforting. We sometimes must act when we do not really have firm convictions about what is right. We feel the pull of different arguments and considerations. In such a situation we may indeed ask the advice of others. We may even be swayed – and not unreasonably – if those we respect favor one course more than the other. We may hope that they are "seeing something" we have missed in our thinking about the case. Of course, we would not just trust anyone in such a situation. And there are risks to our seeking out only those who usually see things our way. But our procedure relies on the presumption that we are not the only morally perspicacious agents in the world: others can get it right too. It is then reasonable to get the views of more people. Though it does not follow that the majority is right, it is not unreasonable to rely on it under the constraints I have described.

REFERENCES

Barry, Brian. 1979. "Is Democracy Special?" In P. Laslett and J. Fishkin, eds., *Philosophy, Politics and Society*, 5th Series, pp. 156–71. New Haven: Yale University Press.

Beitz, Charles. 1989. *Political Equality*. Princeton: Princeton University Press.

Nord, Eric. 1993. "The Relevance of Health State after Treatment in Prioritising between Different Patients," *Journal of Medical Ethics* 19:1(March 1993):37–42.

Chapter 16

Wide reflective equilibrium in practice

In 1992 through 1993, when I was a fellow in the Program in Ethics and the Professions at Harvard, I was quite astounded to learn from other fellows that the field of bioethics was in a state of methodological upheaval, fractured along many fault lines, much like Los Angeles but without the sunny climate. They portrayed an intellectual war zone, reminiscent of evolutionary theory or paleontology, where there are many bones to pick. When I expressed my surprise, I was chided. How "out of it" could I be? Had I had not heard that "principlism" (a position held by Beauchamp and Childress[1]) had been routed "from above" by advocates of "theory" (like Clouser and Gert[2] and Green[3]) and, more effectively, ambushed "from below" by contextualists (like Hoffmaster[4]) and their allies, the casuists (like Jonsen and Toulmin[5])? Had I not heard that "theory" was out, that "deductivism" and other "top-down" approaches were defeated in favor of "bottom-up" ones? The battle was so advanced that new rescue efforts for old fortifications had already been mounted, like Richardson's "specifying norms"[6] or DeGrazia's "specified principlism."[7] I was abashed. I had not noticed that I was working in a war zone and that defending or applying a moral principle put me at risk of taking a sniper's bullet.

Though I am loathe to make excuses for not being "with it," let me offer three to start with. One is really a confession: I do not read the bioethics literature as widely as I should, except for what bears most directly on the problems on which I am working. More important, I thought "doing ethics" involved familiarity with all these method-ological weapons, not just one or some of them. And I also thought that we do ethics to solve many different kinds of problems and that the methods we use plausibly vary with the problems we want to solve and the interests we have in solving them. So much for my naiveté, though I shall return to defend its charm later. Nevertheless, my mor-bid interest was stimulated – perhaps I was just shamed – into taking a closer look at the war zone. The battle reports promised to be at least as interesting as the *New York Times* and might rival *USA Today* or CNN News, but that's pushing it.

A BRIEF REPORT FROM THE BATTLE ZONE
IN THE LAND OF BIOETHICS

Occupying the Middle Kingdom, a series of fortified hills, are the forces of the "principlists." Overlooking the Middle Kingdom there is a more ethereal high ground that is occupied by roving bands of Uplanders who are often dubbed "theorists." Down in the valley are the Lowlanders, "contextualists" and "casuists" and various others, who distrust high places and like the feel of each blade of grass between their bare toes. Somewhat prophetically, the original topographical map for this land was sketched by Beauchamp and Childress.[8] It looked like this:

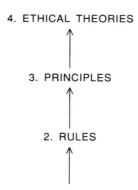

The upward ascending arrows in the original diagram may have originally only indicated *height*, since it was just a crude topographical map. The problems arise when Beauchamp and Childress say that justification flows downward, in a direction opposite to their arrows. Thus we would justify particular judgments by subsuming them under rules, and rules by subsuming them under principles, and so on. The current battle, as I understand it, interprets the arrows to mean *priority* or *dominance*: do theories or principles govern the terrain of ethics, or do particular judgments in context? The fight is about what directions the arrows should point.

The principlists who occupy the Middle Kingdom include some of the earliest settlers of this land, and they played an active role in recruiting others to toil and live here as well. Their doctrine was consolidated in an early training manual for such recruits,[9] and this has caused considerable mischief. (The manual has been substantially revised, and its most recent edition is reasonably eclectic.) It is easy for recruits to elevate the kind of simplified instruction involved in a training manual into dogma, much like cadets in a military academy. Some years later its central principles – autonomy, beneficence, nonmaleficence, and justice – have been contemptuously referred to as the "Georgetown mantra." In any case, large numbers of cadre toil in the fields surrounding the Middle Kingdom; their missives and other communications often invoke the mantra.

There is considerable dispute about how we should interpret these principles and their role in governing the land. Like most leaders and prophets, Beauchamp and Childress have said things about them that can be interpreted in various ways. (Ambiguity allows you to be right more often.) Despite the directional arrows in the original map, and despite the claim that justification flows downward from the heights, Beauchamp[10] also insists that theory plays a role at all levels of work in bioethics and that theory does not arise in a vacuum but out of myriad cases. Had the arrows been bidirectional from the start, allowing each level to influence but not govern the others, and capturing more accurately the nature of justification in ethics, much of the current bloodshed could have been avoided.

More confusing is Beauchamp and Childress' view (in early editions of the manual) that their principles are really neutral between various theories and that bioethicists can (sometimes? often? always?) start working their way downward from the principles, ignoring the greater heights occupied by competing ethical theories. As might be expected, this claim is sharply disputed by Uplanders like Clouser and Gert.[11] Beauchamp and Childress are misleading here: we need work in ethical theory to resolve disputes about priorities among principles as well as about their limits and scope (the point is clarified in the new edition of the manual). Clouser and Gert complain that a smorgasbord or "anthology" approach to theory is adopted and that no effort is made to resolve theoretical disputes so that one dominant theory can then be used to resolve disputes about principles, rules, and cases. There is no doubt that Gert has his own theory in mind for that role.

A more charitable gloss on what Beauchamp and Childress are saying is that sometimes we can agree on mid-level principles and rules, even while we disagree about theory, and, given the pressure to produce practical judgments in real time, not seeking more agreement than we need is good practical advice. A training manual ought to be explicit, however, about whether it is giving tactical or strategic advice. In any case, we should not confuse the pragmatics of good tactical advice with an account of the legitimacy, in this case, of the authority of principles. Here I lodge a complaint against both the Uplanders and the principlists: the appeal to ethical theory is valuable even when it is not one dominant theory we are drawing on but the systematic consideration of issues that bear on the selection of principles and evaluation of cases. More on this later.

I have already noted one line of attack by the Uplander theorists, but they have focused their mortars on other Middle Kingdom targets as well, close to the heart of the mantra. Clouser and Gert[12] argue that the "principles" intoned in the mantra are not really general moral principles but "chapter headings" for a "discussion of some concepts which are often only superficially related to each other." Their point is most persuasive in the case of the "principle" of justice cited by Beauchamp and Childress. No single principle is really articulated; we get a checklist of considerations. These chapter headings cannot generate specific rules for guiding action in particular cases, and resolving disputes about how concerns about autonomy and beneficence conflict, for example, necessarily engages us in appeals to theory. Green[13] makes similar points. decrying the lack of interest in theoretical issues spawned by the prominence within the field of "principlism."

More strenuous and varied than the attacks on principlism by the Uplanders is the multifront campaign launched by the Lowlanders. Lowlanders find their bearings best, they insist, by reading the trail signs in front of them, not by looking to high and distant landmarks. They are much better at finding their way through the trees than at surveying whole forests. They complain that advocates of rules or principles or theories ignore the details and texture of real cases. We should not, they insist, force cases to fit the rubric of simple principles. The real moral terrain is much more finely textured than that. A careful diagnosis of the pitfalls, rough brush, and swamps is needed before we can reliably find our way in bioethics. Principles – and theories – are of necessity highly idealized and simplified and, when we pay attention to them, we become impatient of providing a truly close diagnosis of a problem. When Middle Kingdomers, invoking their mantra, cast the simple white beam of principle on the ground from on high, attempting to illuminate our path, they cast shadows that hide crucial complexities and may even blind us to the roots and snarls in our way.

The Lowlanders' campaign attacks the appeal to principles at a vulnerable point. To show that a particular principle ought to govern a particular case may require showing that the morally salient features of that case fall under that principle. But careful examination of many aspects of the situation may be needed to decide what the morally salient features are. The problem is compounded when a case seems to fall under conflicting principles. It seems that there is some basis for alliance between the Uplanders and Lowlanders, but the battle lines are more complex. (In the most recent edition of their manual, Beauchamp and Childress concede ground, agreeing that the original diagram applies only in the simplest cases, when there are no conflicting principles.)[14]

The Lowlanders may be right that sometimes close examination of cases can produce agreement about what counts as right action. But this close examination must employ some views about how to convert details or "data" into real evidence for a conclusion. We do insist on reasons. We want to treat relevantly similar cases in similar ways. We need some way of determining what counts as similar in the relevant ways. We need to know when to discount differences and when to rest weight on them. We need, in effect, more systematic accounts of what we are doing. But that is exactly what reason giving, appeals to principle, and the development of moral theory was supposed to do: provide us with a basis for converting observations into evidence for a view. The hard work of ethics lies not just in its observations and diagnosis of the particular case but in figuring out what counts as relevant moral reasons for treating situations the way we should.

To one degree or another, the Lowlanders' emphasis on context and case feeds an antitheory inclination and not just an antiprinciplist stance. They are no doubt right that sometimes, after deliberation, we may agree on what to do about particular cases when we are far from seeing how appeals to ethical theory or even to principles can help. They then suggest that by accumulating agreement around cases we can reason our way "analogically" toward some modest principles. Arras[15] notes that this causistical approach may not be so theory free as it claims, that it may quite conventionally, in unnoticed ways, accept without question important features of our social institutions and practices. Unnoticed theory is still theory, but unnoticed it is unexamined. Unexamined assumptions underlying our agreement may not, after all, be justifiable.

It is not surprising then that the two-front attack on principlism is not a coordinated one after all. The Uplanders may welcome the assault by the Lowlanders on the Middle Kingdom, but the Lowlanders are just as suspicious of the theorists as they are of the principlists. Like the principlists, the Lowlanders fear that theory turns idle wheels and does not contribute to moral decisions in real time. So the Uplanders, too, have little patience and offer no true alliance with the Lowlanders, whatever tribe of contextualist or casuist they belong to.

Justice and justification

A PEACE PROPOSAL

Is there a Nobel Peace Prize in the offing here? Can peace be brought to this land? Are there points of agreement that we could use to leverage further agreements? Is there a basis for cooperation? Could there be a division of moral labor that would allow all to cooperate in a joint endeavor? Or at least to live in peace, pursuing their own efforts and contributing individually to our knowing better what we ought to do?

One proposal aimed at bridging the gap between principlists and contextualists is Richardson's[16] suggestion that the real work of practical ethics lies in "specifying norms." Acknowledging the point of careful diagnosis of a situation and sensitivity to context, while at the same time insisting that norms or principles must provide us with a bridge between cases, Richardson describes how we must successively qualify our principles or "specify" the norms we use so that they better fit or apply to particular cases. We must work back and forth between cases or cases and principles, carrying out this refinement of the principle. We get proper specification when we arrive at an equilibrium between the texture of the case and our moral beliefs about it and the qualifications we need on the principle or principles we had thought should apply to it. This is a version of what has been called narrow reflective equilibrium – we revise our principles and judgments about cases until we achieve an equilibrium. DeGrazia[17] endorses this approach, calling it "specified principlism," adding the suggestion, perhaps in an appeal to the Uplanders, that we construe ethical theory as the various branching specifications of principles that result when we carry out this process extensively. There is merit in this Richardson–DeGrazia proposal, but I think the picture it involves of theory is still impoverished. I believe work in ethics must seek a very wide reflective equilibrium that erodes many of the distinctions about the levels of terrain in the kingdom of bioethics.

Justification in ethics rests, I have long thought, on a broad coherentist approach involving beliefs at many levels.[18] Though we may be committed to some views quite firmly, no beliefs are beyond revision. It is important that we see how diverse these types of beliefs are. I include here our beliefs about particular cases; about rules and principles and virtues and how to apply or act on them; about the right-making properties of actions, policies, and institutions; about the conflict between consequentialist and deontological views; about partiality and impartiality and the moral point of view; about motivation, moral development, strains of moral commitment, and the limits of ethics; about the nature of persons; about the role or function of ethics in our lives; about the implications of game theory, decision theory, and accounts of rationality for morality; about the ways we should reply to moral skepticism and moral disagreement; and about moral justification itself. As is evident from this broad and encompassing list, the elements of moral theory are diverse.

When I suggest that "theory" must be appealed to, I do not mean some particular comprehensive view, like Kant's or Mill's, that takes a particular stand on some of these areas, though some might accept such theories. I mean our appeal to some or all of those elements involved in the process of giving a systematic account of moral beliefs and practices. These elements are involved in the effort to achieve *wide reflective equilibrium*, the coherence of our beliefs about many of these matters. Wide reflective equilibrium is actually endorsed as an account of justification by various of the disputants, including Beauchamp, DeGrazia, and Green; key elements in it are appealed to by Hoffmaster and to some extent by Jonsen and Toulmin. This suggests that there may be some common ground after all, provided it can be used and shared appropriately.

"Doing ethics" involves trying to solve very different kinds of problems answering to rather different interests we may have, some quite practical, others more theoretical. Sometimes we want to know what to do in this case or in developing this policy or designing this institution. Sometimes our problem is in understanding the relationship between this case, policy, or institution and others and making sure we adopt an approach consistent with what we are convinced we ought to do elsewhere. Sometimes our problem is to provide a systematic account of some salient element in our approach to thinking about cases, such as an account of the nature of rights or virtues or consequences. We can sometimes presume considerable agreement on some aspects of the problem but not others, so the practical problem may be how to leverage agreement we already have to reduce areas of disagreement. *There is no one thing we do that is always central to solving an ethical problem for there is no one paradigmatic ethical problem.*

Putting these points about justification together with this claim that there are many types of ethical problems, I conclude doing ethics may require doing many different kinds of things. Sometimes it may require doing many of them at once. Sometimes we can narrow our effort.

Much of the methodological dispute comes from ignoring these first and second points. It comes from looking at one kind of problem and one kind of effort and insisting it is the primary problem or effort and that other methodologies are wrong not to see its primacy. My peace proposal thus constitutes a kind of plea for tolerance. It is an effort to see the kernel of truth in many approaches while refusing to treat the kernel as the whole ear of corn. Ethics, or bioethics, should not be top down or bottom up. Or rather, how bottom up or top down it should be may depend on the problem and our purpose in solving it. My comments in what follows will be an attempt to illustrate this plea with examples. I use examples from my own work not because I think it is the best work, nor because it is even the best illustration of my point, but only because I am most familiar with it and confident about the motivation behind it. (In any case, I will at least avoid the problem of misinterpreting others.)

Like many of the disputants in the battle zone, I will decry the division between "practical ethics" and "ethical theory." I thus join ranks with participants from every camp, including Beauchamp, Green, Hoffmaster, and others. Specifically, I believe that the "purism" that pervades many of the best Ph.D. programs is unjustifiable and damaging. Good work in ethics tests theory and forces its development by trying to solve practical problems and showing what guidance theory can give. So too, efforts to solve practical problems often can make little progress without some guidance from theory. Ideally, people who do ethics should have rigorous training in both areas of problem solving. Unfortunately, "mainstream" purists often do not want to get their hands dirty with practical problems, preferring the more tractable, idealized "philosophers'" thought experiments. Too many people in bioethics and other areas of practical ethics do not want to fill their heads with "theory" that may seem to turn no wheels, at least for their purposes, or that does not interest clinicians or policymakers. Given the diverse disciplines that lead people into bioethics – law, theology, medicine, philosophy – it is not surprising that many have little training in ethical theory and find it difficult to acquire it. My plea for toleration is coupled with a plea for rigor and comprehensiveness in training in ethics. Nevertheless, with a judicious focus on problems, good work can often result even without the kind of rigorous, comprehensive training that is ideal. There is plenty of room for a division of moral labor.

I doubt these remarks provide the basis for a Nobel Peace Prize, but I do want to illustrate why I think there is common ground that the different combatants must learn to till together. The illustrations that follow highlight kernels of truth that can be culled from the positions defended by various disputants. The suggestion is that they help delineate that common ground.

LANDMARKS IN THE PEACEABLE KINGDOM

1. *We do not have to agree about everything to solve moral problems*

In an early paper Jonsen and Butler[19] introduced the phrase "public ethics" to delimit a type of problem facing bioethics, the application of normative ethics to public policy. Public ethics deals with making particular public moral decisions about specific matters that are pressing and that do not involve profound structural changes in the social order.[20] Because the matters of policy do not involve fundamental changes, some agreement on relevant principles can be expected. By articulating these principles, clarifying policy options in light of them, and then ranking the moral options for policy choices, public ethics has a reasonably specific agenda that can yield results without forcing us to engage in the most abstract philosophical ethics. Indeed, Jonsen and Butler[21] introduce the neologism "infraethics" to describe this level of ethical inquiry and to distinguish it from the more theoretical or "metaethical" inquiry they say is characteristic of normative ethics more generally.

The work of public ethics is modest: it does not seek to challenge or justify more fundamental moral principles, as it might have to do if more fundamental social change were at issue, and so theory plays a modest role. Under the pressure to solve a practical problem in real time, we engage only in as much abstraction as we need to solve the problem. Still, public ethics requires sensitivity to context, for the implications of different policy options and their moral consequences relative to the principles must be made explicit. This characterization of the method involved in public ethics is *problem driven*. It does not purport to be a methodological description of the whole domain of bioethics or of ethics more generally. In that regard it differs from the "principlism" attributed to Beauchamp and Childress.

I want to describe a recent example of public ethics in which I was involved. Dan Brock and I[22] have described the work we did together on the principles and values underlying Clinton's health-care reform proposal.[23] The Ethics Working Group was a diverse group of academics including philosophers, lawyers, doctors, and theologians. We were diverse in our philosophical training and beliefs – for example, some were communitarians who thought in a very religious framework ("stewardship" was their term for resource allocation) and others were quite secular proponents of various views about justice. Had we sought agreement on philosophical fundamentals, we would never have gotten any place. Instead, we were able to agree on fourteen basic "principles and values" that we thought ought to govern health-care reform, including the Clinton proposal. We intended them to serve as a test of the Clinton proposal and alternatives. What we are calling principles here would not pass muster as such in Clouser or Gert's view; but they are not "chapter headings" either. I think of them as "design principles" that capture morally desirable features of health-care institutions.[24]

Agreeing on principles and values without deeper agreement on the underlying theory of justice has its risks and limitations. Specifically, it leaves us less able to resolve disputes that arise when the principles conflict with each other. Can we trade comprehensiveness of benefits in order to secure universality of access? Developing a framework of such principles, however, does give a matrix within which features of institutional design can be assessed for their moral implications relative to the principles. Thus we can note that a long-term phase-in of universal access, especially if it is made contingent on savings generated by reform, constitutes a serious violation of the principles. Similarly, if a reform plan makes the content of their benefit package shrink if savings are inadequate to fund subsidies to low-income individuals, then recasting this constraint on subsidies as a clear sacrifice of the principle assuring comprehensive benefits shows what is morally at stake. Further argument is then needed to resolve disputes about priorities, and some disputes may not be resolved at all if they reflect more fundamental disagreements.

I believe there is value to the ethical work involved in articulating these principles underlying health-care reform, and I think that is true even though my own work much more specifically ties such principles to a specific theory of justice for health care. There is a need for a reasonable division of moral labor: an ethics working group constituted to reflect diversity in the field and in the society as a whole cannot be expected to arrive at complete agreement on underlying theory within the real-time limits set by the task force. Our solution reflects the problem we were set: we had to understand the context well, see the implications of institutional design, and find some framework of principles and values that let us improve areas of agreement where possible.

2. Most problems resist either straightforward "top-down" or "bottom-up" approaches

The HIV epidemic raised two problems that derive from the risk of transmission in medical settings (nosocomial risks). Do physicians have a duty to treat HIV-positive patients despite the risks they impose? Do patients have a right to know the HIV status of their physicians, at least for invasive procedures? I think these problems illustrate the futility of thinking that their ethical resolution could rely solely on a top-down appeal to principle or a bottom-up careful examination of context and case.

In the late 1980s, it was common in the United States to hear some physicians, even through their professional associations, assert that they would not treat AIDS patients. They insisted they had no "duty to treat." They insisted they had never agreed to face those risks, did not want to, and were not obliged to. In effect, they insisted they had not ever consented to take those particular risks, and it did not matter that some other physicians had or would. Some professional associations, like the American Medical Association (AMA), disagreed, at least by 1987. The AMA insisted that physicians were obliged to treat "without regard to risks," that they had a tradition of acting virtuously in the face of epidemics, at least recently, and that refusing to do so in the case of HIV patients was "invidious discrimination."

A careful examination of the context revealed that the risks of transmission to physicians were very low but not risks that could be ignored. In fact, the estimated risks could vary considerably with the type of medical activity and the incidence of HIV in the local patient population. An obligation to face any risk whatsoever, like that asserted by the AMA, was indefensible. But even if obligations to take risks in general arose out of voluntary acts, like undergoing the training and identifying with the role of being a physician, then how could we accommodate the variability of this risk? The solution to the problem is to claim that physicians undertake a package of obligations when they enter that professional role, including an obligation to face some standard level of risk. Obligations to take much greater risks would require further, more specific consent. Refusal to face standard risks – and HIV risks seemed standard if HVB (hepatitis B) risks did – would then seem like invidious discrimination, if directed only against HIV patients. Role-based obligations come in clusters or packages, and individuals adopting these roles and assuming these obligations are not free to custom design their consent and thus their obligations.[25]

This proposal has some resemblance to the Richardson–DeGrazia view about specifying norms. I had modified the principles about consent and about physician obligations to respond to the specifics of risk taking in these situations. But the analysis of professional obligations that facilitated the modification (or clarification) involved doing a piece of theoretical work, not "theory" in the sense of invoking some overarching general theory, like Kant's or Mill's, but a careful analysis of the nature of obligations, facilitated by interesting work by others developing a virtue-based account of professional obligations.[26]

A second example to make the same point involves the conflicting right claims that HIV-infected health-care workers and patients can make. The issue came to public attention in the glare of the discovery that a Florida dentist had infected (perhaps deliberately, we may now suspect) five or six patients. A campaign was launched by one victim to require physician disclosure of HIV status, following compulsory testing, with the removal of infected practitioners. The AMA argued that physicians must "do no harm" and inferred that this meant they should disclose their status to patients or remove themselves from invasive procedures. The Centers for Disease Control passed regulations that seemed to capitulate to the public fears: the regulations, still in place, called for infected practitioners to refrain from engaging in "exposure-prone" procedures. On the other side, advocates for infected health-care workers insisted these workers had rights, like all handicapped workers, to be allowed to work unless they imposed "significant" risks on fellow workers or patients. Since the risks of transmission were minuscule – between 1 in 40,000 and 1 in 400,000 from a known infected surgeon, and only 1 in 20,000,000 from any surgeon – these did not constitute significant risks.

Which right claim should be given priority? Doesn't context help? What context? Knowing these levels of risk does not help us in the way we might think. Although it might seem irrational to worry about these risks when we standardly ignore greater ones in medical contexts, it is not really irrational for patients to want to find out a surgeon's status and to switch surgeons at no cost to themselves. Nor should we follow the AMA in thinking that "do no harm" means that these physicians have abandoned the protection of the rights of handicapped workers. Presumably, physicians should avoid imposing harms it is not worth the risk of imposing, keeping the benefits in mind. So these right claims seem intractably juxtaposed, and it is not at all obvious simply working back and forth between principle and case how we should "specify the norm" or modify the principles in narrow reflective equilibrium. Nor is it obvious that protecting equality of opportunity or protecting patient autonomy should be given priority over the other.

The solution comes from invoking both a piece of theory and a careful diagnosis of the details of the case.[27] The unconstrained exercise of patient rights here has the effect, on plausible assumptions about the costs and effects of different strategies of risk reduction, of setting up a many-person prisoners' dilemma. Each person is made less safe by a system that gives full reign to patients' rights to know and to switch, since the resources needed to carry out that strategy, rational from each patient's point of view, are an ineffective way of reducing transmission risks. An analysis and proposed solution like this one requires both careful diagnosis of the context and appropriate invocation of a piece of theory.

3. The standard model of "applied ethics" – plugging facts into principles – does not work in the peaceable kingdom

Nearly all disputants agree that the term "applied ethics" is terribly misleading. It suggests that there is a supply of ready-at-hand, general moral theories or principles and that the task of finding out what to do in particular cases consists of specifying the "facts" that would connect

344

the general principle to a specific case. No doubt this picture may have been influenced by positivist views about scientific laws: in order to get predictions from laws we simply need to specify the relevant observations. In the philosophy of science, we long ago rejected this view, acknowledging among other things that an extensive body of auxiliary theories must be brought to bear before we can decide just what "data" will count as evidence for a theory or as predictions that follow from it. We do not simply plug data points into formulae. Similarly in ethics, we need a much more sophisticated view of the relationship between general principles and particular cases. How general principles really can guide action is much more complicated than the "applied ethics" picture allows. I illustrate the point with two examples.

When I began thinking about justice and health-care delivery, having spent much of the 1970s working on problems in the general theory of justice, I thought it should be easy to "apply" to health care principles like those argued for by Rawls. I was in the grip of the false picture of "applied ethics." Rawls' principles, I was aware, were developed under a special, idealizing assumption: that fully functional people should specify principles of fair cooperation. No one was ill or disabled. I was immediately stymied.[28] Should health care be governed by a principle aimed at making those who were worst off maximally well off? Or did Rawls' theory need to add a new primary social good, health care? Or would some other principle do the job? Looking from the theory "down" to the system of delivery, it was quite unclear what "applying" the principles really meant.

I had to reverse directions to make any progress.[29] I began to think directly about health care and the different kinds of things it does for us. I had to answer questions about why we might think some of those functions had special moral importance. I had to think about cases in which we felt that assisting people with medical services was an obligation and when we thought assisting them was not. Gradually, I focused on the generalization that disease and disability impairs the range of opportunities open to us, whereas health-care services that we think we are obliged to offer to people protects that range of opportunities. What emerged was the claim that a general principle assuring fair equality of opportunity should govern the design of health-care systems. But even here the account of fair equality of opportunity had to be broadened from its focus on access to jobs and offices. To extend Rawls' theory meant not simply plugging in the facts but modifying the theory in modest and reasonable ways. My procedure required developing an account of what health care does for us and its importance that was sensitive to the wide variety of things health care does and captured many of our intuitive judgments and practices, such as insurance coverage. Only then did it become clear how to connect general principles – appropriately modified – to the world of institutions.

My second example shows that these lessons do not sink in quickly. Once I had developed an account of justice for health care that appealed to the fair equality of opportunity principle, I thought that principle would actually be able to guide us in some detail in designing institutions that allocated health-care resources equitably. I thought it would tell us how, under resource constraints, we should limit access to beneficial services. I have since concluded that the gap between principle and guidance in institutional design is quite wide and that we do not yet know how to fill it. Again, it was by examining actual cases of rationing decisions that it became apparent general principles fell short of offering adequate guidance. Let me explain briefly.

The fair equality of opportunity principle gives some guidance about rationing. Quite generally, it implies that under resource constraints, we should use our resources in ways that most effectively protect the range of opportunities open to us, focusing on services that maintain normal functioning. More specifically, it supports a distinction between treatment and enhancement, though that is a more complicated story to which I shall return shortly. It also supports a distinction between proven and unproven treatments, though just how the line should be drawn is a further issue. But how much priority should we give to treating those whose opportunities are most impaired by disease or disability? How much "opportunity cost" should we impose on those who are less ill in order to help those most ill or disabled? Giving full priority – maximizing benefits for the worst off – seems implausible. So does giving no priority to them. Is there a principled position in between? We have no philosophical account of one, and the equal opportunity principle fails to guide us. Similarly, how much weight should we give to getting the best outcomes, measured in health benefits, from resources? Giving full priority to achieving best outcomes may mean that we deny some people equal or fair chances at some benefits. Here, too, either extreme seems implausible: we intuitively reject always going for best outcomes or always going for equal chances at some benefit. But we have no principled way of determining an intermediary policy.

These "unsolved" rationing problems show just how indeterminate the equal opportunity principle is.[30] It fails to guide our action at a crucial point, where we must design institutions and policies to embody general principles under resource constraints. The problem is perfectly general. The same problem arises outside health care, for example, when we try to allocate educational resources or legal aid services. We encounter the same unsolved rationing problems.

One way out is to try to appeal to fair procedures for making the relevant choices about institutional design. But we have given little attention to what counts as a fair procedure for solving this kind of problem.[31] The implication of this analysis is that we must revise considerably our view about the nature of general distributive principles: they cannot guide action as we might have hoped. It could be that the predominant lesson is that many general principles must fall short of guiding action without an acceptable process for making determinate choices that fall within a class of outcomes acceptable in light of the general principles. But this is a feature of general theory ignored in the literature.

One lesson from these examples is that work in ethical theory is enriched in deep ways by forcing the question of how the theory guides action into very specific areas of practice. It is much too easy for "pure" theory to think it offers guidance when it does not. We discover the problem only when we test the theory against practice. To put the point contentiously, "applied ethics" makes an essential contribution to "ethical theory." Put more clearly, we fail to do our best work at either level if we do not see them as part of the same project.

4. Impatience with the limits of theory should not drive us to think that an examination of context alone can guide us

Several years ago, James Sabin and I began examining how clinicians made decisions about what is "medically necessary" mental health care. We asked clinicians to describe what they found to be "hard cases" in their own practice. We found a clear tension in the judgments made by different practitioners – sometimes the tension was strongly felt within a single practitioner.[32] Some "hard-line" clinicians strongly held the view that their services were aimed at treating diagnosable disorders; more "expansive" clinicians were inclined to use their skills to reduce any kind of unhappiness they encountered. They arrived at quite different judgments about what was "medically necessary," moving in quite different ways on many particular cases. When they disagreed about particular cases, it was not so much about the "facts" of the case, though "expansive" clinicians were often willing to broaden diagnostic categories to try to fit their inclinations about particular patients, and "hard-line" clinicians were somewhat more disposed to hold patients "responsible" for attitudes and behaviors that expansive clinicians tended to view as symptoms of an underlying disorder.

Our analysis suggests that different clinicians have internalized somewhat different views about the goals and limits of medicine. These views can be connected to rather different theoretical stances or "glosses" on the notion of equality of opportunity. For example, the hard-line clinicians make judgments that fit quite well with the view that there is a reasonably sharp line that we can draw between treatment and enhancement and that our obligations in health care are to restore people to some notion of "normal functioning." The expansive clinicians seem to think that any limitation on functioning, even if it is part of a normal range, can impose disadvantages on people, and it is the task of medicine to provide people with more equal capabilities to be or achieve whatever they want in life. What this suggested to us is that there was considerable disagreement in practice because that reflected some underlying disagreement at the level of theory about the demands of equality.[33]

It seems impossible, just by comparing cases, to resolve the dispute among these clinicians about what should be viewed as medically necessary treatment. To resolve the dispute, we must give some arguments that show why one view of the demands of equality and the goals of medicine is preferable to adopt to the other. We must raise our heads above the level of "context" and "case" to see where to go in this matter. Thinking we can avoid appeal to theory if we can at least agree on cases, after careful diagnosis, is not helpful if there are systematic disagreements on cases that reflect related disagreements in theory. Conversely, to repeat a point made earlier, considering the cases involved here can lead to clarification and modification of the underlying theory.[34]

5. *There is moral surprise in the peaceable kingdom*

The process of ethical inquiry can lead us to change our minds about what we think is right. We may begin with a view about what is right in a particular case or type of case and discover that we cannot sustain that view on more careful consideration of other cases and relevant theory. We may begin with a piece of theory that we can no longer support. Surprise can occur at any level. We are surprised because we discover even our firmly held views are revisable. I mention briefly three examples, two of which I already noted.

When I first began thinking about health-hazard regulation in the workplace, I believed it should be easy to defend the criterion underlying standards in U.S. law, specifically, the requirement that exposure to harmful toxins should be reduced "to the extent it is technologically feasible" to do so. Deep in my heart, I was for worker safety and health and had few compunctions about government regulation, even if it imposed significant costs on employers. When I asked myself, however, just why it was reasonable to restrict the options of workers to take some risks for hazard pay, I found it more difficult to explain my initial view.[35] Suppose we provided workers with adequate information about the risks they faced and suppose that we internalize the costs of the health risks we imposed on these workers. Suppose we can approximate the costs of internalization by cleaning up the workplace to the point that it is cost beneficial to do so. Cleaning it up further costs more than we save in health-care costs. Why not let workers negotiate for hazard-pay extra costs between a cost–benefit standard and the technological feasibility criterion? Is insisting on the higher level of health protection unjustifiably paternalistic?

I was able to justify the higher standard, after considering in some detail the context, only under the following condition. The array of choices open to typical workers facing such hazard-pay negotiation would have to be an unfairly restricted set of choices. That might well be true in the United States, though it is unlikely that the U.S. Congress would admit that as a reason for its legislating such a stiff criterion. In a more just society, if these workers had a fair or just range of choices open to them, then the strict criterion would seem unjustifiably paternalistic. This outcome surprised me.

I already indicated two other examples of surprise. In the controversy about HIV-infected professionals, I found my view shifted twice.[36] At first, I thought the risks were so low – so "insignificant" – that any restriction on infected workers was a violation of their rights as handicapped workers. But after I persuaded myself that it was indeed rational for individuals to avoid even small risks if they could do so at no cost to themselves by finding out their physician's HIV status and switching if necessary, I could not see how to avoid the force of the AMA or CDC positions. My view has now returned to opposing restrictions, but for very different reasons than I originally had. Am I morally indecisive? Overly intellectual? The surprise to me is that the shift in what I believed right in these cases was dramatic and based on reasoned deliberation.

A final surprise to me was the discovery that general distributive principles could fall so short of guiding decisions about institutional design, as my discussion about rationing suggests. I have been forced quite dramatically to rethink what kinds of moral arguments must be brought to bear on questions of rationing and institutional design. I now think we must pay much more attention to problems of fair process and to refinements of democratic theory.

PEACE IN OUR TIMES?

My point in developing these examples is to highlight why the strife we now see seems so useless and avoidable. Let me conclude by indicating the points I think form a basis for a cooperative division of moral labor in ethics.

(1) There is not one kind of ethical problem but many, and different problems require somewhat different approaches.

(2) Because there are many types of problems and a division of moral labor is reasonable, many people from many different disciplines and training backgrounds can expect to make important contributions in bioethics.

(3) As contextualists, casuists, and other "lowlanders" argue, it is essential to develop a careful diagnosis of a moral issue and to be leery of forcing it prematurely into the mold provided by ready-at-hand principles.

(4) As principlists and theorists of various clans insist, we must provide reasons for our moral views that allow us to see relationships among cases and begin to assure ourselves we have consistent approaches and coherent accounts of what we are doing.

(5) Most ethical problem-solving cannot therefore be either top down or bottom up but must be multifaceted and responsive to the demands of both context and theory.

(6) The diverse appeals to theoretical considerations we need to make in solving problems should not be confused with the adoption of some particular comprehensive moral view; some may accept such views, but most people have much more eclectic and diverse conceptions of theory.

(7) Though we begin with firm views on some issues and matters of theory, we must hold all our views to be revisable in the light of good arguments and in an effort to seek the widest coherence in our beliefs.

(8) Reasonable people can end up disagreeing on moral matters: disagreement is not a sign of ignorance, evil, or irrationality. We have no infallible faculty or method for resolving disagreements or arriving at moral truths, and moral progress depends on our having respect for the sources of disagreement and a commitment to finding arguments that prove persuasive.

No doubt there are further elements that should be included here, but these are necessary elements in any peace settlement.

NOTES

1 Tom L. Beauchamp and James F. Childress, *Principles of Biomedical Ethics* (New York: Oxford University Press, 1979, 1983, 1989, 1994).

2 K. Danner Clouser and Bernard Gert, "A Critique of Principlism," *Journal of Medicine and Philosophy* 15 (1990):219–36.

3 R. M. Green, "Method in Bioethics: A Troubled Assessment," *Journal of Medicine and Philosophy* 15 (1990):179–97.

4   Barry Hoffmaster, "The Theory and Practice of Applied Ethics," *Dialogue* 30 (1991):213–34.
5   Albert R. Jonsen and Stephen Toulmin, *The Abuse of Casuistry: A History of Moral Reasoning* (Berkeley: University of California Press, 1988).
6   Henry Richardson, "Specifying Norms as a Way to Resolve Concrete Ethical Problems," *Philosophy and Public Affairs* 19:4(Fall 1990):279–310.
7   David DeGrazia, "Moving Forward in Bioethical Theory: Theories, Cases, and Specified Principlism," *Journal of Medicine and Philosophy* 17(1990):511–39.
8   Tom L. Beauchamp and James F. Childress, *Principles of Biomedical Ethics* (1979) p. 5, (1994) p. 15.
9   Beauchamp and Childress, *Principles of Biomedical Ethics*, 1979.
10 Tom L. Beauchamp, "On Eliminating the Distinction between Applied Ethics and Ethical Theory," *Monist* 67(1984):515–31.
11 Clouser and Gert, "A Critique of Principlism," p. 231.
12 Clouser and Gert, "A Critique of Principlism," p. 221.
13 Green, "Method in Bioethics," p. 188ff.
14 Beauchamp and Childress, *Principles of Bioethics*, 1994, p. 16.
15 John Arras, "Getting Down to Cases: The Revival of Casuistry in Bioethics," *Journal of Medicine and Philosophy* 16:(1991):29–51; see p. 39.
16 Richardson, "Specifying Norms," p. 280ff.
17 DeGrazia, "Moving Forward," p. 512.
18 Norman Daniels, "Wide Reflective Equilibrium and Theory Acceptance in Ethics," *Journal of Philosophy* 76:5(May 1979):256–82; "Reflective Equilibrium and Archimedean Points," *Canadian Journal of Philosophy*, 10:1(March 1980):83–103; see Chapters 2 and 3 in this book.
19 Albert R. Jonsen and Lewis H. Butler, "Public Ethics and Policy Making," *Hastings Center Report* 5(August 1975):19–31.
20 Jonsen and Butler, "Public Ethics," p. 22; they cite Daniel Callahan, *Abortion: Law, Choice and Morality* (New York: Macmillan, 1970), p. 341, for introducing the related notion, "moral policy."
21 Jonsen and Butler, "Public Ethics," p. 24.
22 Dan Brock and Norman Daniels, "Ethical Foundations of the Clinton Administration's Proposed Health Care System," *JAMA*, 271:15(April 20, 1994):1189–96.
23 White House Domestic Policy Council, *The President's Health Security Plan* (New York: Times Books, 1993).
24 See Norman Daniels, *Seeking Fair Treatment: From the AIDS Epidemic to National Health Care Reform* (New York: Oxford University Press, 1995), ch. 8.
25 Norman Daniels, "Duty to Treat or Right to Refuse?" *Hastings Center Report* 21:2(March–April 1991):36–46; see also Daniels, *Seeking Fair Treatment*, ch. 2.
26 See A. Zuger and S. M. Miles, "Physicians, AIDS, and Occupational Risk," *JAMA* 258(1987):14:1924–28; and J. Arras, "The Fragile Web of Responsibility: AIDS and the Duty to Treat," *Hastings Center Report* 18(suppl. 1988):10–20.
27 Norman Daniels, "HIV-Infected Health Care Professionals: Public Threat

or Public Sacrifice?" *Milbank Quarterly* 70:1(1992):3–42; and Norman Daniels, "HIV-Infected Professionals, Patient Rights, and the Switching Dilemma," *JAMA* 267:10(March 11, 1992):1368–71; and Norman Daniels, *Seeking Fair Treatment*, ch. 3.

28 Norman Daniels, "Rights to Health Care and Distributive Justice: Programmatic Worries," *Journal of Medicine and Philosophy* 4:2(1979):174–91.

29 See Norman Daniels, *Just Health Care* (Cambridge: Cambridge University Press, 1985).

30 See Norman Daniels, "Rationing Fairly: Programmatic Considerations," *Bioethics* 7:2–3:224–33; see Chapter 15, this book.

31 See "Fair Procedures and Just Rationing," Postscript to Chapter 15, this book.

32 J. Sabin and N. Daniels, "Determining 'Medical Necessity' in Mental Health Practice: A Study of Clinical Reasoning and a Proposal for Insurance Policy," *Hastings Center Report* 24:6(November–December 1994):5–13; see Chapter 11, this book.

33 A. Sen, "Justice: Means versus Freedoms," *Philosophy and Public Affairs* 19 (Spring 1990):111–21; A. Sen, *Inequality Reexamined* (Cambridge: Harvard University Press, 1992); G. A. Cohen, "On the Currency of Egalitarian Justice," *Ethics* 99:4(1989):906–44; R. Arneson, "Equality and Equality of Opportunity for Welfare," *Philosophical Studies* 54(1988):79–95; and N. Daniels, "Equality of What? Welfare, Resources, or Capabilities? *Philosophy and Phenomenological Research* 50 (suppl. fall 1990):273–96; (see Chapter 10, this book); J. Rawls, *Political Liberalism* (New York: Columbia University Press, 1993).

34 See Rawls, *Political Liberalism*, pp. 182–85, and Daniels, "Equality of What?"

35 Daniels, *Just Health Care*, ch. 7.

36 Daniels, *Seeking Fair Treatment*, ch. 3.

Index

353

Index

Bedau, H. A., 316n.12
Beigel, A., 249n.3
Beitz, C., 329, 330
Bias
 age (health care), 195–96
 in estimates of physical impairment, 323
 racial (prudential life-span policies),
  263–64
Bioethics, 333–34, 350
 and ethical theory, 340
 "principlists" vs. "theorists" in, 333,
  334–38
 and public ethics, 340–41
Biomedical model, 185–87, 213–14
Bipolar disorder case, 233–35, 236
Birth cohorts, equity between, 258–59,
  269, 278–81
Blaming the victim, difficulty in
  eradicating ideologies of, 93
Block, N., 45n.33, 315n.3
Boorse, C., 204nn.12,13,16,17, 229n.21
Botha, P. W., 117
Boundaries between persons
 and personal identity, 295–300
 and prudential life-span account, 284
 as standard assumption, 285
Boundaries between public and
  nonpublic, 150, 157, 158–60, 171–
  72, 173–74
Bowles, S., 206n.35, 315n.3
Boyd, R., 45nn.32,33, 168
Boyle, P. J., 250n.27
Brandt, R., 5, 29, 43n.13, 81–82, 84–99,
  99n.1, 100nn.7,10,11,
  101nn.12,13,14,15,16,17,18,20,21,
  102n.22, 115, 116, 118n.12, 203n.8,
  230n.41, 293
Branson, R., 205n.29
Braybrooke, D., 184, 185, 189, 203nn.10,11
Brink, D., 10
British National Health Service and age-
  based rationing, 272
Brock, D., 14, 272, 276, 318, 319, 341,
  351n.23
Broome, J., 319
Brown, P., 207n.43
Buchanan, A., 280, 282n.1
Burdens of judgment, 8, 147, 156, 158,
  167, 171
Butler, Joseph, 287
Butler, L. H., 340, 341, 351nn.19,20,21
Byerly, H. C., 45n.33

Callahan, D., 14, 204n.14, 250n.27, 271,
  272, 277, 351n.20
Callow, A., 104
Capabilities
 as egalitarian target, 208, 209–10, 256

and equality of opportunity, 251–56
and merit, 14 (see also Meritocracy)
and primary goods, 210–18, 229–30n.30
Capability model of medical necessity,
  242, 243–44, 246, 255–56
Caplan, A., 42n.5
Capron, A., 325n.3
Caste system in India, 117, 118n.9
Casuistry and bioethics controversy, 16,
  333, 334, 337, 350
Cherniak, C., 10, 101n.13
Child abuse case, 241
Childress, J. F., 333, 334, 335, 336, 337,
  341, 350n.1, 351nn.8,9,14
Chomsky, N., 78n.8
Claim about compensation, 295–96
Clinton health care proposal, 246, 341
Clouser, K. D., 333, 335, 336, 341, 350n.2,
  351nn.11,12
Coady, C. A. J., 141n.10
Cognitive psychotherapy, Brandt on, 5,
  87–91, 92, 100n.8
Cohen, G. A., 208, 209, 210, 218, 219, 221–
  22, 223, 224, 225, 227, 228n.3,
  230nn.34,35,43,44,46, 231n.48,
  352n.33
Cohen, J., 7, 10, 12, 64n.30, 109, 112,
  118n.6, 147, 148, 155, 156, 165, 166,
  173, 205n.28, 230n.31, 254, 255
Cohen, L. M., 280
Cohen, R. S., 143n.36, 206n.35, 315n.3
Coherence, 2, 21
 and justification, 33, 36, 38–39, 45n.29,
  48, 60–62, 153, 167–68, 338
Compensation, claim about, 295–96
Complete-lives egalitarianism, 264–65, 266
Complex proceduralism, 329
Consensus, overlapping, 8, 149, 150, 151,
  155, 164, 166, 170–71, 172, 226, 227
Constitutional essentials
 and politicization of justice, 148, 151
 and public reason, 156
 U.S. in agreement on, 173
Constructivism
 and political conception of justice, 226–
  27
 and wide reflective equilibrium, 45n.30
Contract
 and expectations, 309
 and Walzer on shared meanings, 112
Contract in Rawls' theory, 23, 47–48, 50,
  56, 99–100n.5, 138
 Brandt on, 92
 and incommensurability, 110
 as prudential (Lyons), 97
 "rigging" charge against, 7, 24, 42n.9,
  47, 48, 59–60, 61–62, 65n.49, 161
 in schematic representation, 51

354

Index

Jecker, N., 263
Johnson, C., 207n.43
Jonsen, A. R., 333, 339, 340, 341, 351nn.5,19,20,21
Judgments, moral. *See* Moral judgments
Justice
 and democracy, 324
 and egalitarian concerns, 252
 and equal opportunity principle, 195
 and health care, 12
 as local, 103–4
  and South African *Apartheid* intervention, 103–4, 117
  Walzer's arguments on, 104–12
  and Walzer's internalism, 112–17
 vs. productivity, 309
 "target" of, 12
 theory of, 252, 253
Justice as fairness, 7–8, 9
 as Archimedean point, 144
 and boundaries between persons, 285
 and Difference Principle, 153, 206n.35, 208, 213, 215, 216, 230n.36
 and health care, 224
 justice as priority in, 147
 and personal identity, 9, 127
 philosophical arguments on, 157
 and pluralism, 146–48
 politicization of, 10, 14–15, 148–50, 153–60, 161, 173, 226–27 (*see also* Political conception of justice)
 and primary social goods, 209
 and public reason, 14–15
 and pure procedural justice, 50
 and relativism, 116
 in schematic representation, 51
 vs. utilitarianism, 7, 53, 156
 in wide reflective equilibrium, 153, 171
 See also Contract in Rawls' theory
Justification, 21, 41n.1
 Brandt on, 86, 91–99, 115
 coherentist view of, 33, 36, 38–39, 45n.29, 48, 60–62, 153, 167–68, 338
 and democracy, 329–31
 full, 149, 162, 164, 165, 167
 for nonmoral theories, 41n.1, 153
 under politicization of justice, 151, 152
 pro tanto, 149, 162, 164
 and two-tiered view of moral theory, 21
 Walzer on, 112, 116
 and wide reflective equilibrium, 2, 21, 40, 59–62, 153
Justification Thesis (Walzer), 106–7

Kagan, S., 286
Kamm, F., 14, 272, 318, 319, 322, 325n.1

Kant, I., and Kantian views, 36, 53–54, 55, 57, 60, 116, 127–28, 137, 148, 150, 155, 339, 343
Kaplan, R. M., 323
Karel, R. B., 249n.3
Katz, J., 78n.4, 79n.17
Kramer, Peter D., 250n.15
Kripke, S., 141n.16, 142n.32
Krock, A., 206n.35

Lappé, M. A., 249n.8
Levinson, D. J., 250n.21
Lewis, D., 141n.6
Lewis, H. D., 43n.12
Liberalism. See Political Liberalism
Life plans, 111
 and normal opportunity range, 187
Linguistics (syntactics)
 and narrow equilibrium, 4, 41n.4, 62–63n.11, 66, 67–70
 and wide equilibrium, 4, 66, 71–72, 79nn.16,17
Lloyd, S. A., 164
Locke, J., 156, 287
Logics, alternative, 72–73
Long-term care in prudential life-span account, 270–71
Lost Administrator case, 238, 244
Luck, option vs. brute, 219
Luzara, V. A., 45n.33
Lycan, W., 43n.15, 78n.13
Lyons, D., 48, 62n.8, 97

McCloskey, J. H., 184, 185, 189, 203–4n.11
MacCorquodale, K., 45n.33
McCreadie, C., 207n.44
McFarland, B., 250n.27
MacGreggor, F. C., 204n.18
McKerlie, D., 13, 264, 265, 266, 268, 277
Macklin, R., 204n.12
McMurrin, S., 228n.6
Managed care and mental health coverage, 232
Manning, W. G., 250n.11
Manton, K. G., 270
Marxist theory, plasticity of person in, 120, 137
Maximin meritocracy, 311, 313, 314
Maximin rule, 273–74, 319
Meadean Measure, 109
Medicaid
 and intergenerational equity, 257, 258
 and medical necessity, 232
Medical necessity, 232–33
 and insurance allocations, 232, 246–47, 248
 and mental health, 232

358

Index

Social theory, general, 51, 63n.13, 64n.32, 128, 145
Soldo, G. J., 270
South Africa, opposition to Apartheid in, 103–4, 117
Species-typical functional organization, 185, 213
Species-typical normal functioning
and disease, 185–87
and needs, 184–85
and normal opportunity range, 187–88
See also Normal functioning
Spheres Thesis (Walzer), 8, 105–6
Spitzer, R. L., 250n.20
Stability condition, 23, 50, 146, 147–48, 149–50, 166–67, 173
Standard of living preservation principle, 262
Stich, S., 3, 10
Sturgeon, N., 99n.2
Subjective criterion of well-being, 182–83
Subjectivism, 21
Sullivan, L., 319, 322–23
Syntactic theory. *See* Linguistics

Tastes
and egalitarian claims, 190, 211, 218–23
life-hampering, 221–22
See also Preferences
Theory acceptance
coherence constraints on, 33
and Plasticity Thesis, 137
and two-tiered theory, 21
and wide reflective equilibrium, 66, 137, 140
See also Justification
Theory of health-care needs, 179–80
insurance-scheme market objection to, 180–81
Theory of Justice, A (Rawls), 2, 144, 145, 146, 150–51, 152, 153, 154, 155, 156–58, 159–60, 161, 165, 166, 168. *See also* Rawls' theory
Theory of justice, equality vs. other concerns in, 252, 253
Theory of the person. *See* Person, theory of
Thomson, D., 279
Toulmin, S., 333, 339, 351n.5
Tradition
and Brandt on moral justification, 91–94
individual's detachment from, 110, 112, 115–16
Transfer schemes and birth-cohort equity, 279
Troyer, J., 315n.4, 315–16n.12

Unhappy Husband case, 235–36, 247, 248
Utilitarianism
criticism and justification of, 3–4, 25–26
and justice as fairness, 7, 53, 156
and moral judgments, 3–4, 81
and personal identity, 9, 25, 60, 127–28
and fairness of distribution (Parfit), 125–26, 127, 136, 142n.25
status quo bias of, 94
and *Theory of Justice*, 146
universal concern of, 294
Utilitarian meritocracy, 311, 313
Utility, 3
discounted, 289–94
expected, 289
Utility function of individual, 289

Van Evra, J. W., 143n.36
Veatch, R., 205n.29, 272, 276
Veil of ignorance, 155
for health-care rationing, 274
Veil of ignorance, thick, 50, 51, 57, 58–59, 193
Brandt on, 94, 101n.15
and rationing, 319
Veil of ignorance, thinned, 193
Vernier, P., 207n.43
Veto provision, 56–57, 96
Vogel, R. J., 270

Walzer, M., 8, 104–17, 118nn.3,9, 318
Watson, T., 257
Webber, R., 206n.35
Welfare (well-being)
as "advantage," 228n.3
vs. alleviation of illness, 235
as egalitarian target, 208, 219, 220–23, 225
local measures of, 287–94
and primary goods, 211–13
satisfaction as (Rawls), 101n.19
satisfactions vs. truncated scale of, 189–91
subjective vs. objective criteria of, 182–83
Welfare model of medical necessity, 242, 244–45, 246
Well-ordered society, 52–54, 63n.15, 128, 163
Westermarck, E. A., 107
White, S., 9, 146, 296, 300
WHO (World Health Organization) on disease, 186
Wide reflective equilibrium. *See* Reflective equilibrium, wide
Williams, B., 25, 118n.7, 139, 141nn.6,10, 142n.33, 143nn.33,42, 205n.25, 228n.5

For EU product safety concerns, contact us at Calle de José Abascal, 56–1°, 28003 Madrid, Spain or eugpsr@cambridge.org.

www.ingramcontent.com/pod-product-compliance
Ingram Content Group UK Ltd.
Pitfield, Milton Keynes, MK11 3LW, UK
UKHW042134130625
459647UK00003B/29